T0309141

Skin Diseases: Eczema, Psoriasis and Related Conditions

Skin Diseases: Eczema, Psoriasis and Related Conditions

Editor: Marcello McCloskey

AMERICAN
MEDICAL PUBLISHERS
www.americanmedicalpublishers.com

Cataloging-in-Publication Data

Skin diseases : eczema, psoriasis and related conditions / edited by Marcello McCloskey.
  p. cm.
Includes bibliographical references and index.
ISBN 978-1-63927-805-3
1. Skin--Diseases. 2. Eczema. 3. Psoriasis. 4. Dermatology. 5. Skin--Diseases--Diagnosis.
6. Skin--Diseases--Treatment. I. McCloskey, Marcello.
RL72 .S55 2023
616.5--dc23

American Medical Publishers,
41 Flatbush Avenue,
1st Floor, New York,
NY 11217, USA

ISBN 978-1-63927-805-3 (Hardback)

Contents

Preface

Over the recent decade, advancements and applications have progressed exponentially. This has led to the increased interest in this field and projects are being conducted to enhance knowledge. The main objective of this book is to present some of the critical challenges and provide insights into possible solutions. This book will answer the varied questions that arise in the field and also provide an increased scope for furthering studies.

The conditions that affect the skin are called as skin diseases. There are various types of skin diseases and disorders, such as acne, eczema, alopecia areata, epidermolysis bullosa, hidradenitis suppurativa (HS), ichthyosis, pachyonychia congenita, etc. Eczema and psoriasis are common chronic inflammatory skin diseases. Both psoriasis and eczema result in red, itchy scaly patches on the skin. Psoriasis is related to rheumatologic (psoriatic arthritis), cardiovascular, metabolic, hepatic, and psychiatric diseases whereas, eczema is related to higher rates of mental health symptoms and disorders that include depression, anxiety, attention-deficit (hyperactivity) disorder, and sleep dysregulation. Both are caused by a complex interplay between skin-barrier disruption, immune dysregulation, host genetics and environment triggers. Common treatment options for eczema and psoriasis include topical treatments often used as monotherapy in mild to moderate disease. In moderate to severe cases, topical treatment is combined with systemic, biologic, or phototherapy. This book unravels the recent studies on skin diseases. It will serve as a valuable source of reference on eczema, psoriasis and related conditions for graduate and post graduate students.

I hope that this book, with its visionary approach, will be a valuable addition and will promote interest among readers. Each of the authors has provided their extraordinary competence in their specific fields by providing different perspectives as they come from diverse nations and regions. I thank them for their contributions.

Editor

1

Derailed Ceramide Metabolism in Atopic Dermatitis (AD): A Causal Starting Point for a Personalized (Basic) Therapy

Markus Blaess [1] and **Hans-Peter Deigner** [1,2,*]

[1] Institute of Precision Medicine, Medical and Life Sciences Faculty, Furtwangen University, Jakob-Kienzle-Strasse 17, 78054 Villingen-Schwenningen, Germany

[2] EXIM Department, Fraunhofer Institute IZI Leipzig, Schillingallee 68, 18057 Rostock, Germany

* Correspondence: Hans-Peter.Deigner@hs-furtwangen.de

Abstract: Active rebuilding, stabilizing, and maintaining the lipid barrier of the skin is an encouraging disease management and care concept for dry skin, atopic dermatitis (eczema, neurodermatitis), and psoriasis. For decades, corticosteroids have been the mainstay of topical therapy for atopic dermatitis; however, innovations within the scope of basic therapy are rare. In (extremely) dry, irritated, or inflammatory skin, as well as in lesions, an altered (sphingo)lipid profile is present. Recovery of a balanced (sphingo)lipid profile is a promising target for topical and personalized treatment and prophylaxis. New approaches for adults and small children are still lacking. With an ingenious combination of commonly used active ingredients, it is possible to restore and reinforce the dermal lipid barrier and maintain refractivity. Lysosomes and ceramide de novo synthesis play a key role in attenuation of the dermal lipid barrier. Linoleic acid in combination with amitriptyline in topical medication offers the possibility to relieve patients affected by dry and itchy skin, mild to moderate atopic dermatitis lesions, and eczemas without the commonly occurring serious adverse effects of topical corticosteroids or systemic antibody administration.

Keywords: atopic dermatitis; lysosomotropic compounds; apoptosis; lysosome; ceramide metabolism; amitriptyline; ceramide de novo synthesis; antioxidants; linoleic acid; sphingolipid profile

---

1. Introduction

Atopic dermatitis (AD), atopic eczema, or neurodermatitis is a chronic or chronic relapsing, non-contagious skin disease. Morphology and localization is age-dependent pronounced differently and frequently accompanied by severe itching [1–3]. Consensus-based European guidelines for treatment of AD are usually associated with sometimes serious adverse events that reduce patient compliance or adherence to treatment and increase the risk of bacterial or virus infections [3,4]. Glucocorticoids, which cause changes in skin structure, are limited in duration of use. With atrophy of the skin at the forefront and in the intertrigenes (armpit, groin), there is an additional risk of superinfections and of triggering rosacea, steroid acne in the face, development of telangiectasias, and spontaneous scars [3,4]. Permanent daily treatment is not recommended. Topical calcineurin inhibitors tacrolismus and pimecrolimus cause transient warmth, tingling, or a burning sensation at the application site during the first days of application and increase the risk of bacterial or viral skin infections [3,4].

Basic therapy for disturbed skin barrier function and emollient therapy of AD includes the topical application of active, compound-free ointment bases with an occlusion effect, which is intended to prevent water loss from outer layers of the skin (e.g., through liquid paraffin or ceresin as an occludent) and improvement in retaining moisture (e.g., through urea as humectant) or the addition of extra water into dry skin using hydrophilic creams. Fatty ointments for dry skin or hydrating oil-in-water emulsions on less dry skin are used. However, many patients do not respond in the expected manner, becoming frustrated with the efficacy of the drugs and fearful of adverse effects [5].

The major goal of any advanced disease management concept is to improve therapeutic effectiveness, increase patient satisfaction with treatment, and minimize adverse effects. Symptomatic therapy (inflammation: glucocorticoids; itching: H_1-receptor antagonists or local anesthetics (polidocanol)) are often unable to restore skin integrity. Thus, a precise knowledge of the role of lysosomes in the pathological derailment of ceramide metabolism in AD enables an advanced disease management concept that may replace some common topical (basic) therapies in the near future. The transition from symptomatic to causal topical treatment will provide patients with long-term relief of their symptoms.

Starting from the altered ceramide profile and the appearance of C_{16}-ceramide in the skin of AD patients, we try to point out the underlying causes and to describe how these alterations can be eliminated by topical therapy in order to restore the original complexion. Our modular disease management concept renders humectants and occludents unnecessary. Targeting one of the AD root causes and AD pathogenesis at an early stage, our suggested therapy is well-suited for patients independent of acute or chronic infections. Our therapeutic approach is applicable to all age groups with just fractional adverse effects.

2. Ceramides and Altered Sphingolipid Profile in AD

Ceramide is a general term for certain well-characterized sphingolipid metabolites and second messengers involved in numerous biological processes in the cell. They consist of a backbone (dihydrosphingosine (sphinganine) [dS] sphingosine [S], phytosphingosine [P], or 6-hydroxy-sphingosine [H]) and a fatty acid residue (non-hydroxy fatty acid [N], α-hydroxy fatty acid [A], or esterified ω-hydroxy fatty acid [EO]) (Figure 1A). The combination of fatty acid and backbone results in 12 subclasses of ceramide fractions of the stratum corneum.

Cell cycle-relevant C_{16}-ceramide and $C_{24:1}$-ceramide (backbone: sphingosine, residue: non-hydroxy fatty acid) belong to subclass NS, representing 7% of total ceramide of the skin (Figure 1B). Subclasses NH (23%), NP (22%), AP (16%), and AH (15%) represent the majority of dermal ceramides. Cellular ceramides typically have fatty acid residues that range from 16 to 26 carbon atoms; in the stratum corneum; ceramides of up to 32 carbon atoms exist [6].

Figure 1. Backbones of dermal ceramides, cell cycle-relevant ceramides, and ceramides in basic ceramide replacement therapy. (**A**) Ceramide fractions of the stratum corneum are classified into 12 subclasses. The identifier is made up of the backbone (sphingosine [S], phytosphingosine [P], or 6-hydroxy-sphingosine [H], and the fatty acid residue (non-hydroxy fatty acid [N], α-hydroxy fatty acid [A] or esterified ω-hydroxy fatty acid [EO]). (**B**) Cell cycle-relevant ceramides C_{16} and $C_{24:1}$ belong to the subclass NS (7% of dermal ceramide). Subclasses NH (23%), NP (22%), AP (16%), and AH (15%) are the most prominent ceramides in the stratum corneum. In AD, the AP subclass is significantly increased; in psoriasis, the AP, NP, and EOP subclasses are significantly lowered [6]. (**C**) Various creams for the treatment of affected skin areas comprise ceramide 1 (EOP) (N-(27-stearoyloxy-heptacosanoyl)-phytosphingosine), ceramide 3 (NP) (ceramide NP, N-oleoylphytosphingosine), and ceramide 6 (AP) (ceramide AP, N-(2-hydroxytetracosanoyl)-phytosphingosine for substitution therapy.

2.1. Role of Ceramides in Cells and Skin Development

Ceramides are not only a key molecule in sphingolipid metabolism that can be modified in cells (Figure 2), but are also important signaling molecules that are able to regulate vital cellular functions [7]. As cellular messengers, they are able to halt the cell cycle (G0/G1 and G2/M arrest) and promote apoptosis [8–10]. The length of the fatty acid residue is decisive for the function or individual effect of each ceramide. Ceramides, in particular C_{16}-ceramide, are strongly increased in apoptotic cells and play a crucial role in apoptosis [11]. On the contrary, (very) long-chain ceramides ($>C_{20}$) are not pro-apoptotic, and are therefore responsible for the epidermal barrier function [12].

In epidermal keratinocytes, ceramide is synthesized and released into the extracellular matrix of the stratum corneum. There, ceramides are an essential element of the extracellular lipid matrix and play an critical role in the formation of the most important natural barrier to water loss and the penetration of various compounds into the skin [12,13]. During keratinocyte maturation, total ceramide increases from 3.8 ± 0.2% (stratum basale/spinosum) to 18.1 ± 0.4% (stratum corneum). Inflammatory skin diseases are accompanied by a shift in the proportion of ceramide subclasses. In AD, the subclass AP is increased; in psoriasis, the subclasses AP, NP, and EOP are lowered [6]. Various care products attempt to compensate alterations in affected areas by local ceramide replacement therapy using ceramide 1 (EOP), ceramide 3 (NP), and ceramide 6 (AP) (Figure 1C).

Figure 2. Ceramide metabolism in keratinocytes. Active pathways are marked with black arrows and inactive pathways are marked with white arrows. The objective of the ceramide metabolism-centered therapeutic concept is to use appropriate compounds to maintain lysosomal NADH-dependent redox chain, V-ATPase activity, and very long-chain ceramide *de novo* synthesis at the endoplasmic reticulum to prevent formation of pro apoptotic C_{16}-ceramide in lysosomes.

2.2. (Sphingo)Lipid Profile of Sensitive and Inflammatory Skin and Lesions of Patients with AD

Experimental findings in patients with AD display a change in the composition of skin lipids (Table 1). In skin lesions, the content of saturated free fatty acids with very long carbon chains $\geq C_{24}$) is significantly reduced, whereas short-chain free fatty acids—in particular, palmitic acid ($C_{16:0}$) and stearic acid ($C_{18:0}$)—are increased. Analysis of the fatty acid residues of ceramides showed substantially increased amounts of short-chain ceramides (<42 carbon atoms, especially C_{16}-ceramide and C_{18}-ceramide [NS]; on the contrary, long-chain ceramides (>42 carbon atoms, e.g., $C_{24:1}$-ceramide) were significantly reduced [6,14–16]. Significantly altered distribution was observed predominantly in skin lesions and in non-lesional skin areas of patients with AD. Among the short-chain ceramides, C_{16}-ceramide (C34-ceramide) in particular is increased. The level of C_{16}-ceramide is the highest in the lesions of patients with AD compared to the skin of healthy individuals [14]. An increase in free palmitic acid indicates an increased degradation of lipids containing palmitic acid from cell membranes of keratinocytes and/or release from palmitoyl-CoA of fatty acid biosynthesis. Mouse models of mice that develop AD also show these changes in ceramide profile [13,17].

Table 1. Most significant anomalies in the (sphingo)lipid profile of inflammatory skin and in lesions of atopic dermatitis patients.

Ceramides	Ceramides + Free Fatty Acids	Free Fatty Acids
Short chain ceramides, in particular C_{16}-ceramide [NS], are elevated in inflammatory skin and lesions	Free fatty acids and ceramides with very long chains ($\geq C_{24}$) are significantly reduced.	Short-chain free fatty acids palmitic acid ($C_{16:0}$) and stearic acid ($C_{18:0}$) are elevated.

2.3. Impaired Maturation and Premature Apoptosis of Keratinocytes

Apoptosis (controlled cell death) is the most important regulatory element in the control of cell populations, organ formation, histological structures, skin, and the related dermal lipid barrier [18]. In contrast to healthy skin, C_{16}-ceramide is elevated in the vulnerable skin areas and lesions of AD patients and in AD mouse models [13,14,17], suggesting that (premature) apoptosis has been induced there. A disorder in the application of this highly specific tool may explain the incomplete maturation of keratinocytes, the defective lipid barrier, and the subsequent inflammatory process. Due to premature apoptosis, a high percentage of keratinocytes in lesions or severely reddened, irritated, or inflammatory skin do not reach full maturity, including the ceramide content required to form a stable cell cluster as a barrier against moisture loss. Figure 3 illustrates how C_{16}-ceramide can be selectively produced in impacted cells. Oxidative stress (lack of NAD(P)H and GSH) in cells not only triggers lysosomal C_{16}-ceramide formation, but also prevents the synthesis of very long-chain ceramides at the endoplasmic reticulum (Figures 3 and 4).

Figure 3. Ceramide metabolism and selective C_{16}-ceramide synthesis in keratinocytes in atopic dermatitis lesions and sensitive/inflammatory skin (compartmentalized model of ceramide synthesis). Active pathways are marked with black arrows, less active and inactive pathways are marked with white arrows. Oxidative stress in keratinocytes results in the dysfunction of lysosomal V-ATPase. Ceramide hydrolase activity of acidic ceramidase (aCERase) loses activity and becomes inactive. In contrast, C_{16}-ceramide is selectively re-synthesized by the reverse ceramide synthase activity of aCERase and accumulated in the lysosome. At the same time, very long-chain ceramide *de novo* synthesis is blocked due to insufficient NADPH. NADPH is an essential cofactor for very long-chain-3-oxoacyl-CoA synthases (ELOVL) for the synthesis of very long-chain acyl-CoAs ($\geq C_{18}$).

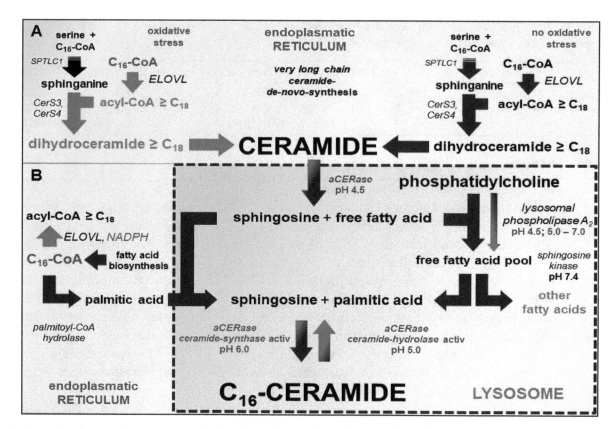

Figure 4. Linkage between synthesis of very long-chain fatty acids and very long-chain ceramides at the endoplasmatic reticulum and substrate supply of reverse ceramide synthase activity of aCERase for selective C_{16}-ceramide synthesis in lysosomes. Active pathways at standard conditions are marked with black arrows, inactive pathways are marked with red arrows. Black and red arrows indicate pathways with diminished activity. **(A)** Very long-chain fatty acid synthesis at standard conditions (highlighted in green) and a lack of NADPH (oxidative stress) (highlighted in red). In cells lacking NADPH, C_{16}-CoA is not converted to acyl-CoA $\geq C_{18}$ and accessible to other reactions. **(B)** The potential sources of palmitic acid for the selective lysosomal synthesis of C_{16}-ceramide by reverse ceramide synthase activity of aCERase are: hydrolysis of accumulating C_{16}-CoA (palmitoyl-CoA hydrolase), hydrolysis of phosphatidylcholine (lysosomal phospholipase A_2), and sphingomyelin of cell membranes. Lysosomal phospholipase A_2 has residual activity, even at pH values up to 7.0.

2.4. The Two Different pH-Dependent Enzymatic Activities of aCERase

Interestingly, lysosomal acidic ceramidase (aCERase) exhibits two different enzymatic activities dependent on the lysosomal pH: the well-known ceramide hydrolase activity (optimum pH 4.0–5.0) and a little-known ATP-independent reverse ceramide synthase activity (revaCERase) (optimum pH 5.5–6.5). revaCERase preferentially reacts palmitic acid (C_{16}) and stearic acid (C_{18}) with sphingosine [19,20]. Unlike ceramide synthases (CerS), no activation of fatty acid via acyl-CoA is required. Sphingomyelin of cell membranes contains a high amount of palmitic acid and only very little stearic acid [21,22]. Therefore, the selectivity of the re-synthesis between C_{16}-ceramide and C_{18}-ceramide is due to the availability of each fatty acid in the lysosome. The objective of a well-suited therapy is to stabilize the physiological pH value of lysosomes in keratinocytes.

2.5. aCERase: Shift from Ceramidase to revaCERase Activity in Lysosomes

Acidic pH (4.6–4.8) in lysosomes is predominantly generated and maintained by the vacuolar H^+-ATPase (V-ATPase). The lysosomal redox chain is the second proton pump transporting protons into the lumen of lysosomes. V-ATPase uses ATP, the lysosomal redox chain uses NADH from cytoplasm as an energy source [23,24]. The catalytically active subunit (73 kDa) of V-ATPase contains a conserved region (P-LOOP) with two cysteines at positions 254 and 532, which are capable of forming disulfide bonds, thus inactivating the active site of V-ATPase. The thiol–disulfide equilibrium depends on the redox potential of the cytoplasm [23]. An excessive drop of cytosolic redox potential leads to the formation of the disulfide bond between Cys 254 and Cys 532, blocking the catalytically active ATPase site. Once formed, the disulfide bond is quite stable under physiological conditions. Physiological glutathione (GSH) concentrations in the cytoplasm are incapable of reconstituting both cysteines and recovering full V-ATPase activity [25]. A consequence of the failure of V-ATPase is the inversion of CERase activity: ceramide hydrolysis vanishes, while revaCERase activity selectively generates C_{16}-ceramide in the lysosome, and triggers the premature apoptosis of keratinocytes (Figures 3 and 4).

C_{16}-ceramide is formed of sphingosine and palmitic acid. Besides the hydrolysis of membranous sphingomyelin, the sources of the required palmitic acid are the hydrolysis of accumulating C_{16}-CoA (by palmitoyl-CoA hydrolase) and the hydrolysis of phosphatidylcholine (by lysosomal phospholipase A_2) (Figure 4B).

3. New Therapy Concept: Active Adjustment of Ceramide Metabolism

Within these findings, a new therapeutic target for the therapy of AD can be identified: reinforcement of the dermal lipid barrier by the active normalization of (sphingo)lipid metabolism and very long chain acyl-CoA biosynthesis in keratinocytes. As a key molecule in the sphingolipid metabolism, ceramides are likewise a product and starting material of various enzymatic modifications in cells. Target-oriented normalization of the altered ceramide metabolism in keratinocytes is a promising approach for effective and patient-friendly treatment and prophylaxis of AD and likely of psoriasis vulgaris as well.

4. Addressed Therapeutic Targets in Keratinocytes

1. Biosynthesis of Ceramides

The first therapeutic target is the biosynthesis of ceramides. The *de novo* synthesis of individual ceramides is performed by ceramide synthases 1–6 (CerS1–CerS6) at the endoplasmic reticulum. The type of synthesized ceramide(s) depends primarily on the fatty acid specificity (acyl-CoA specificity) of the CerSs that are present, the availability of different acyl-CoAs for incorporation as fatty acid side chain, and palmitoyl-CoA for the assembly of the sphingosine backbone [26,27]. Notably, a successful therapeutic approach has to ensure the availability of the required very long-chain acyl-CoAs (C_{24} to C_{30}) (Figure 2). Keratinocytes in the epidermis of mice predominantly contain CerS3 (24%) and CerS4 (55.4%); CerS3 converts C_{18}-CoA to C_{32}-CoA and CerS4 C_{18}-CoA to C_{22}-CoA. Furthermore, according to recent studies, $C_{24:0}$-CoA and $C_{24:1}$-CoA are being incorporated [26,28]. Due to a lack of specificity for palmitoyl-CoA, both CerS3 and CerS4, which are predominantly present in skin, are not the reasonable point of origin of the pronounced increase of C_{16}-ceramide in AD patient skin.

Ceramides with phytosphingosine backbone are formed by sphingolipid-C4-monooxygenase (hDES2) from ceramides with sphingosine backbone [29]. Phytosphingosine ceramide composition is closely related to ceramide *de novo* synthesis. Therefore, the normalization of sphingosine ceramide biosynthesis results in the normalization of phytosphingosine ceramides as well.

2. Composition of Free Fatty Acids

The second therapeutic target is closely linked to ceramide *de novo* synthesis and addresses alterations in the composition of free fatty acids due to impairment in very long-chain fatty acid biosynthesis. Very long–chain fatty acids ($\geq C_{24}$) are substantially reduced, while shorter fatty acids, in particular palmitic acid ($C_{16:0}$) and stearic acid ($C_{18:0}$), are increased [15]. Both fatty acids are preferably released by palmitoyl-CoA hydrolase (long-chain fatty-acyl-CoA hydrolase), unless their corresponding acyl-CoAs are processed by very long-chain-3-oxoacyl-CoA synthases (ELOVL1–ELOVL7) to obtain more elongated acyl-CoAs. Of the well-known ELOVLs, ELOVL7 (preferably C_{16}–C_{22} acyl-CoA), ELOVL3 (especially C_{18} acyl-CoA) and ELOVL6 (chain extension C_{16}-CoA to C_{18}-CoA) are of particular interest. Although NADPH is not a cofactor of ELOVLs, NADPH activates the enzymatic activity of ELOVL6 and ELOV7 up to 10-fold. 3-ketoacyl-CoA reductase is responsible for the downstream reduction step in which NADPH is an enzyme cofactor, and activates ELOVL6 threefold [30]. Therefore, the abundant availability cytosolic NADPH is important for ELOVL elongation activity and the assembly of very long-chain ceramides. In cells lacking NADPH, C_{16}-CoA is not converted to acyl-CoA $\geq C_{18}$ and is accessible to other reactions such as hydrolysis by palmitoyl-CoA hydrolase (Figure 4).

3. Availability of NADPH

Ensuring the availability of reduction equivalents (NAD(P)H) is the third therapeutic target, which is closely linked to the composition of free fatty acids (second target). NADPH is a powerful cellular reductant that is linked via mitochondrial nicotinamide nucleotide transhydrogenase (NNT) with NAD^+, which is a mitochondrial proton acceptor and oxidant. NNT connects the hydride transfer between NADH and $NADP^+$ (to NADPH and NAD^+) across the inner mitochondrial membrane. Under physiological conditions, energy originates from the mitochondrial proton gradient. NAD^+ is more than just an electron acceptor in mitochondrial energy generation. NAD^+ acts as a substrate in mono(ADP)-ribosylation and poly(ADP)-ribosylation reactions of proteins and histones in the nucleus of cells as well. Ribosylation reactions are involved in cell regulation and the repair of single-strand breaks of DNA. Additional metabolites, including nicotinamide, free mono(ADP)-ribose, and poly(ADP)-ribose, can be derived from NAD^+ [31].

ATP synthesis in mitochondria, glutathione (GSH) regeneration, and intracellular redox potential are directly linked to the availability of NAD^+ and $NADH/NAD^+$ levels. The involvement of NAD^+ in these regulatory processes requires a constant re-synthesis of NAD^+ to avoid exhaustion of the intracellular NAD^+ pool. The availability of sufficient GSH is in turn necessary to neutralize reactive oxygen species (ROS) or reactive carbonyl species (RCS) to prevent DNA single-strand breaks.

4. Specific Generation of C_{16}-ceramide

The fourth therapeutic target is the root cause of the specific generation of C_{16}-ceramide in the skin of patients with AD and apoptotic cells. Unlike ceramides C_{18} to C_{24}, it is not formed by *de novo* synthesis at the endoplasmic reticulum. CerS3 and CerS4 present in skin exhibit no selectivity for palmitoyl-CoA, which is required for the synthesis of C_{16}-Ceramide [26]. The origin of C_{16}-ceramide is located in the lysosome. Under physiological conditions, sphingomyelin from the cell membrane is degraded in the lysosome by acidic sphingomyelinase (aSMase) to phosphocholine and ceramide. In turn, the resulting ceramide is directly hydrolyzed by aCERase to sphingosine and free fatty acid. In AD patients, predominant sphingomyelins 16:0-SM and 24:1-SM are increased [21], indicating the inhibition of degradation by lysosomal enzymes aSMase and aCERase. Membranous sphingomyelin is ruled out as being of (C_{16}-) ceramide origin.

5. Therapy Objectives for Treatment and Prophylaxis

Critical pro-apoptotic C_{16}-ceramide in the skin of AD patients originates from a different cellular compartment than the (very) long-chain ceramides ($>C_{20}$), which are responsible for establishing the dermal lipid barrier. The objectives of successful active adjustment of the ceramide metabolism are:

1. Inhibition of forming C_{16}-ceramide in lysosomes.
2. Stabilization of very long-chain fatty acid-CoA synthesis ($\geq C_{18}$) for very long-chain ceramide *de novo* synthesis.
3. Protecting lysosomal V-ATPase from inactivation (formation of the disulfide bond between Cys 254 and Cys 532) and stabilizing the ceramidase activity of aCERase.
4. Modulating expression of AD-relevant gene.
5. Enrichment of very long-chain ceramides of *de novo* synthesis.

6. Implementation of Therapy Objectives

1.   Inhibition of forming C_{16}-ceramide in lysosomes.

The synthesis of C_{16}-ceramide in lysosomes can be blocked by lysosomotropic compounds. Well-known antidepressants imipramine, desipramine, and amitriptyline, together with the carbazole NB06 belong to this class of compounds (Figure 5) [32]. Lysosomotropic compounds are characterized by raising the lysosomal pH above 6 or higher. Thus, lysosomal enzymes are inactivated, and the lysosomal substrate supply of revaCERase is capped. Lysosomotropy is a physico-chemical property of a compound and is independent of a specific therapeutic indication. Inhibition of the formation of C_{16}-ceramide likewise prevents premature apoptosis [11,32–34]. An overview of lysosomotropic compounds and their field of indication can be found in [35,36].

Figure 5. Lysosomotropic compounds amitriptyline, imipramine, sertraline, and the model compound NB 06 [32,36].

Lysosomotropy leads to an inhibition of the aCERase hydrolase activity by increasing the pH value. Very long-chain ceramides from *de novo* synthesis will no longer be degraded in the lysosome and will accumulate [33]. Although the lysosomal pH value is within the optimum range of revaCERase activity, only small amounts of C_{16}-ceramide are formed due to a lack of substrate palmitic acid.

2.   Stabilization of very long-chain fatty acid-CoA synthesis ($\geq C_{18}$) for very long-chain ceramide *de novo* synthesis and

3.   Protecting lysosomal V-ATPase from inactivation and stabilizing the ceramidase activity of aCERase

Stabilization of the synthesis of very long-chain ceramides and the protection of lysosomal V-ATPase as well as the stabilization of aCERase function are closely linked via NAD^+ and NADPH. It is important to stabilize or reduce cytosolic redox potential to, or to below, a level that protects both cysteines of V-ATPase from oxidation and ensures sufficient amounts of NADPH and ATP for the individual reduction steps of the *de novo* synthesis of very long-chain ceramides and the lysosomal proton pumps.

One of the topical active compounds that can be used to implement the therapeutic concept is linoleic acid (Figure 6). Linoleic acid can serve as a radical scavenger or is available via linoleate $\Delta12$-cis-$\Delta11$-trans-isomerase for the β-oxidation of fatty acids to recover reduction equivalents (NADH/NADPH) and/or energy (ATP). In general, the use of gamma-linolenic acid (evening primrose seed oil) is also feasible, but nerve-sensitizing prostaglandins (e.g., PGD2 and PGE2) can easily be formed via arachidonic acid, thus increasing itching. The maintenance of lysosomal pH ensures the stability of the ceramide hydrolase functionality of aCERase. No C_{16}-ceramide that induces apoptosis can be formed.

linoleic acid	gamma linolenic acid	arachidonic acid
((9Z,12Z)-octadeca-9,12-dienoic acid	(6Z,9Z,12Z)-octadeca-6,9,12-trienoic acid	(5Z,8Z,11Z,14Z)-icosa-5,8,11,14-tetraenoic acid

Figure 6. Fatty acids to protect the lysosomes and stabilize very long-chain ceramide *de novo* synthesis. Gamma-linolenic acid can be converted into dihomo-gamma-linolenic acid by elongation and subsequent oxidation to arachidonic acid by acyl lipid (8–3) desaturase. Arachidonic acid itself is a substrate of COX2 (PTGS2), which is inducible by oxidative stress. The resulting prostaglandin PGH2 and its derivatives can sensitize neurons. Linoleic acid first has to be converted into gamma linolenic acid by linoleoyl-CoA desaturase before it can be metabolized toward arachidonic acid. This can be a key advantage if itching or prostaglandin-mediated inflammatory reactions occur due to the application of creams containing gamma-linolenic acid.

4. Modulating expression of AD-relevant genes

Another important objective is the modulation of cytokines and interleukins involved in the development of AD. Anti-apoptotic lysosomotropic compounds not only interfere with classical lysosomal metabolic processes such as proteolysis and degradation of membrane lipids, but also have a modulating effect on the release or formation (transcription at gene level or maturation) of cytokines and interleukins such as CXCL3, CXCL2, CCL4, CCL20, CXCL10, PTX3, PTGS2, ICAM1, IL23A, IL6, and TNFalpha, which are involved in a variety of biological processes (apoptosis, lipid metabolism, cytokine secretion, cell activation, cell death, cell adhesion, cell differentiation, cell stimulation, and cell proliferation) [32]. In contrast to antibodies, small lysosomotropic chemical compounds such as NB 06 or amitriptyline can be used as local therapeutics for inflammatory skin or lesions. Thus, the self-perpetuating inflammatory process in keratinocytes can be interrupted.

5. Enrichment of very long-chain ceramides of *de novo* synthesis

A spin-off effect of lysosomotropic compounds is the accumulation of very long-chain ceramides by the inhibition of the ceramidase activity of aCERase [32]. However, this requires the formation of very long-chain ceramide in ceramide *de novo* synthesis. Obviously, the enrichment is closely linked to a stable, or with reduction equivalents stabilized, very long-chain ceramide *de novo* synthesis. Without an adequate supply of redox equivalents by linoleic acid, an enrichment using the lysosomotropic compounds amitriptyline or NB 06 is meaningless. C_{16}-CoA, being unable to be converted through the lack of NADPH through ELOVL6 and ELOVL7, is hydrolyzed to palmitic acid and thus together with sphingosine is available in the lysosome for C_{16}-ceramide synthesis. Due to the lysosomotropic compound, the pH in the lysosome is elevated to 6, which is in the optimum range of activity of the revaCERase (ceramide synthase activity). Now, there is no lack of substrates, and C_{16}-ceramide can be formed.

While the preliminary stages of AD may be treated effectively with mere lysosomotropic compounds, the prevention of C_{16}-ceramide increase in keratinocytes using lysosomotropic compounds alone is insufficient, and even risky, in moderate to severe forms and acute exacerbations, as they may provoke severe but reversible adverse effects (acute generalized exanthematous pustulosis) [37]. Sertraline is a lysosomotropic compound that is similar to amitriptyline [36], which exhibits lysosomotropic properties in keratinocytes if orally administered (50 mg per day). Therefore, it is obvious that the lysosomotropy of sertraline plays an important role in the development of the severe adverse effects that have been reported. A lack of redox equivalents NADPH and GSH in combination with pharmacologically-induced lysosomotropy is linked to the severe adverse effect that is observed. This implies that only the combination of a recovery of reduction equivalents (linoleic acid) and lysosomotropic active compound (amitriptyline) can result in an efficient accumulation of very long-chain ceramides in affected skin.

7. Therapeutic Concept

The customizable therapeutic concept consists of two modules: therapy and prophylaxis. The therapy combines two components: 1. lysosome protection and stabilization of very long-chain ceramide *de novo* synthesis, and 2. lysosomotropic and anti-apoptotic treatment of keratinocytes. Depending on the severity, treatment consists of a combination of components 1 and 2 (lesions, mild to moderate AD) or merely component 1 (initial redness, (mild) itching, feeling of tension). Prophylaxis is typically performed with component 1. Prophylaxis, on the other hand, has no time limit, and is also useful and recommended even after symptoms have subsided. Exclusive treatment with component 2 is insufficient and may cause itching and pustules, as previously described in Section 6.

On the basis of the suggested foundations listed in the European guidelines for treatment of AD, a light, moisturizing oil-in-water emulsion without the addition of urea and glycerin is used as the foundation of the cream. Fatty or occlusion-promoting foundations were excluded, since a poor release of active compounds is to be expected.

Therapeutic targets, the implementation of therapy objectives, and the active compound(s) applied for each purpose are summarized in Figure 7.

	Therapeutic target	Implementation of therapy objectives	Active compound
1	Synthesis of C_{16}-ceramide in lysosomes of keratinocytes	Inhibition of substrate supply of revaCERase	amitriptyline
		or	
		Protection of lysosomal V-ATPase	linoleic acid
2	Stabilizing *de-novo* synthesis of very long-chain ceramides (ELOVL)	Stabilization of synthesis of acyl CoAs ($\geq C_{18}$) for *de-novo* synthesis of very long-chain ceramides	linoleic acid
	Normalizing composition of free fatty acids	Stabilization of synthesis of acyl-CoAs ($\geq C_{18}$)	linoleic acid
3	Reduction equivalents (NADPH, GSH) for stabilizing functionality of lysosomal V-ATPase	Protection of lysosomal V-ATPase from inactivation (formation of disulfide bond) and stabilization of aCERase functionality	linoleic acid
4	Normalization of gene expression of AD-relevant genes	Modulating gene expression of AD-relevant genes	amitriptyline
5	Enrichment of very long-chain ceramides of *de-novo* synthesis	Inhibition of C_{16}-ceramide formation **and** hydrolysis of very long-chain ceramides of *de-novo* synthesis in lysosomes	amitriptyline linoleic acid

Figure 7. Derived therapeutic targets and the implementation of therapy objectives to reduce keratinocytes with disturbed maturation and premature apoptosis in the stratum corneum of AD patients. Therapeutic targets are listed in chronological order in Sections 5 and 6.

8. Personalized Therapy

The therapeutic concept presented can be easily customized in its composition and adapted to the individual requirements of patients. Variations in the composition of the cream can be: the concentration of linoleic acid, the concentration of the lysosomotropic compound, and its combination and the lysosomotropic compound itself, if additional pharmacological effects are advantageous. The suitable choice of foundation can be guided by the requirements of the individual patient, as is currently common with individual formulations. However, the basis should not be too rich (oily). Starting from a standard formulation, adjustments can easily be made for individual prescriptions. Semi-solid preparations are easy to prepare in pharmacies.

The verification of therapy success (response to therapy) can be performed by comparing the ceramide profiles of samples obtained from intact skin, reddened skin, and lesions in addition to the usual scores (e.g., EASI-score). Alternatively, a gene expression profile of specific genes (e.g., PTG2, CXCL10, IL23A, or IL8) is also appropriate.

A crucial factor for the duration of treatment is the time frame of approximately 28 days that the skin requires for complete regeneration. In more severe or chronic cases, the therapeutic effect may only occur after a half or full regeneration cycle of the epidermis (due to the therapeutic target skin).

9. Does the Concept Work?

Dissatisfaction with therapy, frustration, and speculation about the root causes of the disease are well-known problems in the treatment of AD patients. Many therapeutic approaches address the disease symptomatically, including inflammation-glucocorticoids, itching-H_1 receptor antagonists or local anesthetics (polidocanol), and fail to alleviate painful itching and restore skin integrity. A typical example is mild AD and chronic AD on the crook of the arm and wrists with spontaneous worsening. Various topical therapy recommendations following the European guidelines for treating AD have been tried (emollient therapy, basic therapy, and glucocorticoids), but severely itching areas on the crook of the arm and wrists have not improved over three years. However, neither the restoration of lesional skin nor the full recovery of skin integrity was achieved with the European guidelines for treating AD. This was the major reason to validate the ceramide metabolism rested therapy concept in an off-label use [38]. With a combination of amitriptyline (lysosomotropic and anti-apoptotic) and linoleic acid (lysosome protection and very long-chain ceramides *de novo* synthesis stabilization) in therapy and linoleic acid in prophylaxis, the lesions vanished completely after approximately 60 days (two regeneration cycles of the skin), and have not recurred since then due to the frequent application of the prophylactic cream containing linoleic acid.

10. Conclusions

Despite new target-oriented anti-inflammatory IL4RA, IL13, IL31RA and IL23 antibodies [39] for severe cases, a holistic concept for the topical treatment of AD and regeneration of the skin's barrier function at the cellular level is still lacking. With our paper, we wish to initiate a discussion about this topic and break new ground in the therapy and prophylaxis of AD and psoriasis. The possibility of a personalized therapy and the individual manufacture of creams provide new therapeutic tools that are beneficial to patients.

The modular and personalized therapy concept described can be used as a valuable complementary treatment option to restore the skin, strengthen the lipid skin barrier, and prevent dry skin as a precursor of AD. It is well-suited for patients with local lesions and independent of acute or chronic infections. A systemic effect by one of the active compounds and the detection in blood is unlikely. The combination of linoleic acid with amitriptyline offers the opportunity to treat dry and itchy skin as well as mild to moderate AD without the serious side effects of corticosteroids and prevent recurrence. Therefore, the described therapeutic approach is applicable for all age groups.

Acknowledgments: We gratefully acknowledge the contributions of Petra and Peter Bauer in organizing the "sea-view office" on the Adriatic Sea, creating a pleasant and very inspiring work environment. We thank Edith Walther for her tremendous technical support in performing elaborate cell experiments and sample preparation in the initial stages of conceptual work, the staff at Riesling Apotheke (Ellerstadt, Germany) and especially Heike Hildebrand and Markus Wollny for their tremendous support. Without them, this strategy in the prophylaxis and treatment of dry and itchy skin and AD would not have been possible. Funding by the Institute of Precision Medicine and the Institute for Applied Research (IAF), Furtwangen University, VS-Schwenningen, Germany), is gratefully acknowledged.

Abbreviations

aCERase	lysosomal acidic ceramidase
acyl-CoA	fatty acid-coenzyme A
AD	atopic dermatitis
EASI score	eczema area and severity index score
ELOVL	very longchain-3-oxoacyl-CoA synthases
CerS	ceramide synthases
GSH	glutathione
revaCERase	reverse ceramide synthase activity of aCERase
V-ATPase	vacuolar H^+-ATPase

References

1. Williams, H.C. Atopic Dermatitis. *N. Engl. J. Med.* **2005**, *352*, 2314–2324. [CrossRef] [PubMed]
2. Paller, A.S.; Kabashima, K.; Bieber, T. Therapeutic pipeline for atopic dermatitis: End of the drought? *J. Allergy Clin. Immunol.* **2017**, *140*, 633–643. [CrossRef] [PubMed]
3. Werfel, T.; Aberer, W.; Ahrens, F.; Augustin, M.; Biedermann, T.; Diepgen, T.; Fölster-Holst, R.; Gieler, U.; Heratizadeh, A.; Kahle, J.; et al. Leitlinie Neurodermitis [atopisch es Ekzem; atopische Dermatitis] Entwicklungsstufe: S2k. *J. Dtsch. Dermatol. Ges.* **2016**, *14*, e1–e75. [CrossRef] [PubMed]
4. Wollenberg, A.; Barbarot, S.; Bieber, T.; Christen-Zaech, S.; Deleuran, M.; Fink-Wagner, A.; Gieler, U.; Girolomoni, G.; Lau, S.; Muraro, A.; et al. Consensus-based European guidelines for treatment of atopic eczema (atopic dermatitis) in adults and children: Part I. *J. Eur. Acad. Dermatol. Venereol.* **2018**, *32*, 657–682. [CrossRef] [PubMed]
5. Patel, N.U.; D'Ambra, V.; Feldman, S.R. Increasing Adherence with Topical Agents for Atopic Dermatitis. *Am. J. Clin. Dermatol.* **2017**, *18*, 323–332. [CrossRef] [PubMed]
6. van Smeden, J.; Janssens, M.; Gooris, G.S.; Bouwstra, J.A. The important role of stratum corneum lipids for the cutaneous barrier function. *Biochim. Biophys. Acta* **2014**, *1841*, 295–313. [CrossRef] [PubMed]
7. Pettus, B.J.; Chalfant, C.E.; Hannun, Y.A. Ceramide in apoptosis: An overview and current perspectives. *Biochim. Biophys. Acta BBA-Mol. Cell Biol. Lipids* **2002**, *1585*, 114–125. [CrossRef]
8. Gómez-Muñoz, A. Ceramide 1-phosphate/ceramide, a switch between life and death. *Biochim. Biophys. Acta BBA-Biomembr.* **2006**, *1758*, 2049–2056. [CrossRef]
9. Lee, J.Y.; Leonhardt, L.G.; Obeid, L.M. Cell-cycle-dependent changes in ceramide levels preceding retinoblastoma protein dephosphorylation in G2/M. *Biochem. J.* **1998**, *334*, 457–461. [CrossRef]
10. Van Brocklyn, J.R.; Williams, J.B. The control of the balance between ceramide and sphingosine-1-phosphate by sphingosine kinase: Oxidative stress and the seesaw of cell survival and death. *Comp. Biochem. Physiol. B Biochem. Mol. Biol.* **2012**, *163*, 26–36. [CrossRef]
11. Thomas, R.L.; Matsko, C.M.; Lotze, M.T.; Amoscato, A.A. Mass Spectrometric Identification of Increased C16 Ceramide Levels During Apoptosis. *J. Biol. Chem.* **1999**, *274*, 30580–30588. [CrossRef] [PubMed]
12. Hoopes, M.I.; Noro, M.G.; Longo, M.L.; Faller, R. Bilayer Structure and Lipid Dynamics in a Model Stratum Corneum with Oleic Acid. *J. Phys. Chem. B* **2011**, *115*, 3164–3171. [CrossRef] [PubMed]
13. Kanoh, H.; Ishitsuka, A.; Fujine, E.; Matsuhaba, S.; Nakamura, M.; Ito, H.; Inagaki, N.; Banno, Y.; Seishima, M. IFN-γ Reduces Epidermal Barrier Function by Affecting Fatty Acid Composition of Ceramide in a Mouse Atopic Dermatitis Model. *J. Immunol. Res.* **2019**, *2019*, 1–10. [CrossRef] [PubMed]

14. Janssens, M.; van Smeden, J.; Gooris, G.S.; Bras, W.; Portale, G.; Caspers, P.J.; Vreeken, R.J.; Hankemeier, T.; Kezic, S.; Wolterbeek, R.; et al. Increase in short-chain ceramides correlates with an altered lipid organization and decreased barrier function in atopic eczema patients. *J. Lipid Res.* **2012**, *53*, 2755–2766. [CrossRef] [PubMed]

15. van Smeden, J.; Janssens, M.; Kaye, E.C.J.; Caspers, P.J.; Lavrijsen, A.P.; Vreeken, R.J.; Bouwstra, J.A. The importance of free fatty acid chain length for the skin barrier function in atopic eczema patients. *Exp. Dermatol.* **2014**, *23*, 45–52. [CrossRef]

16. Ishikawa, J.; Narita, H.; Kondo, N.; Hotta, M.; Takagi, Y.; Masukawa, Y.; Kitahara, T.; Takema, Y.; Koyano, S.; Yamazaki, S.; et al. Changes in the Ceramide Profile of Atopic Dermatitis Patients. *J. Investig. Dermatol.* **2010**, *130*, 2511–2514. [CrossRef]

17. Franco, J.; Ferreira, C.; Paschoal Sobreira, T.J.; Sundberg, J.P.; HogenEsch, H. Profiling of epidermal lipids in a mouse model of dermatitis: Identification of potential biomarkers. *PLoS ONE* **2018**, *13*, e0196595. [CrossRef]

18. Huppertz, B.; Frank, H.-G.; Kaufmann, P. The apoptosis cascade-morphological and immunohistochemical methods for its visualization. *Anat. Embryol. (Berl.)* **1999**, *200*, 1–18. [CrossRef]

19. He, X.; Okino, N.; Dhami, R.; Dagan, A.; Gatt, S.; Schulze, H.; Sandhoff, K.; Schuchman, E.H. Purification and Characterization of Recombinant, Human Acid Ceramidase. Catalytic reactions and interactions with acid sphingomyelinase. *J. Biol. Chem.* **2003**, *278*, 32978–32986. [CrossRef]

20. Okino, N.; He, X.; Gatt, S.; Sandhoff, K.; Ito, M.; Schuchman, E.H. The Reverse Activity of Human Acid Ceramidase. *J. Biol. Chem.* **2003**, *278*, 29948–29953. [CrossRef]

21. Berdyshev, E.; Goleva, E.; Bronova, I.; Dyjack, N.; Rios, C.; Jung, J.; Taylor, P.; Jeong, M.; Hall, C.F.; Richers, B.N.; et al. Lipid abnormalities in atopic skin are driven by type 2 cytokines. *JCI Insight* **2018**, *3*, e98006. [CrossRef] [PubMed]

22. Leidl, K.; Liebisch, G.; Richter, D.; Schmitz, G. Mass spectrometric analysis of lipid species of human circulating blood cells. *Biochim. Biophys. Acta BBA-Mol. Cell Biol. Lipids* **2008**, *1781*, 655–664.

23. Pillay, C.S.; Elliott, E.; Dennison, C. Endolysosomal proteolysis and its regulation. *Biochem. J.* **2002**, *363*, 417–429. [CrossRef] [PubMed]

24. Gille, L.; Nohl, H. The Existence of a Lysosomal Redox Chain and the Role of Ubiquinone. *Arch. Biochem. Biophys.* **2000**, *375*, 347–354. [CrossRef] [PubMed]

25. Nishi, T.; Forgac, M. The vacuolar (H+)-ATPases-nature's most versatile proton pumps. *Nat. Rev. Mol. Cell Biol.* **2002**, *3*, 94–103. [CrossRef] [PubMed]

26. Grösch, S.; Schiffmann, S.; Geisslinger, G. Chain length-specific properties of ceramides. *Prog. Lipid Res.* **2012**, *51*, 50–62. [CrossRef] [PubMed]

27. Laviad, E.L.; Albee, L.; Pankova-Kholmyansky, I.; Epstein, S.; Park, H.; Merrill, A.H.; Futerman, A.H. Characterization of Ceramide Synthase 2: tissue distribution, substrate specificity, and inhibition by sphingosine 1-phosphate. *J. Biol. Chem.* **2008**, *283*, 5677–5684. [CrossRef]

28. Tidhar, R.; Zelnik, I.D.; Volpert, G.; Ben-Dor, S.; Kelly, S.; Merrill, A.H.; Futerman, A.H. Eleven residues determine the acyl chain specificity of ceramide synthases. *J. Biol. Chem.* **2018**, *293*, 9912–9921. [CrossRef]

29. Mizutani, Y.; Kihara, A.; Igarashi, Y. Identification of the human sphingolipid C4-hydroxylase, hDES2, and its up-regulation during keratinocyte differentiation. *FEBS Lett.* **2004**, *563*, 93–97. [CrossRef]

30. Naganuma, T.; Kihara, A. Two Modes of Regulation of the Fatty Acid Elongase ELOVL6 by the 3-Ketoacyl-CoA Reductase KAR in the Fatty Acid Elongation Cycle. *PLoS ONE* **2014**, *9*, e101823. [CrossRef]

31. Hassa, P.O.; Haenni, S.S.; Elser, M.; Hottiger, M.O. Nuclear ADP-Ribosylation Reactions in Mammalian Cells: Where Are We Today and Where Are We Going? *Microbiol. Mol. Biol. Rev.* **2006**, *70*, 789–829. [CrossRef] [PubMed]

32. Blaess, M.; Bibak, N.; Claus, R.A.; Kohl, M.; Bonaterra, G.A.; Kinscherf, R.; Laufer, S.; Deigner, H.-P. NB 06: From a simple lysosomotropic aSMase inhibitor to tools for elucidating the role of lysosomes in signaling apoptosis and LPS-induced inflammation. *Eur. J. Med. Chem.* **2018**, *153*, 73–104. [CrossRef] [PubMed]

33. Blaess, M.; Le, H.; Claus, R.; Kohl, M.; Deigner, H.-P. Stereospecific induction of apoptosis in tumor cells via endogenous C16-ceramide and distinct transcripts. *Cell Death Discov.* **2015**, *1*, 15013. [CrossRef] [PubMed]

34. Deigner, H.-P.; Claus, R.; Bonaterra, G.A.; Gehrke, C.; Bibak, N.; Blaess, M.; Cantz, M.; Metz, J.; Kinscherf, R. Ceramide induces aSMase expression: Implications for oxLDL-induced apoptosis. *FASEB J.* **2001**, *15*, 807–814. [CrossRef] [PubMed]

35. Kornhuber, J.; Tripal, P.; Reichel, M.; Terfloth, L.; Bleich, S.; Wiltfang, J.; Gulbins, E. Identification of New Functional Inhibitors of Acid Sphingomyelinase Using a Structure–Property–Activity Relation Model. *J. Med. Chem.* **2008**, *51*, 219–237. [CrossRef] [PubMed]

36. Kornhuber, J.; Tripal, P.; Reichel, M.; Mühle, C.; Rhein, C.; Muehlbacher, M.; Groemer, T.W.; Gulbins, E. Functional Inhibitors of Acid Sphingomyelinase (FIASMAs): A Novel Pharmacological Group of Drugs with Broad Clinical Applications. *Cell. Physiol. Biochem.* **2010**, *26*, 9–20. [CrossRef] [PubMed]

37. Thédenat, B.; Loche, F.; Albes, B.; Marguery, M.C.; Bazex, J. Acute Generalized Exanthematous Pustulosis with Photodistribution Pattern Induced by Sertraline. *Dermatology* **2001**, *203*, 87–88. [CrossRef] [PubMed]

38. Blaess, M.; Wenzel, F.; Csuk, R.; Deigner, H.-P. Topical off-label use of amitriptyline and linoleic acid to restore ceramide rheostat in atopic dermatitis lesions-a case report. *Pharm.* **2019**, *74*. [CrossRef]

39. Guttman-Yassky, E.; Krueger, J.G.; Lebwohl, M.G. Systemic immune mechanisms in atopic dermatitis and psoriasis with implications for treatment. *Exp. Dermatol.* **2018**, *27*, 409–417. [CrossRef] [PubMed]

Pathophysiology of Atopic Dermatitis and Psoriasis: Implications for Management in Children

Raj Chovatiya [1] and Jonathan I. Silverberg [2,*]

[1] Department of Dermatology, Northwestern University Feinberg School of Medicine, Chicago, IL 60611, USA; raj.chovatiya@gmail.com

[2] Department of Dermatology, George Washington University School of Medicine, Washington, DC 20037, USA

* Correspondence: jonathanisilverberg@gmail.com

Abstract: Atopic dermatitis (AD) and psoriasis are chronic inflammatory skin diseases associated with a significant cutaneous and systemic burden of disease as well as a poor health-related quality of life. Here, we review the complex pathophysiology of both AD and psoriasis and discuss the implications for treatment with current state-of-the-art and emerging topical and systemic therapies. Both AD and psoriasis are caused by a complex combination of immune dysregulation, skin-barrier disruption, genetic factors, and environmental influences. Previous treatments for both diseases were limited to anti-inflammatory agents that broadly suppress inflammation. Emerging insights into relevant pathways, including recognition of the role of T-helper type 2 driven inflammation in AD and T-helper 1 and 17 driven inflammation in psoriasis, have led to a therapeutic revolution. There are a number of novel treatment options available for AD and psoriasis with many more currently under investigation.

Keywords: atopic dermatitis; psoriasis; inflammation; cytokine; skin-barrier; topical therapy; systemic therapy; biologic therapy

1. Introduction

Atopic dermatitis (AD) and psoriasis are chronic, inflammatory skin diseases associated with considerable morbidity. Though both AD and psoriasis were once considered to be skin-limited disorders, emerging evidence suggests a substantial systemic burden of disease. AD is associated with higher rates of mental health symptoms and disorders, including depression, anxiety, and attention-deficit (hyperactivity) disorder, sleep dysregulation, other atopic disorders (e.g., asthma, hay fever), cardiovascular disease, stroke, and obesity [1–7]. Psoriasis is associated with rheumatologic (psoriatic arthritis), cardiovascular, metabolic, hepatic, and psychiatric disease [8–11]. Both AD and psoriasis are strongly associated with poor health-related quality of life (QOL), high direct and indirect costs of care, and significant societal cost—highlighting a need for optimal disease control [12–15].

AD and psoriasis are caused by a complex interplay between skin-barrier disruption, immune dysregulation, host genetics, and environment triggers [16,17]. Both diseases result in chronic, systemic inflammation with increased circulating populations of leukocytes, lymphocytes, cytokines, and chemokines (predominantly Th2 pathways in AD vs. Th1 and Th17 pathways in psoriasis) [18,19]. Previously, therapeutic options for AD and psoriasis, particularly extensive and/or severe disease, were limited to topical and non-targeted systemic immunosuppressants that had poor efficacy, safety and/or tolerability. In recent years, a better understanding of the underlying pathologic mechanisms in both conditions has led to a revolution in the development of novel, targeted therapies.

This manuscript reviews the pathophysiology of AD and psoriasis, current and novel therapeutics, and implications for management in children.

2. Atopic Dermatitis

Atopic dermatitis affects up to 15–20% of children and 1–10% of adults worldwide [20]. Approximately two-thirds of affected children present by two years of age, and 80% present by five years of age [21]. AD is a heterogeneous disorder associated with variable symptoms (e.g., pain, sleep disturbance, depression, anxiety), signs (e.g., papules, plaques, xerosis, erosions, oozing/weeping, lichenification, prurigo nodules, lichenoid papules, follicular accentuation), distributions (e.g., flexural, extensor, head and neck, hands, trunk), age of onset (e.g., pediatric, adult) and persistence (e.g., transient, intermittent, persistent) [4,5,22–34]. While some clinical characteristics are more common in children (e.g., ventral wrist dermatitis), others are more common in adults (e.g., hand and foot dermatitis, nipple eczema, thinning of the eyebrows, modification of disease course by emotional or environmental factors) [24].

AD is characterized by dysfunction in both non-immune and immune components of the skin-barrier. Despite this general framework, there is continued debate as to the exact etiology. The "outside-in" hypothesis posits that physical changes in the epidermal structure (e.g., keratinocytes, proteins, lipids, pH) drive immune dysregulation, whereas the "inside-out" hypothesis suggests that aberrant immune activity (e.g., leukocytes, lymphocytes, cytokines, antimicrobial peptides) alters the skin-barrier [35]. Despite the incongruity in the sequence of events, both models agree upon many of the same common mechanisms that result in chronic inflammation.

2.1. Pathophysiology

2.1.1. The Outside-In Hypothesis

The physical barrier function of the epidermis is crucial for protection against pathogens, allergens, toxins, and other irritants and maintenance of appropriate skin hydration. According to the outside-in hypothesis, a compromise in the complex matrix of epidermal keratinocytes, proteins, and/or lipids predisposes the epidermis to external insults, transepidermal water loss (TEWL) and reduced skin hydration, resulting in immune dysregulation and inflammation [36]. Previous studies found that lesional skin from AD patients had significant barrier dysfunction compared to healthy controls. Moreover, even previously inflamed and non-lesional skin continues to show barrier disruption [37].

Further evidence for importance of barrier dysfunction in AD is provided by loss-of-function mutations in the filaggrin gene (FLG) [38,39]. The outermost skin-barrier is composed of the cornified envelope, a highly cross-linked, flexible, insoluble structure composed of corneocytes, lipids, involucrin, loricrin, and filaggrin. Filaggrin, cleaved from its precursor profilaggrin, plays a key role in aligning and securing corneocytes, protein fibrils, and lamellar sheets [40]. Loss-of-function mutations in FLG confer increased risk of developing AD, earlier onset, persistent disease, other atopic disorders, and infection [41–43]. The processing of profilaggrin to filaggrin produces polycarboxylic acids (e.g., urocanic acid, pyrrolidone-5-carboxylic acid) known as natural moisturizing factors (NMFs) These NMFs promote hydration of the skin. A decrease in NMFs as a result of impaired profilaggrin cleavage decreases osmotic draw and results in increased TEWL [44].

NMFs and other acidic metabolites, including free fatty acids, function more broadly in decreasing skin surface pH [45]. Acidic skin pH (4–6) is important for appropriate expression, confirmation, and modification of epidermal proteins [46], inhibition (e.g., proteases) and activation (e.g., lipases) of enzymes that are critical for barrier function [47,48], and regulation of nonpathogenic skin flora [49]. Patients with AD have significantly higher pH in both lesional and non-lesional skin [50,51].

Tight junctions are epidermal protein complexes composed of claudins and occludins that are designed to seal off intercellular space, control permeability to solutes, water, pathogens, antigens, and allergens, and maintain cell polarity [52]. Functional impairment of tight junctions has been observed in patients with AD and results in skin-barrier dysfunction [53–55].

A variety of external and environmental factors have also been shown to contribute to skin-barrier impairment in AD patients, including in utero exposures [56], bacterial dysbiosis [57], harsh climate [58], water hardness [59,60], airborne pollutants [61–63], tobacco smoke [64], personal care products (i.e., irritants and pruritogens) [65–67], and, in certain cases, contact allergens [68]. Kantor and Silverberg have recently reviewed the topic of environmental risk factors in AD [69].

Thus, a variety of factors contribute to dysfunction of the physical epidermal barrier, resulting in keratinocyte damage, enhanced antigen and allergen penetration, and increased microbial signaling, ultimately resulting in immune cell activation, cytokine production, and inflammation.

2.1.2. The Inside-Out Hypothesis

According to the inside-out hypothesis of AD, dysregulation of the immune system results in disruption of the keratinocyte barrier and inflammation [70]. General support for this model is provided by the fact that many patients with AD have genetic polymorphisms in cytokines, chemokines, and receptors (including IL-4, IL-13, IL-18, IL-22, IL-31, CCL5, and CD14) [71–74], and treatment of human epidermal keratinocytes with many of these same mediators recapitulates the atopic dermatitis phenotype [75].

The innate immune system is composed of soluble and cellular effectors that utilize germline-encoded pattern recognition receptors (PRRs). Genetic polymorphisms in Toll-like receptors (TLRs), one such family of PRRs, confers increased risk of AD and staphylococcus aureus (SA) infection [76,77]. Antimicrobial peptides (AMPs), a diverse group of soluble, amphipathic, cationic proteins, are decreased in the skin of atopics and associated with increased TEWL, fatty acid loss, increased pH, and colonization with SA [78–80]. Various subsets of CD11c+ and CD1a+ dendritic cells (DCs), which specialize in antigen uptake and presentation to lymphocytes, are increased in number and activity in patients with AD and contribute to T-cell activation and polarization [81,82]. Type 2 innate lymphoid cells (ILCs) also show increased activity in AD patients and contribute to DC activation by producing IL-5 and IL-13 [83]. Keratinocyte-derived IL-25, IL-33, and thymic stromal lymphopoietin (TSLP) are increased in atopic skin and contribute to activation of DCs, type 2 ILCs, and type 2 inflammation. Though eosinophils and mast cells can both be elevated in the skin and blood of AD patients, they likely play a lesser role in the pathogenesis of AD [84].

The adaptive immune system is composed of antigen-specific lymphocytes (T-cells, B-cells) that utilize long-lasting, specific memory to direct the host immune response. Previously, AD was thought to be a disease of Th1/Th2 imbalance; however, more recent data suggest a biphasic T-cell response with additional roles played by Th17 and Th22 cells [85]. All stages of AD (early through late) are dominated by Th2 cell activity, as evidenced by increased production of the type 2 cytokines and chemokines IL-4, IL-5, IL-10, IL-13, IL-31, and CCL5 [86]. This group of mediators is involved in allergic responses, B-cell class-switching to IgE, impairment of terminal keratinocyte differentiation (through inhibition of filaggrin, loricrin, and involucrin), and downregulation of AMPs, all of which lead to increased skin permeability to exogenous antigens and pathogens [75,87]. Later stages of AD show upregulation of Th1 activity, resulting in higher levels of IFN-γ and ultimately keratinocyte apoptosis [88]. Th17 cells, a subset of T-cells defined by production of IL-17 and IL-22, appear to be increased in number but decreased in activity in AD (unlike psoriasis). Their role in pathogenesis still remains unclear. Th22 cells, a more recently described subset of T-cells that show an increased number and activity in AD lesions, produce high levels of IL-22 that may induce epidermal hyperplasia and terminal keratinocyte differentiation [89].

2.2. Treatments

2.2.1. Topical Treatments

Topical therapies are typically the first-line treatment modality for AD. They are often used as monotherapy in mild to moderate disease and in combination with systemic, biologic, or phototherapy in moderate to severe cases. Moisturizers and emollients restore the dysfunctional epidermal barrier by reducing TEWL and in certain formulations, replacing and supplementing lipids [90]. Emollients include thicker, occlusive vehicles like petrolatum and thinner, more spreadable vehicles such as creams and lotions, which are generally less effective sealants. Topical corticosteroids (TCS) act broadly to suppress the activity of innate and adaptive immune cells. Numerous randomized controlled trials (RCTs) demonstrated efficacy for both reactive and proactive treatment protocols [91]. While TCS are overall safe, efficacious, and well tolerated for a wide spectrum of disease, adverse effects (AEs) of their chronic use include skin atrophy, fragility, striae, poor wound healing, local immunosuppression, and potential systemic absorption leading to adrenal insufficiency. Topical calcineurin inhibitors (TCIs), including tacrolimus and pimecrolimus, inhibit calcineurin signaling thereby inhibiting T-cell activation. TCIs are most often used in areas of thinner skin (e.g., eyelids, axillae, genitals) that have a higher risk of AEs from TCS. They are less commonly used as first-line therapy owing to high cost, activity comparable to low potency TCS [92], slower onset than TCS, application site reactions (e.g., stinging, burning) and an FDA-issued black box warning for potential malignancy. Long-term manufacturer sponsored registries for pimecrolimus and tacrolimus have found no evidence of increased malignancy to-date [92]. As such, TCIs are still recommended for topical treatment of AD in infants, children and adults [91].

2.2.2. Systemic Treatments

Systemic corticosteroids, unlike TCS, universally suppress immune activity. While effective in the short-term and as a bridge therapy, their long-term use is limited by a poor AE profile including hyperglycemia, diabetes, weight gain, insomnia, cardiovascular disease, osteoporosis and osteonecrosis, adrenal insufficiency, gastroesophageal reflux, and immune suppression [93,94]. Systemic immunosuppressants, including cyclosporine A, methotrexate, azathioprine, and to a lesser extent, mycophenolate mofetil, demonstrated efficacy for moderate to severe AD in a variety of RCTs [95]. While more specific than systemic corticosteroids, given their relatively broad effects on immune function, systemic immunosuppressants still have a broad AE profile and are often poorly tolerated and not ideal options for long-term treatment.

2.2.3. Phosphodiesterase-4 Inhibition

In 2016, the FDA approved the first topical phosphodiesterase-4 (PDE-4) inhibitor (crisaborole) for use in mild-to-moderate AD in children and adults. PDE-4 is responsible for degrading cAMP in immune cells, which promotes the expression of pro-inflammatory cytokines like IFN-γ and IL-17 and inhibits production of anti-inflammatory cytokines such as IL-10 [96]. Two phase III, double-blind, placebo controlled RCTs in adults and children showed that crisaborole was significantly more effective than vehicle with no major AEs other than application site reactions (e.g., stinging) [97]. Other topical PDE-4 inhibitors are currently in phase I, II, and II development [98]. Apremilast, an oral PDE-4 inhibitor that is approved for the treatment of moderate-to-severe psoriasis, has also been studied in AD. A recent phase II showed no difference compared to vehicle at lower doses and modest (but statistically significant) improvement in AD at higher doses [99]. However, higher doses of apremilast were associated with a high rate of treatment emergent AEs resulting in its discontinuation during the trial [99].

2.2.4. IL-4 And IL-13 Inhibition

In 2017, the FDA approved dupilumab, a fully human monoclonal antibody for the treatment of AD. Dupilumab targets IL4Ra, a receptor subunit protein shared by both type I and type II receptors for IL-4 and/or IL-13. In phase II and III double-blind, placebo controlled RCTs, patients with moderate to severe AD treated with dupilumab showed significant improvement in a number of primary and secondary outcomes including clinician reported outcomes (e.g., Eczema Area and Severity Index (EASI), SCORing Atopic Dermatitis (SCORAD), body surface area (BSA) involvement, investigators global assessment (IGA)) and patient-reported outcomes (e.g., pruritus numeric rating scale (NRS), Patient-Oriented Eczema Measure (POEM), and Dermatology Life Quality Index (DLQI)) [100–103]. Dupilumab demonstrated an excellent safety profile with mainly mild or moderate AEs, including injection site reactions and ocular AEs (dry eye, eye pruritus, blepharitis, conjunctivitis, keratitis), with no increases of infection or malignancy overall, and lower rates of bacterial skin infection compared to placebo.

There are currently ongoing studies examining the impact of monoclonal antibodies targeting IL-13 (lebrikizumab and tralokinumab), which are even more specific than targeting IL4 and IL13 for AD [104]. Lebrikizumab in combination with TCS showed promising results in a phase II study with significant improvement in the proportion of patients achieving ≥50% reduction in EASI from baseline (EASI-50) at 12 weeks compared to placebo [105]. Tralokinumab in combination with mid-potency TCS was effective in a phase II RCT in adults and showed significant improvement in EASI, DLQI, SCORAD, and NRS-itch scores with a significant proportion of patients achieving EASI-50 and EASI-75 at 12 weeks compared to placebo [106].

2.2.5. Il-31 Inhibition

Nemolizumab, a humanized monoclonal antibody targeting the IL-31 receptor (a major signaling pathway for itch in AD), is currently in development. A phase I double-blind, placebo controlled RCT showed that a single dose of nemolizumab in AD patients resulted in significant improvement in visual analog scale (VAS)-itch, sleep and decreased use of TCS compared to placebo [107]. A phase II double-blind placebo controlled RCT demonstrated that nemolizumab 0.5 mg/kg every four weeks significantly improved VAS-itch, EASI, and IGA in adults with AD [108]. The results of phase III studies are pending.

2.2.6. Janus Kinase Inhibition

IL-4, IL-13, IL-31, and other important cytokines in the pathogenesis of AD signal through extracellular receptors that activate intracellular Janus kinases (JAKs) [109,110]. Activation of JAKs results in downstream activation of mitogen-activated protein kinases (MAPKs), phosphoinositide 3-kinases (PI3Ks), and signal transducers and activators of transcription (STATs). Multiple JAK inhibitors are currently approved therapy for treatment of rheumatoid arthritis, psoriatic arthritis, and ulcerative colitis. Emerging data showed potential efficacy for AD. A case series of six adults with moderate to severe AD treated off-label with tofacitinib (an oral JAK 1 and 3 inhibitor) showed significant improvements in pruritus and mean SCORAD [111]. A phase II double-blind, placebo controlled RCT of adults with mild-to-moderate AD demonstrated that topical tofacitinib ointment versus vehicle resulted in significant reduction in EASI, BSA, and Physician's Global Assessment (PGA). A number of other topical and/or oral JAK inhibitors are currently under investigation for treatment of AD. A phase II double-blind, placebo controlled RCT with baricitinib (an oral selective JAK 1 and 2 inhibitor) in combination with TCS showed improvement in inflammation and pruritus with significantly more patients achieving EASI-50 at 16 weeks compared to placebo [112]. A phase II double-blind, placebo controlled RCT with upadacitinib (an oral JAK 1 inhibitor) monotherapy showed a significant decrease in EASI and NRS itch scores at 16 weeks (primary endpoint) and 32 weeks (long-term extension) [113]. Additional long-term studies are underway to better understand the efficacy and safety profile of JAK inhibitors.

3. Psoriasis

Psoriasis is estimated to affect 2–3% of the global population, corresponding to >125 million individuals [114,115]. Though most affected individuals present during adulthood between 18–39 or after the age of 50, approximately one-third of patients experience their first episode of psoriasis under the age of 20 [17,114]. Psoriasis is an immune-mediated disease characterized by cycles of sustained inflammation and remission, uncontrolled keratinocyte proliferation, and impaired keratinocyte differentiation. Inflammation is driven by dysregulation in both the innate and adaptive immunity, and influenced by genetic factors. Plaque psoriasis is characterized by well-demarcated, erythematous, scaly plaques on the trunk and extensor surfaces of the limbs. Inverse psoriasis affects the intertrigenous skin with erythematous, occasionally erosive patches and plaques. Guttate psoriasis is more common in children and adolescents, and is characterized by droplet sized scaly plaques that can be triggered by group A streptococcal infection. Nearly one-half of childhood cases of psoriasis may first present in this way. Pustular psoriasis, occurring in both local and generalized forms, presents with innumerable, coalescing, sterile pustules. While psoriasis can manifest with a variety of morphologies, all subtypes share several important features: (1) hyperplasia of the epidermis (i.e., acanthosis), (2) incomplete keratinization with retention of nuclei (i.e., parakeratosis), (3) newly generated, tortuous superficial blood vessels (i.e., neovascularization), and (4) a dense inflammatory infiltrate composed of DCs, macrophages, neutrophils, and T-cells [116].

3.1. Pathophysiology

3.1.1. Dysregulated Immune Activity

The initiation phase of psoriasis consists of an external insult to the epidermis, such as trauma (e.g., Koebner phenomenon), medication (e.g., β-blocker, ACE-inhibitor, lithium), and/or infection (e.g., group A streptococcus) [115]. Following keratinocyte damage, two important events occur to activate the innate immune system: (1) keratinocytes dramatically upregulate the production of AMPs including S100, β-defensins, and LL-37 (i.e., cathelicidin), and (2) damaged keratinocytes release DNA, RNA, and other endogenous danger signals [117,118]. One proposed mechanism for the initiation of psoriasis posits that these AMPs bind to the keratinocyte DNA and RNA and activate plasmacytoid DCs (pDCs), a circulating antigen presenting cell (APC) specialized for recognition of viral pathogens. In particular, LL37 complexes with self-genetic material and binds to TLR7, TLR8, and TLR9, resulting in the secretion of type I interferons (IFN-α and IFN-β) and a break in immunologic tolerance [119–121]. Keratinocytes, which also function as a physical barrier and sensory cell in the innate immunity, produce pro-inflammatory cytokines in response to AMP-nucleic acid complexes, including type I IFNs, TNF-α, IL-1, and IL-6 [122]. Type I IFNs promote myeloid DC (mDC) differentiation, activation, and entry into skin-draining lymph nodes [123]. These cells also secrete a number of pro-inflammatory cytokines, such as TNF-α, IL-12, and IL-23, resulting in the differentiation and activation of activation of Th1, Th17, and Th22 cells.

Without specific therapeutic intervention, activation of adaptive immunity drives the self-sustaining, maintenance phase of inflammation in psoriasis [124]. The initial stage of the adaptive immunity is characterized by Th1 cell activity and concomitant production of type 1 cytokines such as IFN-γ, while Th17 cells (and to a lesser extent, Th22 cells) dominate the later portion of the adaptive immune response with production of IL-17, IL-23, IL-21, and IL-22 [125]. Recent studies focused extensively on the role Th17 cells in the pathogenesis of psoriasis, in part due to their high concentration in psoriatic lesions and significant reduction following anti-TNF-α treatment [126]. Th17 cells are a subset of T-lymphocytes that specialize in epithelial surveillance and defense against extracellular pathogens through production of IL-17, IL-23, and IL-22. The IL-17 family is composed of six members, two of which (IL-17A and IL-17F) appear to be most relevant in psoriasis. IL-17 activates a variety of intracellular kinase cascades in effector cells, including JAK, MAPK, NF-κB, and glycogen synthase kinase 3 β (GSK-3-β) [127]. IL-22 and IL-23 link immune activity and keratinocyte function by inducing keratinocyte proliferation and secretion of AMPs and cytokines [128].

Though TNF-α, IL-17, and IL-23 play a key role in the general pathophysiology of psoriasis, especially plaque psoriasis, there are additional relevant pathways in other variants of psoriasis. IL-1, IL-8, and IL-36 appear to be important for neutrophilic activity in pustular psoriasis [129,130], whereas guttate psoriasis may be driven by streptococcal superantigen mediated activation of TCRs and subsequent molecular mimicry of keratin proteins [131,132].

3.1.2. Genetic Factors

Early epidemiologic studies suggested a genetic component to psoriasis, as patients with psoriasis had higher incidence of disease among first and second-degree relatives compared to the general population, and monozygotic twins had two to threefold higher risk of psoriasis compared to dizygotic twins [133–135]. These findings were later confirmed by genome-wide linkage studies, which have identified over 70 different genetic loci associated with psoriasis [136,137]. However, variability in these loci are thought to only account for about 30% of heritability, suggesting a cumulative effect from multiple mutations with smaller individual effects and/or undetected gene-gene interactions. The nine most highly associated loci are named psoriasis susceptibility 1 through 9 (PSORS1 through PSORS9), with PSORS1 accounting for 35–50% of heritability in psoriasis [136,138]. PSORS1 is located in the major histocompatibility complex (MHC) on chromosome 6p21, spanning a 220 kb segment class I telomeric region of human leukocyte antigen B (HLA-B). This region contains several candidate genes, including *HLA-C* (associated variant HLA-Cw6 [HLA-C*06:02]; an MHC class I protein), *CDSN* (associated variant allele 5; corneodesmin, a protein expressed in the upper epidermis) [139], and *CCHCR1* (associated variant WWCC; a widely expressed protein that is overexpressed in psoriasis) [140]. While exact identification has been technically challenging due to strong linkage disequilibrium, most studies agree that HLA-Cw6 is the susceptibility allele in PSORS1 [141]. Studies of HLA-Cw6 showed several important associations: overall increased risk of psoriasis, especially in white and Chinese populations [141,142]; early-onset and more severe disease, especially in those with positive family history [141,143]; guttate psoriasis and streptococcal pharyngitis, but not pustular psoriasis [143,144]. Other psoriasis susceptibility loci include PSORS2 on chromosome 17q24–q25, which spans the gene for caspase recruitment domain-containing protein 14 (CARD14), a scaffolding protein involved triggering NF-κB activation [145,146]; PSORS4 on chromosome 1q which spans the epidermal differentiation complex [147]; PSORS6 on chromosome 19p13, which spans the gene for tyrosine kinase 2 (TYK2) [148]; PSORS7 on chromosome 1p, which spans the gene for IL-23 receptor (IL-23R) [149].

Genome-wide association studies (GWAS) have largely confirmed the findings from previous linkage studies, including the importance of the PSORS1 and the MHC locus [150–152], while identifying additional risk loci through high resolution analyses of small nucleotide polymorphisms (SNPs) in large sample populations [153,154]. Many of these variants highlight the importance of the immune system in the pathogenesis of psoriasis [155,156]. Numerous GWAS studies identified variants in cytokines, receptors, and signaling pathways that are critical for Th17 cell function: IL-23R (the receptor that binds to IL-23 and promotes activation and expansion of Th17 cells); IL-12B (the shared p40 subunit of IL-23 and IL-12); STAT3 (a signal transducer in the JAK/STAT signaling pathway downstream of several cytokine receptors including IL-23R); and Runx1 (a transcription factor important in Th17 cell differentiation) [153,155–158]. Additional variants were identified in the NF-κB signaling pathway [159,160]. More recently, next-generation sequencing and expression profiling have been combined with linkage and association studies to identify genetic variants with high accuracy, as evidenced by the successful identification of loss-of-function mutation in IL-36 antagonist (IL-36N) as the genetic basis for generalized pustular psoriasis [161,162].

3.2. Treatments

3.2.1. Topical Treatments

As with AD, topical therapies are the first-line treatment for psoriasis, both as monotherapy in mild-to-moderate disease and as combination therapy with oral systemic, biologic, and phototherapy in moderate-to-severe disease. Historically, treatment for psoriasis was limited to topical preparations of anthralin (also known as dithranol), which induces apoptosis of keratinocytes through production of reactive oxygen species, and coal tar, which inhibits production of IL-15 and nitric oxide [163,164]. Though still used today, these therapies have largely been replaced by TCS. Numerous RCTs demonstrated clinical efficacy for both continuous and intermittent treatment of psoriasis with varying potencies of TCS [165,166]. Topical vitamin D analogs (including calcitriol, calcipotriene, and tacalcitol) have broad effects of keratinocyte proliferation, apoptosis, and immunomodulation [167]. Their activity is comparable to mid-potency TCS (without the associated AEs), and is enhanced when combined or alternated with TCS [168,169]. Topical vitamin D analogs have few AEs, and systemic effects on vitamin D, calcium, and parathyroid hormone are extremely rare [170]. The TCIs tacrolimus and pimecrolimus are used off-label to treat psoriasis, particularly in the facial, genital, and intertrigenous areas [171]. While safe and efficacious, their use is limited by their overall potency, which is rated lower than mid-potency TCS and vitamin D analogs [172]. Topical retinoids (vitamin A derivatives) bind to the retinoic acid receptor (RAR) on both keratinocytes and non-immune cells, altering expression of genes important for differentiation, proliferation, and inflammation [173]. Tazarotene was the first retinoid developed for treatment of psoriasis, and, while efficacious, its continuous use is limited by local irritation. In combination with TCS, tazarotene shows increased potency and decreased local AEs [174,175].

3.2.2. Phototherapy

Phototherapy is a therapeutic option for moderate-to-severe psoriasis involving a large BSA (>10%), both as monotherapy and combination therapy. Its utility, however, is practically limited by the requirement to travel to a phototherapy center multiple times weekly or own a home phototherapy unit. The mechanism of phototherapy is believed to be multifactorial, including induction of apoptosis in keratinocytes, APCs, and Th17 cells, and promotion of regulatory T-cell (Treg) activation [176]. Broadband UVB (290–320 nm) was used for nearly a century; however, it has largely been replaced by narrow band UVB (NB-UVB; 311 nm) and excimer laser (308 nm) [177]. NB-UVB has a good safety profile with a low risk for cutaneous malignancy. In contrast, an alternative to UVB-based therapy is psoralen combined with UVA (PUVA). Oral ingestion of 8-methoxsalen is followed by exposure to UVA light, resulting in selective apoptosis of proliferating cells. Once the gold standard for targeted phototherapy, PUVA has fallen out of favor due to its carcinogenic effects and association with squamous cell carcinoma and melanoma of the skin [178,179].

3.2.3. Systemic Therapy

As was previously discussed for AD, systemic immunosuppressants, including methotrexate (the first systemic therapy approved for psoriasis) and cyclosporine A, have shown efficacy in treating moderate-to-severe psoriasis, but are limited by their relative non-specificity and broad AE profile. Acitretin is an oral second-generation retinoid that is approved for the treatment of moderate-to-severe psoriasis and is particularly efficacious for pustular psoriasis, erythrodermic psoriasis, and as an adjunct to phototherapy [180]. Similar to the mechanism of action of tazarotene, it binds to the RAR and regulates transcription of genes important for epidermal proliferation, keratinocyte differentiation, and immune cell production of cytokines. Overall, it appears to be less effective than traditional systemic agents for plaque psoriasis, and has several important AEs including dry skin and mucous membranes, dyslipidemia, elevated liver function tests, and potential teratogenicity [181].

3.2.4. Phosphodiesterase-4 Inhibition

In 2014, the FDA approved apremilast for the treatment of moderate-to-severe psoriasis. As discussed earlier, apremilast is a small molecule inhibitor of the PDE-4 enzyme that reduces the level of pro-inflammatory Th17 cytokines and increases expression of IL-10 [182]. In multiple phase III double-blind, placebo controlled RCTs, patients with moderate-to-severe plaque or palmoplantar psoriasis treated with apremilast showed significant improvement in PASI-50 (Psoriasis Area and Severity Index, ≥50% reduction from baseline), PASI-75, and static investigators global assessment (sIGA) at week 16 [183–186]. AEs include nausea, diarrhea, and weight loss, which can be quite significant and chronic in some patients. Though apremilast does not carry the same immunosuppression risks as biologic therapy, it is overall less efficacious with only approximately 30% of patients achieving PASI-75 scores at week 16.

3.2.5. TNF-α Inhibition

TNF-α inhibitors are the first generation of biologic medications for psoriasis, and they have been successfully used to treat moderate-to-severe psoriasis for over a decade. TNF-α is a pleiotropic, pro-inflammatory cytokine involved in both the innate and adaptive arms of the immune response in psoriasis. However, given its more general role in the immune response, TNF-α inhibitors have a broad AE profile, especially with regard to increased infectious risk (e.g., conversation of tuberculosis from latent to active, reactivation of hepatitis B virus). Etanercept (a recombinant human fusion protein consisting of the TNF-α receptor protein and Fc portion of immunoglobulin IgG1) was first-in-class and approved by the FDA in 2004, followed by infliximab (a human-murine chimeric monoclonal IgG1 antibody against TNF-α) in 2006, adalimumab (the first fully human monoclonal IgG1 antibody against TNF-α) in 2008, and certolizumab (a recombinant humanized IgG1 antibody Fab fragment against TNF-α conjugated to polyethylene glycol) in 2018 [187]. Phase III double-blind, placebo controlled RCTs for etanercept (PASI-75 at week 10–16: 47–49%) [188–190], infliximab (75–80%) [191,192], adalimumab (53–80%) [193–196], and certolizumab (67–83%) [197] demonstrated that biologic therapy with TNF-α inhibitors is efficacious and safe, thus paving the way for additional generations of immunotherapy.

3.2.6. IL-12/IL-23 Inhibition

The FDA approved Ustekinumab for treatment of psoriasis in 2009. Representing the next generation of biologic therapy after TNF-α inhibitors, ustekinumab is a fully human IgG1 monoclonal antibody against the shared p40 subunit of IL-12 and IL-23, thus blocking two distinct pathways of T-cell activity: Th1 and Th17, respectively [187]. Th17 cells, and to a lesser extent Th1 cells, are crucial for orchestrating the chronic, maintenance phase of psoriasis, and, as such, the p40 subunit presents a more specific target for psoriasis compared to TNF-α. Phase III double-blind, placebo controlled RCTs showed a PASI-75 of 65–78% at week 12 with overall good efficacy, safety, and long-term drug survival [198–200]. While infectious complications were the most serious AEs associated with ustekinumab, the overall rate of infections was lower than that seen with TNF-α inhibitors [201].

3.2.7. IL-17 Inhibition

Highlighting an evolving understanding of the immunological basis of psoriasis, the third generation of biologic medications approved by the FDA was the IL-17 inhibitors: secukinumab (a fully human monoclonal IgG1 antibody against IL-17A) in 2015; ixekizumab (a humanized monoclonal IgG4 antibody against IL-17A) in 2016; brodalumab (a human monoclonal IgG2 antibody against IL-17RA) in 2017 [187]. IL-17 is one of the signature cytokines produced by Th17 cells and responsible for amplifying the inflammatory cascade during the chronic phase of psoriasis. Phase III double-blind, placebo controlled RCTs showed high PASI-75 scores at week 12 (secukinumab: 75–87%; ixekizumab: 87–90%; brodalumab: 83–86%) and even significant, measurable PASI-90 and PASI-100 responses compared to placebo, TNF-α inhibitors, and/or ustekinumab [202–207]. Interestingly, even after discontinuation of treatment with secukinumab, approximately 20% maintained their response even after one year, suggesting the possibility of altering homeostatic set points with biologic therapy. Overall, while IL-17 inhibitors were well-tolerated and safe, AEs included upper respiratory infections, nasopharyngitis, and candidal infections, underscoring the important role of Th17 cells in extracellular defense at epithelial surfaces. However, the role of IL-17 inhibition in flaring inflammatory bowel disease (IBD) in those with a personal or family history of IBD is currently under investigation [208].

3.2.8. IL-23 Inhibition

Based on clinical data from ustekinumab patients in conjunction with basic studies showing protective effects of IL-12 in psoriasis [209] and a more important role for IL-12 in Th1 mediated host defense, IL-23 was identified as a more specific target for psoriasis therapy [210]. The latest generation of biologic medications approved by the FDA for use in moderate-to-severe psoriasis are the IL-23 inhibitors: guselkumab in 2017; tildrakizumab in 2018; and risankizumab in 2019, all of which are human monoclonal IgG1 antibodies against the p19 subunit of IL-23 [187]. Primary or secondary endpoints for the phase III double-blind, placebo controlled RCTs of the IL-23 inhibitors were measured with PASI-90 (guselkumab: week 16, 70–85%; tildrakizumab: week 12, 35%; risankizumab: week 16, 72–75%) and PASI-100 scores, representing a remarkable improvement in treatment specificity [211–216]. IL-23 inhibitors showed higher efficacy compared head-to-head with TNF-α inhibitors and/or ustekinumab. As was seen with IL-17 inhibitors, about one-quarter of patients who discontinued therapy with risankizumab after 16 weeks maintained their response even after 48 weeks, again suggesting the possibility for long-term modification of cytokine signaling pathways with biologic therapy. IL-23 inhibitors were well-tolerated and safe, with most AEs related to infection (upper respiratory infection, gastroenteritis, herpes simplex virus, tinea).

3.2.9. Janus Kinase Inhibition

Many of the Th17 and Th1 cytokines involved in the pathogenesis of psoriasis signal through JAK. Oral tofacitinib is currently an FDA-approved therapy for psoriatic arthritis [217,218], and has shown promising findings for the treatment of psoriasis in phase III double-blind, placebo controlled RCTs (PASI-75 at week 16: 40–59%) [219,220]. Topical tofacitinib has also demonstrated efficacy in phase II RCTs for psoriasis [221,222]. However, systemic tofacitinib use is associated with a number of infectious AEs (several of which were observed during trials), and, in 2015, the FDA declined to approve oral tofacitinib for use in moderate-to-severe without additional safety studies. Further investigation of tofacitinib, as well as other oral JAK inhibitors including baricitinib [223] and peficitinib [224], is ongoing.

4. Management in Children

For the treatment of mild-to-moderate AD or psoriasis in children, first-line therapies include TCS and TCI, with the addition of emollients for AD and topical vitamin D analogs for psoriasis. Data supporting their use in monotherapy and/or combination therapy is derived from years of anecdotal clinical experience and studies performed in adults, as RCTs are for these agents are rare in children, especially under the age of 12. TCS use in children is sometimes limited given concern for cutaneous (e.g., atrophy, fragility, striae, infection) and systemic (e.g., hypothalamic–pituitary axis suppression) AEs. While TCIs do not cause atrophy or hypothalamic–pituitary axis suppression, they are associated with application site reactions such as burning or stinging and a theoretical black-box warning by the United States Food and Drug Association for malignancy. Despite these potential AEs, both TCS and TCIs can be used safely and efficaciously in continuous and/or intermittent fashion. Adjunctive treatment with topical vitamin D analogs in children with psoriasis is overall very well tolerated with minimal cutaneous AEs and extremely rare systemic AEs (e.g., hypercalcemia, hypercalciuria) with overuse. Crisaborole was recently added as an additional first-line topical option in AD, and the combination of its relatively specific mode of action, non-steroidal formulation, and promising long-term safety data make it an important addition to the pediatric AD arsenal [225]. However, further studies are needed to better understand crisaborole's efficacy in children, especially in comparison with TCS and TCIs. Common AEs of crisaborole in children include application site burning and/or stinging and, rarely, application site skin infection. For psoriasis, Tazarotene is rarely used in children given the associated skin irritation, while anthralin and coal tar are limited by practical features associated with application: staining of skin and clothing (both agents) and malodor (coal tar).

For the treatment of moderate-to-severe AD or psoriasis in children, treatment options include systemic therapy (most of which are used off-label), phototherapy, and biologic agents. Current guidelines recommend a stepwise approach to treatment in children with moderate-to-severe disease with biologic agents at the top of the therapeutic ladder. Methotrexate is the most frequently used systemic agent in children and has demonstrated reasonable efficacy in prospective and retrospective analyses, though the overall quality of data is low with high inter-study variability [226–231]. Disadvantages include the need for continuous lab monitoring and potential AEs including hepatotoxicity and liver fibrosis (especially with long-term use), hematologic abnormalities, and gastrointestinal symptoms. Cyclosporine A, which is usually reserved for flaring and/or refractory AD and psoriasis, has shown good efficacy in the short-term in several uncontrolled studies; however, there are sparse data on long-term effects in children [229,232]. Furthermore, chronic use of cyclosporine A is associated with a number of severe AEs including infection, malignancy, hypertension, nephrotoxicity, and hepatotoxicity. Acitretin can be effective for children with psoriasis (especially the pustular subtype) but can cause severe dryness of the skin and mucous membranes as well as dyslipidemia [229]. Other systemic therapies have limited data to support use, including mycophenolate mofetil and azathioprine. Both are associated with similar AEs that restrict their use in children, including diarrhea, nausea, vomiting, anemia, leukopenia, immune suppression, and increased risk of infection. Systemic corticosteroids are generally contraindicated for management of AD and psoriasis despite continued inappropriate use especially in childhood AD [233], and they should only be used as bridge therapy, for immediate relief, or when other options are not available. Common side effects of chronic systemic corticosteroid use in children are similar to those in adults and include immune suppression, hyperglycemia, weight gain, insomnia, gastroesophageal reflux, osteonecrosis, and adrenal insufficiency.

For both AD and psoriasis, phototherapy with either NB-UVB or excimer laser can be preferable to systemic immunosuppressive therapy in children given the limited AEs. Uncontrolled studies support its efficacy; however, multiple sessions per week in-office can be challenging for children and caregivers, and there continues to be concern about long-term exposure to UVB light starting in childhood [234–236].

Dupilumab is currently the only biologic agent available for the treatment of AD, though many new biologics are under investigation. The FDA recently expanded dupilumab's indication in 2019 for use in children ≥12 years old with AD, and investigation for use in infants and children with AD is currently ongoing. Long-term safety and efficacy data for dupilumab use in children are eagerly anticipated, with adult open-label extension data supporting its continuous, long-term use [237]. The most common treatment-related AEs observed in both adolescents and adults included injection site reactions, conjunctivitis, and nasopharyngitis. For children with psoriasis, etanercept [238], adalimumab [239], and ustekinumab [240] have been studied in phase III double-blind, placebo controlled RCTs. All three agents showed comparable efficacy and safety to the previous adult trials. Adalimumab showed higher efficacy in head-to-head comparison with methotrexate. Currently, the only FDA-approved biologics in children are etanercept (≥4 years old) and ustekinumab (≥12 years old), with ongoing studies for many of the newer treatment classes. In general, biologic treatment-associated AEs in children with psoriasis are similar to those observed in adults and more favorable compared to classic systemic therapies. Common AEs associated with TNF-α and IL-12/IL-23 inhibitors use in children include injection site reactions, nasopharyngitis, mild upper respiratory infection (similar to those normally seen in children), and headache.

5. Conclusions

Improved understanding of the pathophysiology of AD and psoriasis has led to a revolution in targeted therapy. Targeted treatments have filled many unmet needs for both of these conditions. As additional novel agents are approved, the next goal in management of AD and psoriasis is to optimize specific treatments for individual patients. The next decade of research will be dominated by extensive genetic, molecular, and clinical phenotyping of patients in order to understand which pathologic mechanisms are most relevant. The era for personalized medicine in AD and psoriasis is upon us!

Author Contributions: Data curation, R.C. and J.I.S.; Formal analysis, R.C. and J.I.S.; Writing—original draft, R.C. and J.I.S.; Writing—review and editing, R.C. and J.I.S.

References

1. Silverberg, J.I.; Silverberg, N.B.; Lee-Wong, M. Association between atopic dermatitis and obesity in adulthood. *Br. J. Dermatol.* **2012**, *166*, 498–504. [CrossRef] [PubMed]

2. Silverberg, J.I. Association between adult atopic dermatitis, cardiovascular disease, and increased heart attacks in three population-based studies. *Allergy* **2015**, *70*, 1300–1308. [CrossRef] [PubMed]

3. Yu, S.H.; Silverberg, J.I. Association between Atopic Dermatitis and Depression in US Adults. *J. Investig. Dermatol.* **2015**, *135*, 3183–3186. [CrossRef] [PubMed]

4. Silverberg, J.I.; Garg, N.K.; Paller, A.S.; Fishbein, A.B.; Zee, P.C. Sleep disturbances in adults with eczema are associated with impaired overall health: A US population-based study. *J. Investig. Dermatol.* **2015**, *135*, 56–66. [CrossRef]

5. Yu, S.H.; Attarian, H.; Zee, P.; Silverberg, J.I. Burden of Sleep and Fatigue in US Adults With Atopic Dermatitis. *Dermatitis* **2016**, *27*, 50–58. [CrossRef]

6. Silverberg, J.I.; Simpson, E.L. Association between severe eczema in children and multiple comorbid conditions and increased healthcare utilization. *Pediatric Allergy Immunol.* **2013**, *24*, 476–486. [CrossRef]

7. Strom, M.A.; Fishbein, A.B.; Paller, A.S.; Silverberg, J.I. Association between atopic dermatitis and attention deficit hyperactivity disorder in U.S. children and adults. *Br. J. Dermatol.* **2016**, *175*, 920–929. [CrossRef]

8. Gelfand, J.M.; Neimann, A.L.; Shin, D.B.; Wang, X.; Margolis, D.J.; Troxel, A.B. Risk of myocardial infarction in patients with psoriasis. *JAMA* **2006**, *296*, 1735–1741. [CrossRef]

9. Ludwig, R.J.; Herzog, C.; Rostock, A.; Ochsendorf, F.R.; Zollner, T.M.; Thaci, D.; Kaufmann, R.; Vogl, T.J.; Boehncke, W.-H. Psoriasis: A possible risk factor for development of coronary artery calcification. *Br. J. Dermatol.* **2007**, *156*, 271–276. [CrossRef]

10. Gisondi, P.; Fostini, A.C.; Fossà, I.; Girolomoni, G.; Targher, G. Psoriasis and the metabolic syndrome. *Clin. Dermatol.* **2018**, *36*, 21–28. [CrossRef]

11. Kim, N.; Thrash, B.; Menter, A. Comorbidities in psoriasis patients. *Semin. Cutan. Med. Surg.* **2010**, *29*, 10–15. [CrossRef] [PubMed]

12. Chiesa Fuxench, Z.C.; Block, J.K.; Boguniewicz, M.; Boyle, J.; Fonacier, L.; Gelfand, J.M.; Grayson, M.H.; Margolis, D.J.; Mitchell, L.; Silverberg, J.I.; et al. Atopic Dermatitis in America Study: A Cross-Sectional Study Examining the Prevalence and Disease Burden of Atopic Dermatitis in the US Adult Population. *J. Investig. Dermatol.* **2019**, *139*, 583–590. [CrossRef]

13. Silverberg, J.I. Public Health Burden and Epidemiology of Atopic Dermatitis. *Dermatol. Clin.* **2017**, *35*, 283–289. [CrossRef] [PubMed]

14. Gelfand, J.M.; Feldman, S.R.; Stern, R.S.; Thomas, J.; Rolstad, T.; Margolis, D.J. Determinants of quality of life in patients with psoriasis: A study from the US population. *J. Am. Acad. Dermatol.* **2004**, *51*, 704–708. [CrossRef] [PubMed]

15. De Korte, J.; Sprangers, M.A.; Mombers, F.M.; Bos, J.D. Quality of life in patients with psoriasis: A systematic literature review. *J. Investig. Dermatol. Symp. Proc.* **2004**, *9*, 140–147. [CrossRef]

16. Weidinger, S.; Beck, L.A.; Bieber, T.; Kabashima, K.; Irvine, A.D. Atopic dermatitis. *Nat. Rev. Dis. Primers* **2018**, *4*, 1–20. [CrossRef]

17. Greb, J.E.; Goldminz, A.M.; Elder, J.T.; Lebwohl, M.G.; Gladman, D.D.; Wu, J.J.; Mehta, N.N.; Finlay, A.Y.; Gottlieb, A.B. Psoriasis. *Nat. Rev. Dis. Primers* **2016**, *2*, 16082. [CrossRef]

18. Cai, Y.; Fleming, C.; Yan, J. New insights of T cells in the pathogenesis of psoriasis. *Cell. Mol. Immunol.* **2012**, *9*, 302–309. [CrossRef]

19. Brunner, P.M.; Guttman-Yassky, E.; Leung, D.Y.M. The immunology of atopic dermatitis and its reversibility with broad-spectrum and targeted therapies. *J. Allergy Clin. Immunol.* **2017**, *139*, S65–S76. [CrossRef]

20. Garg, N.; Silverberg, J.I. Epidemiology of childhood atopic dermatitis. *Clin. Dermatol.* **2015**, *33*, 281–288. [CrossRef]

21. Levy, R.M.; Gelfand, J.M.; Yan, A.C. The epidemiology of atopic dermatitis. *Clin. Dermatol.* **2003**, *21*, 109–115. [CrossRef]

22. McKenzie, C.; Silverberg, J.I. The prevalence and persistence of atopic dermatitis in urban United States children. *Ann. Allergy Asthma Immunol.* **2019**, *123*, 173–178.e171. [CrossRef] [PubMed]

23. Kim, J.P.; Chao, L.X.; Simpson, E.L.; Silverberg, J.I. Persistence of atopic dermatitis (AD): A systematic review and meta-analysis. *J. Am. Acad. Dermatol.* **2016**, *75*, 681–687.e611. [CrossRef] [PubMed]

24. Yew, Y.W.; Thyssen, J.P.; Silverberg, J.I. A systematic review and meta-analysis of the regional and age-related differences in atopic dermatitis clinical characteristics. *J. Am. Acad. Dermatol.* **2019**, *80*, 390–401. [CrossRef]

25. Vakharia, P.P.; Silverberg, J.I. Adult-Onset Atopic Dermatitis: Characteristics and Management. *Am. J. Clin. Dermatol.* **2019**, *76*, 958. [CrossRef]

26. Vakharia, P.P.; Chopra, R.; Sacotte, R.; Patel, K.R.; Singam, V.; Patel, N.; Immaneni, S.; White, T.; Kantor, R.; Hsu, D.Y.; et al. Burden of skin pain in atopic dermatitis. *Ann. Allergy Asthma Immunol.* **2017**, *119*, 548–552.e543. [CrossRef]

27. Silverberg, J.I.; Vakharia, P.P.; Chopra, R.; Sacotte, R.; Patel, N.; Immaneni, S.; White, T.; Kantor, R.; Hsu, D.Y. Phenotypical Differences of Childhood- and Adult-Onset Atopic Dermatitis. *J. Allergy Clin. Immunol. Pract.* **2018**, *6*, 1306–1312. [CrossRef]

28. Silverberg, J.I.; Margolis, D.J.; Boguniewicz, M.; Fonacier, L.; Grayson, M.H.; Ong, P.Y.; Chiesa Fuxench, Z.C.; Simpson, E.L.; Gelfand, J.M. Distribution of atopic dermatitis lesions in United States adults. *J. Eur. Acad. Dermatol. Venereol.* **2019**, *33*, 1341–1348. [CrossRef]

29. Silverberg, J.I.; Gelfand, J.M.; Margolis, D.J.; Boguniewicz, M.; Fonacier, L.; Grayson, M.H.; Ong, P.Y.; Chiesa Fuxench, Z.C.; Simpson, E.L. Symptoms and diagnosis of anxiety and depression in atopic dermatitis in U.S. adults. *Br. J. Dermatol.* **2019**, *119*, e3. [CrossRef]

30. Silverberg, J.I.; Gelfand, J.M.; Margolis, D.J.; Boguniewicz, M.; Fonacier, L.; Grayson, M.H.; Chiesa Fuxench, Z.C.; Simpson, E.L.; Ong, P.Y. Pain Is a Common and Burdensome Symptom of Atopic Dermatitis in United States Adults. *J. Allergy Clin. Immunol. Pract.* **2019**. [CrossRef]

31. Silverberg, J.I. Adult-Onset Atopic Dermatitis. *J. Allergy Clin. Immunol. Pract.* **2019**, *7*, 28–33. [CrossRef] [PubMed]

32. Patel, K.R.; Immaneni, S.; Singam, V.; Rastogi, S.; Silverberg, J.I. Association between atopic dermatitis, depression, and suicidal ideation: A systematic review and meta-analysis. *J. Am. Acad. Dermatol.* **2019**, *80*, 402–410. [CrossRef] [PubMed]

33. Li, J.C.; Fishbein, A.; Singam, V.; Patel, K.R.; Zee, P.C.; Attarian, H.; Cella, D.; Silverberg, J.I. Sleep Disturbance and Sleep-Related Impairment in Adults With Atopic Dermatitis: A Cross-sectional Study. *Dermatitis* **2018**, *29*, 270–277. [CrossRef] [PubMed]

34. Cheng, B.T.; Silverberg, J.I. Depression and psychological distress in US adults with atopic dermatitis. *Ann. Allergy Asthma Immunol.* **2019**, *123*, 179–185. [CrossRef] [PubMed]

35. Silverberg, N.B.; Silverberg, J.I. Inside out or outside in: Does atopic dermatitis disrupt barrier function or does disruption of barrier function trigger atopic dermatitis? *Cutis* **2015**, *96*, 359–361. [PubMed]

36. Wolf, R.; Wolf, D. Abnormal epidermal barrier in the pathogenesis of atopic dermatitis. *Clin. Dermatol.* **2012**, *30*, 329–334. [CrossRef]

37. Seidenari, S.; Giusti, G. Objective assessment of the skin of children affected by atopic dermatitis: A study of pH, capacitance and TEWL in eczematous and clinically uninvolved skin. *Acta Derm. Venereol.* **1995**, *75*, 429–433. [CrossRef]

38. Baurecht, H.; Irvine, A.D.; Novak, N.; Illig, T.; Bühler, B.; Ring, J.; Wagenpfeil, S.; Weidinger, S. Toward a major risk factor for atopic eczema: Meta-analysis of filaggrin polymorphism data. *J. Allergy Clin. Immunol.* **2007**, *120*, 1406–1412. [CrossRef]

39. Palmer, C.N.A.; Irvine, A.D.; Terron-Kwiatkowski, A.; Zhao, Y.; Liao, H.; Lee, S.P.; Goudie, D.R.; Sandilands, A.; Campbell, L.E.; Smith, F.J.D.; et al. Common loss-of-function variants of the epidermal barrier protein filaggrin are a major predisposing factor for atopic dermatitis. *Nat. Genet.* **2006**, *38*, 441–446. [CrossRef]

40. O'Regan, G.M.; Sandilands, A.; McLean, W.H.I.; Irvine, A.D. Filaggrin in atopic dermatitis. *J. Allergy Clin. Immunol.* **2009**, *124*, R2–R6. [CrossRef]

41. Mócsai, G.; Gáspár, K.; Nagy, G.; Irinyi, B.; Kapitány, A.; Bíró, T.; Gyimesi, E.; Tóth, B.; Maródi, L.; Szegedi, A. Severe skin inflammation and filaggrin mutation similarly alter the skin barrier in patients with atopic dermatitis. *Br. J. Dermatol.* **2014**, *170*, 617–624. [CrossRef] [PubMed]

42. Szegedi, A. Filaggrin mutations in early- and late-onset atopic dermatitis. *Br. J. Dermatol.* **2015**, *172*, 320–321. [CrossRef] [PubMed]

43. Irvine, A.D.; McLean, W.H.I.; Leung, D.Y.M. Filaggrin mutations associated with skin and allergic diseases. *N. Engl. J. Med.* **2011**, *365*, 1315–1327. [CrossRef] [PubMed]

44. Riethmuller, C.; McAleer, M.A.; Koppes, S.A.; Abdayem, R.; Franz, J.; Haftek, M.; Campbell, L.E.; MacCallum, S.F.; McLean, W.H.I.; Irvine, A.D.; et al. Filaggrin breakdown products determine corneocyte conformation in patients with atopic dermatitis. *J. Allergy Clin. Immunol.* **2015**, *136*, 1573–1580.e1572. [CrossRef]

45. Fluhr, J.W.; Kao, J.; Jain, M.; Ahn, S.K.; Feingold, K.R.; Elias, P.M. Generation of free fatty acids from phospholipids regulates stratum corneum acidification and integrity. *J. Investig. Dermatol.* **2001**, *117*, 44–51. [CrossRef]

46. Fluhr, J.W.; Elias, P.M. Stratum corneum pH: Formation and Function of the 'Acid Mantle'. *Exog. Dermatol.* **2002**, *1*, 163–175. [CrossRef]

47. Jang, H.; Matsuda, A.; Jung, K.; Karasawa, K.; Matsuda, K.; Oida, K.; Ishizaka, S.; Ahn, G.; Amagai, Y.; Moon, C.; et al. Skin pH Is the Master Switch of Kallikrein 5-Mediated Skin Barrier Destruction in a Murine Atopic Dermatitis Model. *J. Investig. Dermatol.* **2016**, *136*, 127–135. [CrossRef]

48. Brattsand, M.; Stefansson, K.; Lundh, C.; Haasum, Y.; Egelrud, T. A proteolytic cascade of kallikreins in the stratum corneum. *J. Investig. Dermatol.* **2005**, *124*, 198–203. [CrossRef]

49. Cork, M.J.; Danby, S.G.; Vasilopoulos, Y.; Hadgraft, J.; Lane, M.E.; Moustafa, M.; Guy, R.H.; Macgowan, A.L.; Tazi-Ahnini, R.; Ward, S.J. Epidermal barrier dysfunction in atopic dermatitis. *J. Investig. Dermatol.* **2009**, *129*, 1892–1908. [CrossRef]

50. Sparavigna, A.; Setaro, M.; Gualandri, V. Cutaneous pH in children affected by atopic dermatitis and in healthy children: A multicenter study. *Skin Res. Technol.* **1999**, *5*, 221–227. [CrossRef]

51. Eberlein-König, B.; Schäfer, T.; Huss-Marp, J.; Darsow, U.; Möhrenschlager, M.; Herbert, O.; Abeck, D.; Krämer, U.; Behrendt, H.; Ring, J. Skin surface pH, stratum corneum hydration, trans-epidermal water loss and skin roughness related to atopic eczema and skin dryness in a population of primary school children. *Acta Derm. Venereol.* **2000**, *80*, 188–191. [CrossRef] [PubMed]

52. Tsukita, S.; Yamazaki, Y.; Katsuno, T.; Tamura, A. Tight junction-based epithelial microenvironment and cell proliferation. *Oncogene* **2008**, *27*, 6930–6938. [CrossRef] [PubMed]

53. Yuki, T.; Tobiishi, M.; Kusaka-Kikushima, A.; Ota, Y.; Tokura, Y. Impaired Tight Junctions in Atopic Dermatitis Skin and in a Skin-Equivalent Model Treated with Interleukin-17. *PLoS ONE* **2016**, *11*, e0161759. [CrossRef] [PubMed]

54. Yuki, T.; Komiya, A.; Kusaka, A.; Kuze, T.; Sugiyama, Y.; Inoue, S. Impaired tight junctions obstruct stratum corneum formation by altering polar lipid and profilaggrin processing. *J. Dermatol. Sci.* **2013**, *69*, 148–158. [CrossRef]

55. De Benedetto, A.; Rafaels, N.M.; McGirt, L.Y.; Ivanov, A.I.; Georas, S.N.; Cheadle, C.; Berger, A.E.; Zhang, K.; Vidyasagar, S.; Yoshida, T.; et al. Tight junction defects in patients with atopic dermatitis. *J. Allergy Clin. Immunol.* **2011**, *127*, 773–786.e7. [CrossRef]

56. Hartwig, I.R.V.; Sly, P.D.; Schmidt, L.A.; van Lieshout, R.J.; Bienenstock, J.; Holt, P.G.; Arck, P.C. Prenatal adverse life events increase the risk for atopic diseases in children, which is enhanced in the absence of a maternal atopic predisposition. *J. Allergy Clin. Immunol.* **2014**, *134*, 160–169. [CrossRef]

57. Nakatsuji, T.; Chen, T.H.; Two, A.M.; Chun, K.A.; Narala, S.; Geha, R.S.; Hata, T.R.; Gallo, R.L. Staphylococcus aureus Exploits Epidermal Barrier Defects in Atopic Dermatitis to Trigger Cytokine Expression. *J. Investig. Dermatol.* **2016**, *136*, 2192–2200. [CrossRef]

58. Engebretsen, K.A.; Johansen, J.D.; Kezic, S.; Linneberg, A.; Thyssen, J.P. The effect of environmental humidity and temperature on skin barrier function and dermatitis. *J. Eur. Acad. Dermatol. Venereol.* **2016**, *30*, 223–249. [CrossRef]

59. Perkin, M.R.; Craven, J.; Logan, K.; Strachan, D.; Marrs, T.; Radulovic, S.; Campbell, L.E.; MacCallum, S.F.; McLean, W.H.I.; Lack, G.; et al. Association between domestic water hardness, chlorine, and atopic dermatitis risk in early life: A population-based cross-sectional study. *J. Allergy Clin. Immunol.* **2016**, *138*, 509–516. [CrossRef]

60. McNally, N.J.; Williams, H.C.; Phillips, D.R.; Smallman-Raynor, M.; Lewis, S.; Venn, A.; Britton, J. Atopic eczema and domestic water hardness. *Lancet* **1998**, *352*, 527–531. [CrossRef]

61. Kathuria, P.; Silverberg, J.I. Association of pollution and climate with atopic eczema in US children. *Pediatric Allergy Immunol.* **2016**, *27*, 478–485. [CrossRef] [PubMed]

62. Kim, J.; Han, Y.; Ahn, J.H.; Kim, S.W.; Lee, S.I.; Lee, K.H.; Ahn, K. Airborne formaldehyde causes skin barrier dysfunction in atopic dermatitis. *Br. J. Dermatol.* **2016**, *175*, 357–363. [CrossRef] [PubMed]

63. Ahn, K. The role of air pollutants in atopic dermatitis. *J. Allergy Clin. Immunol.* **2014**, *134*, 993–999, discussion 1000. [CrossRef] [PubMed]

64. Kantor, R.; Kim, A.; Thyssen, J.P.; Silverberg, J.I. Association of atopic dermatitis with smoking: A systematic review and meta-analysis. *J. Am. Acad. Dermatol.* **2016**, *75*, 1119–1125.e1111. [CrossRef] [PubMed]

65. Gfatter, R.; Hackl, P.; Braun, F. Effects of soap and detergents on skin surface pH, stratum corneum hydration and fat content in infants. *Dermatology* **1997**, *195*, 258–262. [CrossRef]

66. Angelova-Fischer, I.; Dapic, I.; Hoek, A.-K.; Jakasa, I.; Fischer, T.W.; Zillikens, D.; Kezic, S. Skin barrier integrity and natural moisturising factor levels after cumulative dermal exposure to alkaline agents in atopic dermatitis. *Acta Derm. Venereol.* **2014**, *94*, 640–644. [CrossRef] [PubMed]

67. Nassif, A.; Chan, S.C.; Storrs, F.J.; Hanifin, J.M. Abnormal skin irritancy in atopic dermatitis and in atopy without dermatitis. *Arch. Dermatol.* **1994**, *130*, 1402–1407. [CrossRef]

68. Thyssen, J.P.; McFadden, J.P.; Kimber, I. The multiple factors affecting the association between atopic dermatitis and contact sensitization. *Allergy* **2014**, *69*, 28–36. [CrossRef]

69. Kantor, R.; Silverberg, J.I. Environmental risk factors and their role in the management of atopic dermatitis. *Expert Rev. Clin. Immunol.* **2017**, *13*, 15–26. [CrossRef]

70. Czarnowicki, T.; Krueger, J.G.; Guttman-Yassky, E. Skin barrier and immune dysregulation in atopic dermatitis: An evolving story with important clinical implications. *J. Allergy Clin. Immunol. Pract.* **2014**, *2*, 371–379. [CrossRef]

71. Schulz, F.; Marenholz, I.; Fölster-Holst, R.; Chen, C.; Sternjak, A.; Baumgrass, R.; Esparza-Gordillo, J.; Grüber, C.; Nickel, R.; Schreiber, S.; et al. A common haplotype of the IL-31 gene influencing gene expression is associated with nonatopic eczema. *J. Allergy Clin. Immunol.* **2007**, *120*, 1097–1102. [CrossRef] [PubMed]

72. Oiso, N.; Fukai, K.; Ishii, M. Interleukin 4 receptor alpha chain polymorphism Gln551Arg is associated with adult atopic dermatitis in Japan. *Br. J. Dermatol.* **2000**, *142*, 1003–1006. [CrossRef] [PubMed]

73. Novak, N.; Kruse, S.; Potreck, J.; Maintz, L.; Jenneck, C.; Weidinger, S.; Fimmers, R.; Bieber, T. Single nucleotide polymorphisms of the IL18 gene are associated with atopic eczema. *J. Allergy Clin. Immunol.* **2005**, *115*, 828–833. [CrossRef] [PubMed]

74. Hanifin, J.M. Evolving concepts of pathogenesis in atopic dermatitis and other eczemas. *J. Investig. Dermatol.* **2009**, *129*, 320–322. [CrossRef]

75. Malajian, D.; Guttman-Yassky, E. New pathogenic and therapeutic paradigms in atopic dermatitis. *Cytokine* **2015**, *73*, 311–318. [CrossRef]

76. Niebuhr, M.; Langnickel, J.; Draing, C.; Renz, H.; Kapp, A.; Werfel, T. Dysregulation of toll-like receptor-2 (TLR-2)-induced effects in monocytes from patients with atopic dermatitis: Impact of the TLR-2 R753Q polymorphism. *Allergy* **2008**, *63*, 728–734. [CrossRef]

77. Ahmad-Nejad, P.; Mrabet-Dahbi, S.; Breuer, K.; Klotz, M.; Werfel, T.; Herz, U.; Heeg, K.; Neumaier, M.; Renz, H. The toll-like receptor 2 R753Q polymorphism defines a subgroup of patients with atopic dermatitis having severe phenotype. *J. Allergy Clin. Immunol.* **2004**, *113*, 565–567. [CrossRef]

78. Ong, P.Y.; Ohtake, T.; Brandt, C.; Strickland, I.; Boguniewicz, M.; Ganz, T.; Gallo, R.L.; Leung, D.Y.M. Endogenous antimicrobial peptides and skin infections in atopic dermatitis. *N. Engl. J. Med.* **2002**, *347*, 1151–1160. [CrossRef]

79. Hata, T.R.; Gallo, R.L. Antimicrobial peptides, skin infections, and atopic dermatitis. *Semin. Cutan. Med. Surg.* **2008**, *27*, 144–150. [CrossRef]

80. Kobayashi, T.; Glatz, M.; Horiuchi, K.; Kawasaki, H.; Akiyama, H.; Kaplan, D.H.; Kong, H.H.; Amagai, M.; Nagao, K. Dysbiosis and Staphylococcus aureus Colonization Drives Inflammation in Atopic Dermatitis. *Immunity* **2015**, *42*, 756–766. [CrossRef]

81. Johnson-Huang, L.M.; McNutt, N.S.; Krueger, J.G.; Lowes, M.A. Cytokine-producing dendritic cells in the pathogenesis of inflammatory skin diseases. *J. Clin. Immunol.* **2009**, *29*, 247–256. [CrossRef] [PubMed]

82. Guttman-Yassky, E.; Lowes, M.A.; Fuentes-Duculan, J.; Whynot, J.; Novitskaya, I.; Cardinale, I.; Haider, A.; Khatcherian, A.; Carucci, J.A.; Bergman, R.; et al. Major differences in inflammatory dendritic cells and their products distinguish atopic dermatitis from psoriasis. *J. Allergy Clin. Immunol.* **2007**, *119*, 1210–1217. [CrossRef] [PubMed]

83. Hammad, H.; Lambrecht, B.N. Barrier Epithelial Cells and the Control of Type 2 Immunity. *Immunity* **2015**, *43*, 29–40. [CrossRef] [PubMed]

84. Liu, F.-T.; Goodarzi, H.; Chen, H.-Y. IgE, mast cells, and eosinophils in atopic dermatitis. *Clin. Rev. Allergy Immunol.* **2011**, *41*, 298–310. [CrossRef]

85. Leung, D.Y.M.; Boguniewicz, M.; Howell, M.D.; Nomura, I.; Hamid, Q.A. New insights into atopic dermatitis. *J. Clin. Investig.* **2004**, *113*, 651–657. [CrossRef]

86. Gittler, J.K.; Shemer, A.; Suárez-Fariñas, M.; Fuentes-Duculan, J.; Gulewicz, K.J.; Wang, C.Q.F.; Mitsui, H.; Cardinale, I.; de Guzman Strong, C.; Krueger, J.G.; et al. Progressive activation of T(H)2/T(H)22 cytokines and selective epidermal proteins characterizes acute and chronic atopic dermatitis. *J. Allergy Clin. Immunol.* **2012**, *130*, 1344–1354. [CrossRef]

87. Howell, M.D.; Fairchild, H.R.; Kim, B.E.; Bin, L.; Boguniewicz, M.; Redzic, J.S.; Hansen, K.C.; Leung, D.Y.M. Th2 cytokines act on S100/A11 to downregulate keratinocyte differentiation. *J. Investig. Dermatol.* **2008**, *128*, 2248–2258. [CrossRef]

88. Rebane, A.; Zimmermann, M.; Aab, A.; Baurecht, H.; Koreck, A.; Karelson, M.; Abram, K.; Metsalu, T.; Pihlap, M.; Meyer, N.; et al. Mechanisms of IFN-γ-induced apoptosis of human skin keratinocytes in patients with atopic dermatitis. *J. Allergy Clin. Immunol.* **2012**, *129*, 1297–1306. [CrossRef]

89. Nograles, K.E.; Zaba, L.C.; Shemer, A.; Fuentes-Duculan, J.; Cardinale, I.; Kikuchi, T.; Ramon, M.; Bergman, R.; Krueger, J.G.; Guttman-Yassky, E. IL-22-producing "T22" T cells account for upregulated IL-22 in atopic dermatitis despite reduced IL-17-producing TH17 T cells. *J. Allergy Clin. Immunol.* **2009**, *123*, 1244–1252. [CrossRef]

90. Czarnowicki, T.; Malajian, D.; Khattri, S.; Correa da Rosa, J.; Dutt, R.; Finney, R.; Dhingra, N.; Xiangyu, P.; Xu, H.; Estrada, Y.D.; et al. Petrolatum: Barrier repair and antimicrobial responses underlying this "inert" moisturizer. *J. Allergy Clin. Immunol.* **2016**, *137*, 1091–1102.e1097. [CrossRef]

91. Eichenfield, L.F.; Tom, W.L.; Berger, T.G.; Krol, A.; Paller, A.S.; Schwarzenberger, K.; Bergman, J.N.; Chamlin, S.L.; Cohen, D.E.; Cooper, K.D.; et al. Guidelines of care for the management of atopic dermatitis: Section 2. Management and treatment of atopic dermatitis with topical therapies. *J. Am. Acad. Dermatol.* **2014**, *71*, 116–132. [CrossRef] [PubMed]

92. Cury Martins, J.; Martins, C.; Aoki, V.; Gois, A.F.T.; Ishii, H.A.; da Silva, E.M.K. Topical tacrolimus for atopic dermatitis. *Cochrane Database Syst. Rev.* **2015**, *36*, CD009864. [CrossRef] [PubMed]

93. Sidbury, R.; Davis, D.M.; Cohen, D.E.; Cordoro, K.M.; Berger, T.G.; Bergman, J.N.; Chamlin, S.L.; Cooper, K.D.; Feldman, S.R.; Hanifin, J.M.; et al. Guidelines of care for the management of atopic dermatitis: Section 3. *Management and Treatment with Phototherapy and Systemic Agents; J. Am. Acad. Dermatol.* **2014**, *71*, 327–349. [CrossRef] [PubMed]

94. Yu, S.H.; Drucker, A.M.; Lebwohl, M.; Silverberg, J.I. A systematic review of the safety and efficacy of systemic corticosteroids in atopic dermatitis. *J. Am. Acad. Dermatol.* **2018**, *78*, 733–740. [CrossRef] [PubMed]

95. Roekevisch, E.; Spuls, P.I.; Kuester, D.; Limpens, J.; Schmitt, J. Efficacy and safety of systemic treatments for moderate-to-severe atopic dermatitis: A systematic review. *J. Allergy Clin. Immunol.* **2014**, *133*, 429–438. [CrossRef]

96. Jimenez, J.L.; Punzón, C.; Navarro, J.; Muñoz-Fernández, M.A.; Fresno, M. Phosphodiesterase 4 inhibitors prevent cytokine secretion by T lymphocytes by inhibiting nuclear factor-kappaB and nuclear factor of activated T cells activation. *J. Pharmacol. Exp. Ther.* **2001**, *299*, 753–759.

97. Paller, A.S.; Tom, W.L.; Lebwohl, M.G.; Blumenthal, R.L.; Boguniewicz, M.; Call, R.S.; Eichenfield, L.F.; Forsha, D.W.; Rees, W.C.; Simpson, E.L.; et al. Efficacy and safety of crisaborole ointment, a novel, nonsteroidal phosphodiesterase 4 (PDE4) inhibitor for the topical treatment of atopic dermatitis (AD) in children and adults. *J. Am. Acad. Dermatol.* **2016**, *75*, 494–503.e496. [CrossRef]

98. Hanifin, J.M.; Ellis, C.N.; Frieden, I.J.; Fölster-Holst, R.; Stein Gold, L.F.; Secci, A.; Smith, A.J.; Zhao, C.; Kornyeyeva, E.; Eichenfield, L.F. OPA-15406, a novel, topical, nonsteroidal, selective phosphodiesterase-4 (PDE4) inhibitor, in the treatment of adult and adolescent patients with mild to moderate atopic dermatitis (AD): A phase-II randomized, double-blind, placebo-controlled study. *J. Am. Acad. Dermatol.* **2016**, *75*, 297–305. [CrossRef]

99. Simpson, E.L.; Imafuku, S.; Poulin, Y.; Ungar, B.; Zhou, L.; Malik, K.; Wen, H.-C.; Xu, H.; Estrada, Y.D.; Peng, X.; et al. A Phase 2 Randomized Trial of Apremilast in Patients with Atopic Dermatitis. *J. Investig. Dermatol.* **2019**, *139*, 1063–1072. [CrossRef]

100. Simpson, E.L.; Gadkari, A.; Worm, M.; Soong, W.; Blauvelt, A.; Eckert, L.; Wu, R.; Ardeleanu, M.; Graham, N.M.H.; Pirozzi, G.; et al. Dupilumab therapy provides clinically meaningful improvement in patient-reported outcomes (PROs): A phase IIb, randomized, placebo-controlled, clinical trial in adult patients with moderate to severe atopic dermatitis (AD). *J. Am. Acad. Dermatol.* **2016**, *75*, 506–515. [CrossRef]

101. Thaçi, D.; Simpson, E.L.; Beck, L.A.; Bieber, T.; Blauvelt, A.; Papp, K.; Soong, W.; Worm, M.; Szepietowski, J.C.; Sofen, H.; et al. Efficacy and safety of dupilumab in adults with moderate-to-severe atopic dermatitis inadequately controlled by topical treatments: A randomised, placebo-controlled, dose-ranging phase 2b trial. *Lancet* **2016**, *387*, 40–52. [CrossRef]

102. Beck, L.A.; Thaçi, D.; Hamilton, J.D.; Graham, N.M.; Bieber, T.; Rocklin, R.; Ming, J.E.; Ren, H.; Kao, R.; Simpson, E.; et al. Dupilumab treatment in adults with moderate-to-severe atopic dermatitis. *N. Engl. J. Med.* **2014**, *371*, 130–139. [CrossRef] [PubMed]

103. Simpson, E.L.; Bieber, T.; Guttman-Yassky, E.; Beck, L.A.; Blauvelt, A.; Cork, M.J.; Silverberg, J.I.; Deleuran, M.; Kataoka, Y.; Lacour, J.-P.; et al. Two Phase 3 Trials of Dupilumab versus Placebo in Atopic Dermatitis. *N. Engl. J. Med.* **2016**, *375*, 2335–2348. [CrossRef] [PubMed]

104. Tsoi, L.C.; Rodriguez, E.; Degenhardt, F.; Baurecht, H.; Wehkamp, U.; Volks, N.; Szymczak, S.; Swindell, W.R.; Sarkar, M.K.; Raja, K.; et al. Atopic Dermatitis Is an IL-13-Dominant Disease with Greater Molecular Heterogeneity Compared to Psoriasis. *J. Investig. Dermatol.* **2019**, *139*, 1480–1489. [CrossRef] [PubMed]

105. Simpson, E.L.; Flohr, C.; Eichenfield, L.F.; Bieber, T.; Sofen, H.; Taïeb, A.; Owen, R.; Putnam, W.; Castro, M.; DeBusk, K.; et al. Efficacy and safety of lebrikizumab (an anti-IL-13 monoclonal antibody) in adults with moderate-to-severe atopic dermatitis inadequately controlled by topical corticosteroids: A randomized, placebo-controlled phase II trial (TREBLE). *J. Am. Acad. Dermatol.* **2018**, *78*, 863–871.e811. [CrossRef] [PubMed]

106. Wollenberg, A.; Howell, M.D.; Guttman-Yassky, E.; Silverberg, J.I.; Kell, C.; Ranade, K.; Moate, R.; van der Merwe, R. Treatment of atopic dermatitis with tralokinumab, an anti-IL-13 mAb. *J. Allergy Clin. Immunol.* **2019**, *143*, 135–141. [CrossRef] [PubMed]

107. Nemoto, O.; Furue, M.; Nakagawa, H.; Shiramoto, M.; Hanada, R.; Matsuki, S.; Imayama, S.; Kato, M.; Hasebe, I.; Taira, K.; et al. The first trial of CIM331, a humanized antihuman interleukin-31 receptor A antibody, in healthy volunteers and patients with atopic dermatitis to evaluate safety, tolerability and pharmacokinetics of a single dose in a randomized, double-blind, placebo-controlled study. *Br. J. Dermatol.* **2016**, *174*, 296–304. [CrossRef] [PubMed]

108. Ruzicka, T.; Hanifin, J.M.; Furue, M.; Pulka, G.; Mlynarczyk, I.; Wollenberg, A.; Galus, R.; Etoh, T.; Mihara, R.; Yoshida, H.; et al. Anti-Interleukin-31 Receptor A Antibody for Atopic Dermatitis. *N. Engl. J. Med.* **2017**, *376*, 826–835. [CrossRef]

109. Cornelissen, C.; Lüscher-Firzlaff, J.; Baron, J.M.; Lüscher, B. Signaling by IL-31 and functional consequences. *Eur. J. Cell Biol.* **2012**, *91*, 552–566. [CrossRef]

110. Kelly-Welch, A.E.; Hanson, E.M.; Boothby, M.R.; Keegan, A.D. Interleukin-4 and interleukin-13 signaling connections maps. *Science* **2003**, *300*, 1527–1528. [CrossRef]

111. Levy, L.L.; Urban, J.; King, B.A. Treatment of recalcitrant atopic dermatitis with the oral Janus kinase inhibitor tofacitinib citrate. *J. Am. Acad. Dermatol.* **2015**, *73*, 395–399. [CrossRef] [PubMed]

112. Guttman-Yassky, E.; Silverberg, J.I.; Nemoto, O.; Forman, S.B.; Wilke, A.; Prescilla, R.; de la Peña, A.; Nunes, F.P.; Janes, J.; Gamalo, M.; et al. Baricitinib in adult patients with moderate-to-severe atopic dermatitis: A phase 2 parallel, double-blinded, randomized placebo-controlled multiple-dose study. *J. Am. Acad. Dermatol.* **2019**, *80*, 913–921.e919. [CrossRef] [PubMed]

113. Beck, L.; Hong, C.; Hu, X.; Chen, S.; Calimlim, B.; Teixeira, H.; Guttman-Yassky, E. Upadacitinib effect on pruritus in moderate-to-severe atopic dermatitis; from a phase 2b randomized, placebo-controlled trial. *Ann. Allergy Asthma Immunol.* **2018**, *121*, S21. [CrossRef]

114. Parisi, R.; Symmons, D.P.M.; Griffiths, C.E.M.; Ashcroft, D.M.; The Identification and Management of Psoriasis and Associated ComorbidiTy (IMPACT) Project Team. Global epidemiology of psoriasis: A systematic review of incidence and prevalence. *J. Investig. Dermatol.* **2013**, *133*, 377–385. [CrossRef] [PubMed]

115. Lebwohl, M. Psoriasis. *Lancet* **2003**, *361*, 1197–1204. [CrossRef]

116. Rendon, A.; Schäkel, K. Psoriasis Pathogenesis and Treatment. *Int. J. Mol. Sci.* **2019**, *20*, 1475. [CrossRef]

117. Nograles, K.E.; Davidovici, B.; Krueger, J.G. New insights in the immunologic basis of psoriasis. *Semin. Cutan. Med. Surg.* **2010**, *29*, 3–9. [CrossRef]

118. Morizane, S.; Gallo, R.L. Antimicrobial peptides in the pathogenesis of psoriasis. *J. Dermatol.* **2012**, *39*, 225–230. [CrossRef]

119. Lande, R.; Gregorio, J.; Facchinetti, V.; Chatterjee, B.; Wang, Y.-H.; Homey, B.; Cao, W.; Wang, Y.-H.; Su, B.; Nestle, F.O.; et al. Plasmacytoid dendritic cells sense self-DNA coupled with antimicrobial peptide. *Nature* **2007**, *449*, 564–569. [CrossRef]

120. Gregorio, J.; Meller, S.; Conrad, C.; Di Nardo, A.; Homey, B.; Lauerma, A.; Arai, N.; Gallo, R.L.; Digiovanni, J.; Gilliet, M. Plasmacytoid dendritic cells sense skin injury and promote wound healing through type I interferons. *J. Exp. Med.* **2010**, *207*, 2921–2930. [CrossRef]

121. Nestle, F.O.; Conrad, C.; Tun-Kyi, A.; Homey, B.; Gombert, M.; Boyman, O.; Burg, G.; Liu, Y.-J.; Gilliet, M. Plasmacytoid predendritic cells initiate psoriasis through interferon-alpha production. *J. Exp. Med.* **2005**, *202*, 135–143. [CrossRef] [PubMed]

122. Morizane, S.; Yamasaki, K.; Mühleisen, B.; Kotol, P.F.; Murakami, M.; Aoyama, Y.; Iwatsuki, K.; Hata, T.; Gallo, R.L. Cathelicidin antimicrobial peptide LL-37 in psoriasis enables keratinocyte reactivity against TLR9 ligands. *J. Investig. Dermatol.* **2012**, *132*, 135–143. [CrossRef] [PubMed]

123. Nestle, F.O.; Turka, L.A.; Nickoloff, B.J. Characterization of dermal dendritic cells in psoriasis. Autostimulation of T lymphocytes and induction of Th1 type cytokines. *J. Clin. Investig.* **1994**, *94*, 202–209. [CrossRef] [PubMed]

124. Uyemura, K.; Yamamura, M.; Fivenson, D.F.; Modlin, R.L.; Nickoloff, B.J. The cytokine network in lesional and lesion-free psoriatic skin is characterized by a T-helper type 1 cell-mediated response. *J. Investig. Dermatol.* **1993**, *101*, 701–705. [CrossRef] [PubMed]

125. Lowes, M.A.; Kikuchi, T.; Fuentes-Duculan, J.; Cardinale, I.; Zaba, L.C.; Haider, A.S.; Bowman, E.P.; Krueger, J.G. Psoriasis vulgaris lesions contain discrete populations of Th1 and Th17 T cells. *J. Investig. Dermatol.* **2008**, *128*, 1207–1211. [CrossRef] [PubMed]

126. Zaba, L.C.; Cardinale, I.; Gilleaudeau, P.; Sullivan-Whalen, M.; Suárez-Fariñas, M.; Fuentes-Duculan, J.; Novitskaya, I.; Khatcherian, A.; Bluth, M.J.; Lowes, M.A.; et al. Amelioration of epidermal hyperplasia by TNF inhibition is associated with reduced Th17 responses. *J. Exp. Med.* **2007**, *204*, 3183–3194. [CrossRef]

127. Gaffen, S.L. Structure and signalling in the IL-17 receptor family. *Nat. Rev. Immunol.* **2009**, *9*, 556–567. [CrossRef]

128. Zheng, Y.; Danilenko, D.M.; Valdez, P.; Kasman, I.; Eastham-Anderson, J.; Wu, J.; Ouyang, W. Interleukin-22, a T(H)17 cytokine, mediates IL-23-induced dermal inflammation and acanthosis. *Nature* **2007**, *445*, 648–651. [CrossRef]

129. Johnston, A.; Xing, X.; Wolterink, L.; Barnes, D.H.; Yin, Z.; Reingold, L.; Kahlenberg, J.M.; Harms, P.W.; Gudjonsson, J.E. IL-1 and IL-36 are dominant cytokines in generalized pustular psoriasis. *J. Allergy Clin. Immunol.* **2017**, *140*, 109–120. [CrossRef]

130. Tauber, M.; Bal, E.; Pei, X.-Y.; Madrange, M.; Khelil, A.; Sahel, H.; Zenati, A.; Makrelouf, M.; Boubridaa, K.; Chiali, A.; et al. IL36RN Mutations Affect Protein Expression and Function: A Basis for Genotype-Phenotype Correlation in Pustular Diseases. *J. Investig. Dermatol.* **2016**, *136*, 1811–1819. [CrossRef]

131. McFadden, J.; Valdimarsson, H.; Fry, L. Cross-reactivity between streptococcal M surface antigen and human skin. *Br. J. Dermatol.* **1991**, *125*, 443–447. [CrossRef] [PubMed]

132. Leung, D.Y.; Travers, J.B.; Giorno, R.; Norris, D.A.; Skinner, R.; Aelion, J.; Kazemi, L.V.; Kim, M.H.; Trumble, A.E.; Kotb, M. Evidence for a streptococcal superantigen-driven process in acute guttate psoriasis. *J. Clin. Investig.* **1995**, *96*, 2106–2112. [CrossRef] [PubMed]

133. Farber, E.M.; Nall, M.L. The natural history of psoriasis in 5,600 patients. *Dermatologica* **1974**, *148*, 1–18. [CrossRef] [PubMed]

134. Farber, E.M.; Nall, M.L.; Watson, W. Natural history of psoriasis in 61 twin pairs. *Arch. Dermatol.* **1974**, *109*, 207–211. [CrossRef]

135. Lønnberg, A.S.; Skov, L.; Skytthe, A.; Kyvik, K.O.; Pedersen, O.B.; Thomsen, S.F. Heritability of psoriasis in a large twin sample. *Br. J. Dermatol.* **2013**, *169*, 412–416. [CrossRef]

136. Bowcock, A.M.; Krueger, J.G. Getting under the skin: The immunogenetics of psoriasis. *Nat. Rev. Immunol.* **2005**, *5*, 699–711. [CrossRef]

137. Gudjonsson, J.E.; Elder, J.T. Psoriasis: Epidemiology. *Clin. Dermatol.* **2007**, *25*, 535–546. [CrossRef]

138. Trembath, R.C.; Clough, R.L.; Rosbotham, J.L.; Jones, A.B.; Camp, R.D.; Frodsham, A.; Browne, J.; Barber, R.; Terwilliger, J.; Lathrop, G.M.; et al. Identification of a major susceptibility locus on chromosome 6p and evidence for further disease loci revealed by a two stage genome-wide search in psoriasis. *Hum. Mol. Genet.* **1997**, *6*, 813–820. [CrossRef]

139. Allen, M.H.; Veal, C.; Faassen, A.; Powis, S.H.; Vaughan, R.W.; Trembath, R.C.; Barker, J.N. A non-HLA gene within the MHC in psoriasis. *Lancet* **1999**, *353*, 1589–1590. [CrossRef]

140. Asumalahti, K.; Laitinen, T.; Itkonen-Vatjus, R.; Lokki, M.L.; Suomela, S.; Snellman, E.; Saarialho-Kere, U.; Kere, J. A candidate gene for psoriasis near HLA-C, HCR (Pg8), is highly polymorphic with a disease-associated susceptibility allele. *Hum. Mol. Genet.* **2000**, *9*, 1533–1542. [CrossRef]

141. Nair, R.P.; Stuart, P.E.; Nistor, I.; Hiremagalore, R.; Chia, N.V.C.; Jenisch, S.; Weichenthal, M.; Abecasis, G.R.; Lim, H.W.; Christophers, E.; et al. Sequence and haplotype analysis supports HLA-C as the psoriasis susceptibility 1 gene. *Am. J. Hum. Genet.* **2006**, *78*, 827–851. [CrossRef] [PubMed]

142. Fan, X.; Yang, S.; Huang, W.; Wang, Z.-M.; Sun, L.-D.; Liang, Y.-H.; Gao, M.; Ren, Y.-Q.; Zhang, K.-Y.; Du, W.-H.; et al. Fine mapping of the psoriasis susceptibility locus PSORS1 supports HLA-C as the susceptibility gene in the Han Chinese population. *PLoS Genet.* **2008**, *4*, e1000038. [CrossRef] [PubMed]

143. Allen, M.H.; Ameen, H.; Veal, C.; Evans, J.; Ramrakha-Jones, V.S.; Marsland, A.M.; Burden, A.D.; Griffiths, C.E.M.; Trembath, R.C.; Barker, J.N.W.N. The major psoriasis susceptibility locus PSORS1 is not a risk factor for late-onset psoriasis. *J. Investig. Dermatol.* **2005**, *124*, 103–106. [CrossRef] [PubMed]

144. Asumalahti, K.; Ameen, M.; Suomela, S.; Hagforsen, E.; Michaëlsson, G.; Evans, J.; Munro, M.; Veal, C.; Allen, M.; Leman, J.; et al. Genetic analysis of PSORS1 distinguishes guttate psoriasis and palmoplantar pustulosis. *J. Investig. Dermatol.* **2003**, *120*, 627–632. [CrossRef]

145. Tomfohrde, J.; Silverman, A.; Barnes, R.; Fernandez-Vina, M.A.; Young, M.; Lory, D.; Morris, L.; Wuepper, K.D.; Stastny, P.; Menter, A. Gene for familial psoriasis susceptibility mapped to the distal end of human chromosome 17q. *Science* **1994**, *264*, 1141–1145. [CrossRef]

146. Jordan, C.T.; Cao, L.; Roberson, E.D.O.; Pierson, K.C.; Yang, C.-F.; Joyce, C.E.; Ryan, C.; Duan, S.; Helms, C.A.; Liu, Y.; et al. PSORS2 is due to mutations in CARD14. *Am. J. Hum. Genet.* **2012**, *90*, 784–795. [CrossRef]

147. Capon, F.; Semprini, S.; Chimenti, S.; Fabrizi, G.; Zambruno, G.; Murgia, S.; Carcassi, C.; Fazio, M.; Mingarelli, R.; Dallapiccola, B.; et al. Fine mapping of the PSORS4 psoriasis susceptibility region on chromosome 1q21. *J. Investig. Dermatol.* **2001**, *116*, 728–730. [CrossRef]

148. Lee, Y.A.; Rüschendorf, F.; Windemuth, C.; Schmitt-Egenolf, M.; Stadelmann, A.; Nürnberg, G.; Ständer, M.; Wienker, T.F.; Reis, A.; Traupe, H. Genomewide scan in german families reveals evidence for a novel psoriasis-susceptibility locus on chromosome 19p13. *Am. J. Hum. Genet.* **2000**, *67*, 1020–1024. [CrossRef]

149. Veal, C.D.; Clough, R.L.; Barber, R.C.; Mason, S.; Tillman, D.; Ferry, B.; Jones, A.B.; Ameen, M.; Balendran, N.; Powis, S.H.; et al. Identification of a novel psoriasis susceptibility locus at 1p and evidence of epistasis between PSORS1 and candidate loci. *J. Med Genet.* **2001**, *38*, 7–13. [CrossRef]

150. Elder, J.T. Expanded Genome-Wide Association Study Meta-Analysis of Psoriasis Expands the Catalog of Common Psoriasis-Associated Variants. *J. Investig. Dermatol. Symp. Proc.* **2018**, *19*, S77–S78. [CrossRef]

151. Hirata, J.; Hirota, T.; Ozeki, T.; Kanai, M.; Sudo, T.; Tanaka, T.; Hizawa, N.; Nakagawa, H.; Sato, S.; Mushiroda, T.; et al. Variants at HLA-A, HLA-C, and HLA-DQB1 Confer Risk of Psoriasis Vulgaris in Japanese. *J. Investig. Dermatol.* **2018**, *138*, 542–548. [CrossRef] [PubMed]

152. Okada, Y.; Han, B.; Tsoi, L.C.; Stuart, P.E.; Ellinghaus, E.; Tejasvi, T.; Chandran, V.; Pellett, F.; Pollock, R.; Bowcock, A.M.; et al. Fine mapping major histocompatibility complex associations in psoriasis and its clinical subtypes. *Am. J. Hum. Genet.* **2014**, *95*, 162–172. [CrossRef] [PubMed]

153. Yin, X.; Low, H.Q.; Wang, L.; Li, Y.; Ellinghaus, E.; Han, J.; Estivill, X.; Sun, L.; Zuo, X.; Shen, C.; et al. Genome-wide meta-analysis identifies multiple novel associations and ethnic heterogeneity of psoriasis susceptibility. *Nat. Commun.* **2015**, *6*, 6916. [CrossRef] [PubMed]

154. Elder, J.T. Genome-wide association scan yields new insights into the immunopathogenesis of psoriasis. *Genes Immun.* **2009**, *10*, 201–209. [CrossRef] [PubMed]

155. Tsoi, L.C.; Spain, S.L.; Knight, J.; Ellinghaus, E.; Stuart, P.E.; Capon, F.; Ding, J.; Li, Y.; Tejasvi, T.; Gudjonsson, J.E.; et al. Identification of 15 new psoriasis susceptibility loci highlights the role of innate immunity. *Nat. Genet.* **2012**, *44*, 1341–1348. [CrossRef] [PubMed]

156. Tsoi, L.C.; Spain, S.L.; Ellinghaus, E.; Stuart, P.E.; Capon, F.; Knight, J.; Tejasvi, T.; Kang, H.M.; Allen, M.H.; Lambert, S.; et al. Enhanced meta-analysis and replication studies identify five new psoriasis susceptibility loci. *Nat. Commun.* **2015**, *6*, 7001. [CrossRef]

157. Capon, F.; Di Meglio, P.; Szaub, J.; Prescott, N.J.; Dunster, C.; Baumber, L.; Timms, K.; Gutin, A.; Abkevic, V.; Burden, A.D.; et al. Sequence variants in the genes for the interleukin-23 receptor (IL23R) and its ligand (IL12B) confer protection against psoriasis. *Hum. Genet.* **2007**, *122*, 201–206. [CrossRef]

158. Cargill, M.; Schrodi, S.J.; Chang, M.; Garcia, V.E.; Brandon, R.; Callis, K.P.; Matsunami, N.; Ardlie, K.G.; Civello, D.; Catanese, J.J.; et al. A large-scale genetic association study confirms IL12B and leads to the identification of IL23R as psoriasis-risk genes. *Am. J. Hum. Genet.* **2007**, *80*, 273–290. [CrossRef]

159. Hüffmeier, U.; Uebe, S.; Ekici, A.B.; Bowes, J.; Giardina, E.; Korendowych, E.; Juneblad, K.; Apel, M.; McManus, R.; Ho, P.; et al. Common variants at TRAF3IP2 are associated with susceptibility to psoriatic arthritis and psoriasis. *Nat. Genet.* **2010**, *42*, 996–999. [CrossRef]

160. Nair, R.P.; Duffin, K.C.; Helms, C.; Ding, J.; Stuart, P.E.; Goldgar, D.; Gudjonsson, J.E.; Li, Y.; Tejasvi, T.; Feng, B.-J.; et al. Genome-wide scan reveals association of psoriasis with IL-23 and NF-kappaB pathways. *Nat. Genet.* **2009**, *41*, 199–204. [CrossRef]

161. Marrakchi, S.; Guigue, P.; Renshaw, B.R.; Puel, A.; Pei, X.-Y.; Fraitag, S.; Zribi, J.; Bal, E.; Cluzeau, C.; Chrabieh, M.; et al. Interleukin-36-receptor antagonist deficiency and generalized pustular psoriasis. *N. Engl. J. Med.* **2011**, *365*, 620–628. [CrossRef] [PubMed]

162. Onoufriadis, A.; Simpson, M.A.; Pink, A.E.; Di Meglio, P.; Smith, C.H.; Pullabhatla, V.; Knight, J.; Spain, S.L.; Nestle, F.O.; Burden, A.D.; et al. Mutations in IL36RN/IL1F5 are associated with the severe episodic inflammatory skin disease known as generalized pustular psoriasis. *Am. J. Hum. Genet.* **2011**, *89*, 432–437. [CrossRef] [PubMed]

163. McGill, A.; Frank, A.; Emmett, N.; Turnbull, D.M.; Birch-Machin, M.A.; Reynolds, N.J. The anti-psoriatic drug anthralin accumulates in keratinocyte mitochondria, dissipates mitochondrial membrane potential, and induces apoptosis through a pathway dependent on respiratory competent mitochondria. *FASEB J.* **2005**, *19*, 1012–1014. [CrossRef] [PubMed]

164. Arbiser, J.L.; Govindarajan, B.; Battle, T.E.; Lynch, R.; Frank, D.A.; Ushio-Fukai, M.; Perry, B.N.; Stern, D.F.; Bowden, G.T.; Liu, A.; et al. Carbazole is a naturally occurring inhibitor of angiogenesis and inflammation isolated from antipsoriatic coal tar. *J. Investig. Dermatol.* **2006**, *126*, 1396–1402. [CrossRef]

165. Castela, E.; Archier, E.; Devaux, S.; Gallini, A.; Aractingi, S.; Cribier, B.; Jullien, D.; Aubin, F.; Bachelez, H.; Joly, P.; et al. Topical corticosteroids in plaque psoriasis: A systematic review of efficacy and treatment modalities. *J. Eur. Acad. Dermatol. Venereol.* **2012**, *26* (Suppl. 3), 36–46. [CrossRef]

166. Samarasekera, E.J.; Sawyer, L.; Wonderling, D.; Tucker, R.; Smith, C.H. Topical therapies for the treatment of plaque psoriasis: Systematic review and network meta-analyses. *Br. J. Dermatol.* **2013**, *168*, 954–967. [CrossRef]

167. Trémezaygues, L.; Reichrath, J. Vitamin D analogs in the treatment of psoriasis: Where are we standing and where will we be going? *Derm. Endocrinol.* **2011**, *3*, 180–186. [CrossRef]

168. Devaux, S.; Castela, A.; Archier, E.; Gallini, A.; Joly, P.; Misery, L.; Aractingi, S.; Aubin, F.; Bachelez, H.; Cribier, B.; et al. Topical vitamin D analogues alone or in association with topical steroids for psoriasis: A systematic review. *J. Eur. Acad. Dermatol. Venereol.* **2012**, *26* (Suppl. 3), 52–60. [CrossRef]

169. Lebwohl, M.; Siskin, S.B.; Epinette, W.; Breneman, D.; Funicella, T.; Kalb, R.; Moore, J. A multicenter trial of calcipotriene ointment and halobetasol ointment compared with either agent alone for the treatment of psoriasis. *J. Am. Acad. Dermatol.* **1996**, *35*, 268–269. [CrossRef]

170. Gerritsen, M.J.; Van De Kerkhof, P.C.; Langner, A. Long-term safety of topical calcitriol 3 microg g(-1) ointment. *Br. J. Dermatol.* **2001**, *144* (Suppl. 58), 17–19. [CrossRef]

171. Wang, C.; Lin, A. Efficacy of topical calcineurin inhibitors in psoriasis. *J. Cutan. Med. Surg.* **2014**, *18*, 8–14. [CrossRef] [PubMed]

172. Kreuter, A.; Sommer, A.; Hyun, J.; Bräutigam, M.; Brockmeyer, N.H.; Altmeyer, P.; Gambichler, T. 1% pimecrolimus, 0.005% calcipotriol, and 0.1% betamethasone in the treatment of intertriginous psoriasis: A double-blind, randomized controlled study. *Arch. Dermatol.* **2006**, *142*, 1138–1143. [CrossRef] [PubMed]

173. Duvic, M.; Asano, A.T.; Hager, C.; Mays, S. The pathogenesis of psoriasis and the mechanism of action of tazarotene. *J. Am. Acad. Dermatol.* **1998**, *39*, S129–S133. [CrossRef]

174. Gold, L.S.; Lebwohl, M.G.; Sugarman, J.L.; Pariser, D.M.; Lin, T.; Martin, G.; Pillai, R.; Israel, R.; Ramakrishna, T. Safety and efficacy of a fixed combination of halobetasol and tazarotene in the treatment of moderate-to-severe plaque psoriasis: Results of 2 phase 3 randomized controlled trials. *J. Am. Acad. Dermatol.* **2018**, *79*, 287–293. [CrossRef]

175. Lebwohl, M.G.; Breneman, D.L.; Goffe, B.S.; Grossman, J.R.; Ling, M.R.; Milbauer, J.; Pincus, S.H.; Sibbald, R.G.; Swinyer, L.J.; Weinstein, G.D.; et al. Tazarotene 0.1% gel plus corticosteroid cream in the treatment of plaque psoriasis. *J. Am. Acad. Dermatol.* **1998**, *39*, 590–596. [CrossRef]

176. Zhang, P.; Wu, M.X. A clinical review of phototherapy for psoriasis. *Lasers Med. Sci.* **2018**, *33*, 173–180. [CrossRef]

177. Mehta, D.; Lim, H.W. Ultraviolet B Phototherapy for Psoriasis: Review of Practical Guidelines. *Am. J. Clin. Dermatol.* **2016**, *17*, 125–133. [CrossRef]

178. Stern, R.S.; Study, P.F.-U. The risk of melanoma in association with long-term exposure to PUVA. *J. Am. Acad. Dermatol.* **2001**, *44*, 755–761. [CrossRef]

179. Stern, R.S.; Study, P.F.-U. The risk of squamous cell and basal cell cancer associated with psoralen and ultraviolet A therapy: A 30-year prospective study. *J. Am. Acad. Dermatol.* **2012**, *66*, 553–562. [CrossRef]

180. Sbidian, E.; Maza, A.; Montaudié, H.; Gallini, A.; Aractingi, S.; Aubin, F.; Cribier, B.; Joly, P.; Jullien, D.; Le Maître, M.; et al. Efficacy and safety of oral retinoids in different psoriasis subtypes: A systematic literature review. *J. Eur. Acad. Dermatol. Venereol.* **2011**, *25* (Suppl. 2), 28–33. [CrossRef]

181. Lee, C.S.; Koo, J. A review of acitretin, a systemic retinoid for the treatment of psoriasis. *Expert Opin. Pharmacother.* **2005**, *6*, 1725–1734. [CrossRef] [PubMed]

182. Schafer, P. Apremilast mechanism of action and application to psoriasis and psoriatic arthritis. *Biochem. Pharmacol.* **2012**, *83*, 1583–1590. [CrossRef] [PubMed]

183. Reich, K.; Gooderham, M.; Green, L.; Bewley, A.; Zhang, Z.; Khanskaya, I.; Day, R.M.; Goncalves, J.; Shah, K.; Piguet, V.; et al. The efficacy and safety of apremilast, etanercept and placebo in patients with moderate-to-severe plaque psoriasis: 52-week results from a phase IIIb, randomized, placebo-controlled trial (LIBERATE). *J. Eur. Acad. Dermatol. Venereol.* **2017**, *31*, 507–517. [CrossRef] [PubMed]

184. Bissonnette, R.; Haydey, R.; Rosoph, L.A.; Lynde, C.W.; Bukhalo, M.; Fowler, J.F.; Delorme, I.; Gagné-Henley, A.; Gooderham, M.; Poulin, Y.; et al. Apremilast for the treatment of moderate-to-severe palmoplantar psoriasis: Results from a double-blind, placebo-controlled, randomized study. *J. Eur. Acad. Dermatol. Venereol.* **2018**, *32*, 403–410. [CrossRef] [PubMed]

185. Papp, K.; Reich, K.; Leonardi, C.L.; Kircik, L.; Chimenti, S.; Langley, R.G.B.; Hu, C.; Stevens, R.M.; Day, R.M.; Gordon, K.B.; et al. Apremilast, an oral phosphodiesterase 4 (PDE4) inhibitor, in patients with moderate to severe plaque psoriasis: Results of a phase III, randomized, controlled trial (Efficacy and Safety Trial Evaluating the Effects of Apremilast in Psoriasis [ESTEEM] 1). *J. Am. Acad. Dermatol.* **2015**, *73*, 37–49. [CrossRef] [PubMed]

186. Paul, C.; Cather, J.; Gooderham, M.; Poulin, Y.; Mrowietz, U.; Ferrandiz, C.; Crowley, J.; Hu, C.; Stevens, R.M.; Shah, K.; et al. Efficacy and safety of apremilast, an oral phosphodiesterase 4 inhibitor, in patients with moderate-to-severe plaque psoriasis over 52 weeks: A phase III, randomized controlled trial (ESTEEM 2). *Br. J. Dermatol.* **2015**, *173*, 1387–1399. [CrossRef]

187. Kaushik, S.B.; Lebwohl, M.G. Review of safety and efficacy of approved systemic psoriasis therapies. *Int. J. Dermatol.* **2019**, *58*, 649–658. [CrossRef]

188. Tyring, S.; Gottlieb, A.; Papp, K.; Gordon, K.; Leonardi, C.; Wang, A.; Lalla, D.; Woolley, M.; Jahreis, A.; Zitnik, R.; et al. Etanercept and clinical outcomes, fatigue, and depression in psoriasis: Double-blind placebo-controlled randomised phase III trial. *Lancet* **2006**, *367*, 29–35. [CrossRef]

189. Papp, K.A.; Tyring, S.; Lahfa, M.; Prinz, J.; Griffiths, C.E.M.; Nakanishi, A.M.; Zitnik, R.; van de Kerkhof, P.C.M.; Melvin, L.; Group, E.P.S. A global phase III randomized controlled trial of etanercept in psoriasis: Safety, efficacy, and effect of dose reduction. *Br. J. Dermatol.* **2005**, *152*, 1304–1312. [CrossRef]

190. Leonardi, C.L.; Powers, J.L.; Matheson, R.T.; Goffe, B.S.; Zitnik, R.; Wang, A.; Gottlieb, A.B.; Group, E.P.S. Etanercept as monotherapy in patients with psoriasis. *N. Engl. J. Med.* **2003**, *349*, 2014–2022. [CrossRef]

191. Reich, K.; Nestle, F.O.; Papp, K.; Ortonne, J.-P.; Evans, R.; Guzzo, C.; Li, S.; Dooley, L.T.; Griffiths, C.E.M.; EXPRESS Study Investigators. Infliximab induction and maintenance therapy for moderate-to-severe psoriasis: A phase III, multicentre, double-blind trial. *Lancet* **2005**, *366*, 1367–1374. [CrossRef]

192. Menter, A.; Feldman, S.R.; Weinstein, G.D.; Papp, K.; Evans, R.; Guzzo, C.; Li, S.; Dooley, L.T.; Arnold, C.; Gottlieb, A.B. A randomized comparison of continuous vs. intermittent infliximab maintenance regimens over 1 year in the treatment of moderate-to-severe plaque psoriasis. *J. Am. Acad. Dermatol.* **2007**, *56*, 31.e1–31.e15. [CrossRef] [PubMed]

193. Gordon, K.; Papp, K.; Poulin, Y.; Gu, Y.; Rozzo, S.; Sasso, E.H. Long-term efficacy and safety of adalimumab in patients with moderate to severe psoriasis treated continuously over 3 years: Results from an open-label extension study for patients from REVEAL. *J. Am. Acad. Dermatol.* **2012**, *66*, 241–251. [CrossRef] [PubMed]

194. Menter, A.; Tyring, S.K.; Gordon, K.; Kimball, A.B.; Leonardi, C.L.; Langley, R.G.; Strober, B.E.; Kaul, M.; Gu, Y.; Okun, M.; et al. Adalimumab therapy for moderate to severe psoriasis: A randomized, controlled phase III trial. *J. Am. Acad. Dermatol.* **2008**, *58*, 106–115. [CrossRef] [PubMed]

195. Saurat, J.H.; Stingl, G.; Dubertret, L.; Papp, K.; Langley, R.G.; Ortonne, J.P.; Unnebrink, K.; Kaul, M.; Camez, A.; Investigators, C.S. Efficacy and safety results from the randomized controlled comparative study of adalimumab vs. methotrexate vs. placebo in patients with psoriasis (CHAMPION). *Br. J. Dermatol.* **2008**, *158*, 558–566. [CrossRef] [PubMed]

196. Gordon, K.B.; Langley, R.G.; Leonardi, C.; Toth, D.; Menter, M.A.; Kang, S.; Heffernan, M.; Miller, B.; Hamlin, R.; Lim, L.; et al. Clinical response to adalimumab treatment in patients with moderate to severe psoriasis: Double-blind, randomized controlled trial and open-label extension study. *J. Am. Acad. Dermatol.* **2006**, *55*, 598–606. [CrossRef]

197. Gottlieb, A.B.; Blauvelt, A.; Thaçi, D.; Leonardi, C.L.; Poulin, Y.; Drew, J.; Peterson, L.; Arendt, C.; Burge, D.; Reich, K. Certolizumab pegol for the treatment of chronic plaque psoriasis: Results through 48 weeks from 2 phase 3, multicenter, randomized, double-blinded, placebo-controlled studies (CIMPASI-1 and CIMPASI-2). *J. Am. Acad. Dermatol.* **2018**, *79*, 302–314.e306. [CrossRef]

198. Kimball, A.B.; Gordon, K.B.; Fakharzadeh, S.; Yeilding, N.; Szapary, P.O.; Schenkel, B.; Guzzo, C.; Li, S.; Papp, K.A. Long-term efficacy of ustekinumab in patients with moderate-to-severe psoriasis: Results from the PHOENIX 1 trial through up to 3 years. *Br. J. Dermatol.* **2012**, *166*, 861–872. [CrossRef]

199. Papp, K.A.; Langley, R.G.; Lebwohl, M.; Krueger, G.G.; Szapary, P.; Yeilding, N.; Guzzo, C.; Hsu, M.-C.; Wang, Y.; Li, S.; et al. Efficacy and safety of ustekinumab, a human interleukin-12/23 monoclonal antibody, in patients with psoriasis: 52-week results from a randomised, double-blind, placebo-controlled trial (PHOENIX 2). *Lancet* **2008**, *371*, 1675–1684. [CrossRef]

200. Leonardi, C.L.; Kimball, A.B.; Papp, K.A.; Yeilding, N.; Guzzo, C.; Wang, Y.; Li, S.; Dooley, L.T.; Gordon, K.B.; PHOENIX 1 Study Investigators. Efficacy and safety of ustekinumab, a human interleukin-12/23 monoclonal antibody, in patients with psoriasis: 76-week results from a randomised, double-blind, placebo-controlled trial (PHOENIX 1). *Lancet* **2008**, *371*, 1665–1674. [CrossRef]

201. Gordon, K.B.; Papp, K.A.; Langley, R.G.; Ho, V.; Kimball, A.B.; Guzzo, C.; Yeilding, N.; Szapary, P.O.; Fakharzadeh, S.; Li, S.; et al. Long-term safety experience of ustekinumab in patients with moderate to severe psoriasis (Part II of II): Results from analyses of infections and malignancy from pooled phase II and III clinical trials. *J. Am. Acad. Dermatol.* **2012**, *66*, 742–751. [CrossRef] [PubMed]

202. Lebwohl, M.; Strober, B.; Menter, A.; Gordon, K.; Weglowska, J.; Puig, L.; Papp, K.; Spelman, L.; Toth, D.; Kerdel, F.; et al. Phase 3 Studies Comparing Brodalumab with Ustekinumab in Psoriasis. *N. Engl. J. Med.* **2015**, *373*, 1318–1328. [CrossRef] [PubMed]

203. Papp, K.A.; Reich, K.; Paul, C.; Blauvelt, A.; Baran, W.; Bolduc, C.; Toth, D.; Langley, R.G.; Cather, J.; Gottlieb, A.B.; et al. A prospective phase III, randomized, double-blind, placebo-controlled study of brodalumab in patients with moderate-to-severe plaque psoriasis. *Br. J. Dermatol.* **2016**, *175*, 273–286. [CrossRef] [PubMed]

204. Griffiths, C.E.M.; Reich, K.; Lebwohl, M.; van de Kerkhof, P.; Paul, C.; Menter, A.; Cameron, G.S.; Erickson, J.; Zhang, L.; Secrest, R.J.; et al. Comparison of ixekizumab with etanercept or placebo in moderate-to-severe psoriasis (UNCOVER-2 and UNCOVER-3): Results from two phase 3 randomised trials. *Lancet* **2015**, *386*, 541–551. [CrossRef]

205. Gordon, K.B.; Blauvelt, A.; Papp, K.A.; Langley, R.G.; Luger, T.; Ohtsuki, M.; Reich, K.; Amato, D.; Ball, S.G.; Braun, D.K.; et al. Phase 3 Trials of Ixekizumab in Moderate-to-Severe Plaque Psoriasis. *N. Engl. J. Med.* **2016**, *375*, 345–356. [CrossRef] [PubMed]

206. Langley, R.G.; Elewski, B.E.; Lebwohl, M.; Reich, K.; Griffiths, C.E.M.; Papp, K.; Puig, L.; Nakagawa, H.; Spelman, L.; Sigurgeirsson, B.; et al. Secukinumab in plaque psoriasis–results of two phase 3 trials. *N. Engl. J. Med.* **2014**, *371*, 326–338. [CrossRef]

207. Blauvelt, A.; Reich, K.; Tsai, T.-F.; Tyring, S.; Vanaclocha, F.; Kingo, K.; Ziv, M.; Pinter, A.; Vender, R.; Hugot, S.; et al. Secukinumab is superior to ustekinumab in clearing skin of subjects with moderate-to-severe plaque psoriasis up to 1 year: Results from the CLEAR study. *J. Am. Acad. Dermatol.* **2017**, *76*, 60–69.e69. [CrossRef]

208. Hueber, W.; Sands, B.E.; Lewitzky, S.; Vandemeulebroecke, M.; Reinisch, W.; Higgins, P.D.R.; Wehkamp, J.; Feagan, B.G.; Yao, M.D.; Karczewski, M.; et al. Secukinumab, a human anti-IL-17A monoclonal antibody, for moderate to severe Crohn's disease: Unexpected results of a randomised, double-blind placebo-controlled trial. *Gut* **2012**, *61*, 1693–1700. [CrossRef]

209. Kulig, P.; Musiol, S.; Freiberger, S.N.; Schreiner, B.; Gyülveszi, G.; Russo, G.; Pantelyushin, S.; Kishihara, K.; Alessandrini, F.; Kündig, T.; et al. IL-12 protects from psoriasiform skin inflammation. *Nat. Commun.* **2016**, *7*, 13466. [CrossRef]

210. Lee, E.; Trepicchio, W.L.; Oestreicher, J.L.; Pittman, D.; Wang, F.; Chamian, F.; Dhodapkar, M.; Krueger, J.G. Increased expression of interleukin 23 p19 and p40 in lesional skin of patients with psoriasis vulgaris. *J. Exp. Med.* **2004**, *199*, 125–130. [CrossRef]

211. Gordon, K.B.; Strober, B.; Lebwohl, M.; Augustin, M.; Blauvelt, A.; Poulin, Y.; Papp, K.A.; Sofen, H.; Puig, L.; Foley, P.; et al. Efficacy and safety of risankizumab in moderate-to-severe plaque psoriasis (UltIMMa-1 and UltIMMa-2): Results from two double-blind, randomised, placebo-controlled and ustekinumab-controlled phase 3 trials. *Lancet* **2018**, *392*, 650–661. [CrossRef]

212. Reich, K.; Gooderham, M.; Thaçi, D.; Crowley, J.J.; Ryan, C.; Krueger, J.G.; Tsai, T.-F.; Flack, M.; Gu, Y.; Williams, D.A.; et al. Risankizumab compared with adalimumab in patients with moderate-to-severe plaque psoriasis (IMMvent): A randomised, double-blind, active-comparator-controlled phase 3 trial. *Lancet* **2019**. [CrossRef]

213. Reich, K.; Papp, K.A.; Blauvelt, A.; Tyring, S.K.; Sinclair, R.; Thaçi, D.; Nograles, K.; Mehta, A.; Cichanowitz, N.; Li, Q.; et al. Tildrakizumab versus placebo or etanercept for chronic plaque psoriasis (reSURFACE 1 and reSURFACE 2): Results from two randomised controlled, phase 3 trials. *Lancet* **2017**, *390*, 276–288. [CrossRef]

214. Langley, R.G.; Tsai, T.-F.; Flavin, S.; Song, M.; Randazzo, B.; Wasfi, Y.; Jiang, J.; Li, S.; Puig, L. Efficacy and safety of guselkumab in patients with psoriasis who have an inadequate response to ustekinumab: Results of the randomized, double-blind, phase III NAVIGATE trial. *Br. J. Dermatol.* **2018**, *178*, 114–123. [CrossRef]

215. Reich, K.; Armstrong, A.W.; Foley, P.; Song, M.; Wasfi, Y.; Randazzo, B.; Li, S.; Shen, Y.-K.; Gordon, K.B. Efficacy and safety of guselkumab, an anti-interleukin-23 monoclonal antibody, compared with adalimumab for the treatment of patients with moderate to severe psoriasis with randomized withdrawal and retreatment: Results from the phase III, double-blind, placebo- and active comparator-controlled VOYAGE 2 trial. *J. Am. Acad. Dermatol.* **2017**, *76*, 418–431. [CrossRef]

216. Blauvelt, A.; Papp, K.A.; Griffiths, C.E.M.; Randazzo, B.; Wasfi, Y.; Shen, Y.-K.; Li, S.; Kimball, A.B. Efficacy and safety of guselkumab, an anti-interleukin-23 monoclonal antibody, compared with adalimumab for the continuous treatment of patients with moderate to severe psoriasis: Results from the phase III, double-blinded, placebo- and active comparator-controlled VOYAGE 1 trial. *J. Am. Acad. Dermatol.* **2017**, *76*, 405–417. [CrossRef]

217. Mease, P.; Hall, S.; Fitzgerald, O.; van der Heijde, D.; Merola, J.F.; Avila-Zapata, F.; Cieślak, D.; Graham, D.; Wang, C.; Menon, S.; et al. Tofacitinib or Adalimumab versus Placebo for Psoriatic Arthritis. *N. Engl. J. Med.* **2017**, *377*, 1537–1550. [CrossRef]

218. Gladman, D.; Rigby, W.; Azevedo, V.F.; Behrens, F.; Blanco, R.; Kaszuba, A.; Kudlacz, E.; Wang, C.; Menon, S.; Hendrikx, T.; et al. Tofacitinib for Psoriatic Arthritis in Patients with an Inadequate Response to TNF Inhibitors. *N. Engl. J. Med.* **2017**, *377*, 1525–1536. [CrossRef]

219. Papp, K.A.; Krueger, J.G.; Feldman, S.R.; Langley, R.G.; Thaçi, D.; Torii, H.; Tyring, S.; Wolk, R.; Gardner, A.; Mebus, C.; et al. Tofacitinib, an oral Janus kinase inhibitor, for the treatment of chronic plaque psoriasis: Long-term efficacy and safety results from 2 randomized phase-III studies and 1 open-label long-term extension study. *J. Am. Acad. Dermatol.* **2016**, *74*, 841–850. [CrossRef]

220. Papp, K.A.; Menter, M.A.; Abe, M.; Elewski, B.; Feldman, S.R.; Gottlieb, A.B.; Langley, R.; Luger, T.; Thaci, D.; Buonanno, M.; et al. Tofacitinib, an oral Janus kinase inhibitor, for the treatment of chronic plaque psoriasis: Results from two randomized, placebo-controlled, phase III trials. *Br. J. Dermatol.* **2015**, *173*, 949–961. [CrossRef]

221. Papp, K.A.; Bissonnette, R.; Gooderham, M.; Feldman, S.R.; Iversen, L.; Soung, J.; Draelos, Z.; Mamolo, C.; Purohit, V.; Wang, C.; et al. Treatment of plaque psoriasis with an ointment formulation of the Janus kinase inhibitor, tofacitinib: A Phase 2b randomized clinical trial. *BMC Dermatol.* **2016**, *16*, 15. [CrossRef] [PubMed]

222. Ports, W.C.; Khan, S.; Lan, S.; Lamba, M.; Bolduc, C.; Bissonnette, R.; Papp, K. A randomized phase 2a efficacy and safety trial of the topical Janus kinase inhibitor tofacitinib in the treatment of chronic plaque psoriasis. *Br. J. Dermatol.* **2013**, *169*, 137–145. [CrossRef] [PubMed]

223. Papp, K.A.; Menter, M.A.; Raman, M.; Disch, D.; Schlichting, D.E.; Gaich, C.; Macias, W.; Zhang, X.; Janes, J.M. A randomized phase 2b trial of baricitinib, an oral Janus kinase (JAK) 1/JAK2 inhibitor, in patients with moderate-to-severe psoriasis. *Br. J. Dermatol.* **2016**, *174*, 1266–1276. [CrossRef] [PubMed]

224. Papp, K.; Pariser, D.; Catlin, M.; Wierz, G.; Ball, G.; Akinlade, B.; Zeiher, B.; Krueger, J.G. A phase 2a randomized, double-blind, placebo-controlled, sequential dose-escalation study to evaluate the efficacy and safety of ASP015K, a novel Janus kinase inhibitor, in patients with moderate-to-severe psoriasis. *Br. J. Dermatol.* **2015**, *173*, 767–776. [CrossRef] [PubMed]

225. Eichenfield, L.F.; Call, R.S.; Forsha, D.W.; Fowler, J.; Hebert, A.A.; Spellman, M.; Stein Gold, L.F.; Van Syoc, M.; Zane, L.T.; Tschen, E. Long-term safety of crisaborole ointment 2% in children and adults with mild to moderate atopic dermatitis. *J. Am. Acad. Dermatol.* **2017**, *77*, 641–649.e645. [CrossRef] [PubMed]

226. El-Khalawany, M.A.; Hassan, H.; Shaaban, D.; Ghonaim, N.; Eassa, B. Methotrexate versus cyclosporine in the treatment of severe atopic dermatitis in children: A multicenter experience from Egypt. *Eur. J. Pediatrics* **2013**, *172*, 351–356. [CrossRef]

227. Dvorakova, V.; O'Regan, G.M.; Irvine, A.D. Methotrexate for Severe Childhood Atopic Dermatitis: Clinical Experience in a Tertiary Center. *Pediatric Dermatol.* **2017**, *34*, 528–534. [CrossRef]

228. Purvis, D.; Lee, M.; Agnew, K.; Birchall, N.; Dalziel, S.R. Long-term effect of methotrexate for childhood atopic dermatitis. *J. Paediatr. Child Health* **2019**, *155*, 145. [CrossRef]

229. Van Geel, M.J.; Mul, K.; de Jager, M.E.A.; van de Kerkhof, P.C.M.; de Jong, E.M.G.J.; Seyger, M.M.B. Systemic treatments in paediatric psoriasis: A systematic evidence-based update. *J. Eur. Acad. Dermatol. Venereol.* **2015**, *29*, 425–437. [CrossRef]

230. Collin, B.; Vani, A.; Ogboli, M.; Moss, C. Methotrexate treatment in 13 children with severe plaque psoriasis. *Clin. Exp. Dermatol.* **2009**, *34*, 295–298. [CrossRef]

231. Kaur, I.; Dogra, S.; De, D.; Kanwar, A.J. Systemic methotrexate treatment in childhood psoriasis: Further experience in 24 children from India. *Pediatric Dermatol.* **2008**, *25*, 184–188. [CrossRef] [PubMed]

232. Schmitt, J.; Schmitt, N.; Meurer, M. Cyclosporin in the treatment of patients with atopic eczema—A systematic review and meta-analysis. *J. Eur. Acad. Dermatol. Venereol.* **2007**, *21*, 606–619. [CrossRef] [PubMed]

233. Totri, C.R.; Eichenfield, L.F.; Logan, K.; Proudfoot, L.; Schmitt, J.; Lara-Corrales, I.; Sugarman, J.; Tom, W.; Siegfried, E.; Cordoro, K.; et al. Prescribing practices for systemic agents in the treatment of severe pediatric atopic dermatitis in the US and Canada: The PeDRA TREAT survey. *J. Am. Acad. Dermatol.* **2017**, *76*, 281–285. [CrossRef] [PubMed]

234. Jury, C.S.; McHenry, P.; Burden, A.D.; Lever, R.; Bilsland, D. Narrowband ultraviolet B (UVB) phototherapy in children. *Clin. Exp. Dermatol.* **2006**, *31*, 196–199. [CrossRef] [PubMed]

235. Pavlovsky, M.; Baum, S.; Shpiro, D.; Pavlovsky, L.; Pavlotsky, F. Narrow band UVB: Is it effective and safe for paediatric psoriasis and atopic dermatitis? *J. Eur. Acad. Dermatol. Venereol.* **2011**, *25*, 727–729. [CrossRef]

236. Zamberk, P.; Velázquez, D.; Campos, M.; Hernanz, J.M.; Lázaro, P. Paediatric psoriasis–narrowband UVB treatment. *J. Eur. Acad. Dermatol. Venereol.* **2010**, *24*, 415–419. [CrossRef]

237. Deleuran, M.; Thaçi, D.; Beck, L.A.; de Bruin-Weller, M.; Blauvelt, A.; Forman, S.; Bissonnette, R.; Reich, K.; Soong, W.; Hussain, I.; et al. Dupilumab shows long-term safety and efficacy in moderate-to-severe atopic dermatitis patients enrolled in a phase 3 open-label extension study. *J. Am. Acad. Dermatol.* **2019**, *81*. [CrossRef]

238. Paller, A.S.; Siegfried, E.C.; Langley, R.G.; Gottlieb, A.B.; Pariser, D.; Landells, I.; Hebert, A.A.; Eichenfield, L.F.; Patel, V.; Creamer, K.; et al. Etanercept treatment for children and adolescents with plaque psoriasis. *N. Engl. J. Med.* **2008**, *358*, 241–251. [CrossRef]

239. Papp, K.; Thaçi, D.; Marcoux, D.; Weibel, L.; Philipp, S.; Ghislain, P.-D.; Landells, I.; Hoeger, P.; Kotkin, C.; Unnebrink, K.; et al. Efficacy and safety of adalimumab every other week versus methotrexate once weekly in children and adolescents with severe chronic plaque psoriasis: A randomised, double-blind, phase 3 trial. *Lancet* **2017**, *390*, 40–49. [CrossRef]

240. Landells, I.; Marano, C.; Hsu, M.-C.; Li, S.; Zhu, Y.; Eichenfield, L.F.; Hoeger, P.H.; Menter, A.; Paller, A.S.; Taïeb, A.; et al. Ustekinumab in adolescent patients age 12 to 17 years with moderate-to-severe plaque psoriasis: Results of the randomized phase 3 CADMUS study. *J. Am. Acad. Dermatol.* **2015**, *73*, 594–603. [CrossRef]

3

Altered Lipid Metabolism in Blood Mononuclear Cells of Psoriatic Patients Indicates Differential Changes in Psoriasis Vulgaris and Psoriatic Arthritis

Piotr Wójcik [1], Michał Biernacki [1], Adam Wroński [2], Wojciech Łuczaj [1], Georg Waeg [3], Neven Žarković [4] and Elżbieta Skrzydlewska [1,*]

[1]   Department of Analytical Chemistry, Medical University of Bialystok, 15-089 Białystok, Poland
[2]   Dermatological Specialized Center "DERMAL" NZOZ in Bialystok, 15-453 Białystok, Poland
[3]   Institute of Molecular Biosciences, University of Graz, 8010 Graz, Austria
[4]   LabOS, Rudjer Boskovic Institute, Laboratory for Oxidative Stress, 10000 Zagreb, Croatia
*   Correspondence: elzbieta.skrzydlewska@umb.edu.

Abstract: The aim of this study was to investigate possible stress-associated disturbances in lipid metabolism in mononuclear cells, mainly lymphocytes of patients with psoriasis vulgaris (Ps, n = 32) or with psoriatic arthritis (PsA, n = 16) in respect to the healthy volunteers (n = 16). The results showed disturbances in lipid metabolism of psoriatic patients reflected by different phospholipid profiles. The levels of non-enzymatic lipid metabolites associated with oxidative stress 8-isoprostaglandin F2α (8-isoPGF2α) and free 4-hydroxynonenal (4-HNE) were higher in PsA, although levels of 4-HNE-His adducts were higher in Ps. In the case of the enzymatic metabolism of lipids, enhanced levels of endocannabinoids were observed in both forms of psoriasis, while higher expression of their receptors and activities of phospholipases were detected only in Ps. Moreover, cyclooxygenase-1 (COX-1) activity was enhanced only in Ps, but cyclooxygenase-2 (COX-2) was enhanced both in Ps and PsA, generating higher levels of eicosanoids: prostaglandin E1 (PGE1), leukotriene B4 (LTB4), 13-hydroxyoctadecadienoic acid (13HODE), thromboxane B2 (TXB2). Surprisingly, some of major eicosanoids 15-d-PGJ$_2$ (15-deoxy-Δ12,14-prostaglandin J$_2$), 15-hydroxyeicosatetraenoic acid (15-HETE) were elevated in Ps and reduced in PsA. The results of our study revealed changes in lipid metabolism with enhancement of immune system-modulating mediators in psoriatic mononuclear cells. Evaluating further differential stress responses in Ps and PsA affecting lipid metabolism and immunity might be useful to improve the prevention and therapeutic treatments of psoriasis.

Keywords: lipid mediators; psoriasis vulgaris; psoriatic arthritis; lipid peroxidation products; endocannabinoids; eicosanoids

1. Introduction

Psoriasis is a chronic autoimmune disease, the most common form of which is psoriasis vulgaris, characterized by pathological interactions between immune cells, especially lymphocytes, and skin cells, especially keratinocytes. In some patients, psoriasis is characterized by a more severe clinical course, leading to the development of psoriatic arthritis [1]. The cause of the disease remains unknown, although some genetic or environmental factors are associated with the development of psoriasis. Thus, it has been observed that lymphocytes and the cytokines they produce, especially interferon γ (IFNγ) and interleukin 17 (IL-17), affect other cells, leading to chronic inflammation and characteristic symptoms such as cutaneous plaques in psoriasis or arthrosis and loss of movement in psoriatic arthritis. Moreover, the pro-inflammatory phenotype of lymphocytes and other immune cells is observed not only locally in the skin or joints, but also in cells isolated from blood, which confirms that general inflammation is present in psoriasis [2]. However, that can only partially explain the course of the disease, still leaving many questions open in respect to the development of psoriasis or the transition of one form to another. Recent studies on immunological diseases have revealed that their development is often accompanied by oxidative stress and increased metabolism of phospholipids, suggesting that both ROS and lipid mediators play important roles in the pathophysiology of psoriasis [3]. In psoriasis, both systemic and local, oxidative stress and increased metabolism of phospholipids have been demonstrated. Among immune-competent, inflammatory cells of psoriatic patients were observed especially for granulocytes, which increasingly generate lipid peroxidation products, thus modulating their inflammatory activities [4]. Furthermore, it has been shown that activation of lymphocytes is also accompanied by the generation of large amounts of reactive oxygen species (ROS) that are important mediators of cytokine-mediated redox biology [5]. Biological activities of ROS are related to their ability to react with biomolecules, such as phospholipids, in particular polyunsaturated fatty acids (PUFA), which leads to lipid peroxidation and generation of reactive aldehydes, e.g., 4-hydroxynonenal (4-HNE), which is denoted also as a "second messenger of free radicals" [6].

In addition to lipid peroxidation, cellular phospholipids are also metabolized by enzymes, the activities of which are increased in various inflammatory processes. The most important enzymes involved in the generation of lipid mediators are phospholipases, cyclooxygenases (COXs), and lipoxygenases (LOXs) [7]. During this process phospholipases begin biosynthesis of endocannabinoids among which the best known are 2-acyloglycerol (2-AG) and anandamide (AEA). Enhanced levels of them are observed in inflammatory diseases like osteoarthritis or systemic lupus erythematosus [8,9]. Endocannabinoids affect cells mostly by interactions with their receptors, cannabinoid receptors (CB1 and CB2). It is known that activation of CB2 receptor results in anti-inflammatory and anti-oxidative regulation, while activation of CB1 shows pro-inflammatory and pro-oxidative activity [10]. In addition, endocannabinoids have been found to be involved in the development of psoriatic comorbidities. Therefore, it can be assumed that disturbances of the endocannabinoid system may also play a significant role in the course of psoriasis.

Moreover, recent studies suggest, that effect of endocannabinoids action is also dependent on the action of their metabolites [11]. Anandamide is metabolized into arachidonic acid which together with arachidonic acid revealed from phospholipids is further metabolized into eicosanoids by (COXs) and LOX. Among cyclooxygenases COX-2 is believed to be the main enzyme responsible for generation of active lipid mediators during inflammation [12], while arachidonic acid is also a substrate to synthesis of thromboxanes, leukotrienes, and prostaglandins [13].

Since lipid mediators are commonly observed in autoimmune diseases, they are constantly gaining increased attention among researchers focused on autoimmune diseases. Lipid mediators might accordingly be important for studies on diseases with poorly understood pathophysiology and without effective therapy, like psoriasis. As such, the aim of this study was to investigate oxidative lipid modifications in mononuclear cells, mainly lymphocytes isolated from patients suffering from psoriasis vulgaris (Ps) or psoriatic arthritis (PsA).

2. Results

Phospholipids that could distinguish patients with psoriasis vulgaris and psoriatic arthritis were selected by use of multivariate statistics. Twenty phospholipid species with variable importance in projection (VIP $\geq$ 1) were selected, which were driving the separation of examined groups. Principal component analysis (PCA) model (Figure 1) was constructed to check classification of each group. The complete data set with the log transformed and auto-scaled phospholipid variables was used to carry out the analysis. The PCA model, on which each point represents an individual sample, showed that the group of healthy subjects was clearly separated from the patients groups, while the separation between both types of psoriasis almost did not occur. The model captured 78.1% of the total variance. The variation in the variables is represented by two principal components of PC1 (57.7%) versus PC2 (14.7%). It is highly probable that PC1 is associated with the age, while PC2 indicates a positive correlation with disease state. It was observed that the samples from both groups of psoriatic patients showed positive values for PC2, whereas those from healthy subjects presented negative values. Finally, we used partial least squares-discriminate analysis (PLS-DA) (Figure S1) and VIP for estimation of the importance of each phospholipid species which drove the separation of the examined groups (Table 1).

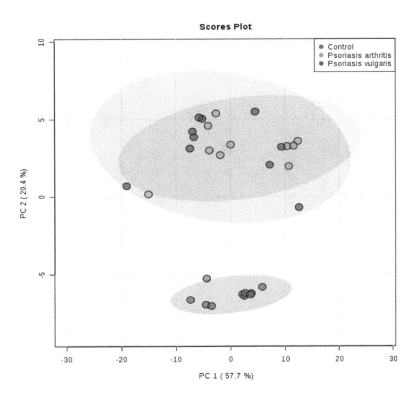

Figure 1. Principal component analysis (PCA) plot of the phospholipid species relative abundance determined by HILIC-LC-MS in lymphocytes of patient with psoriasis vulgaris (n = 10) and psoriatic arthritis (n = 10) as well as healthy subjects (n = 10); 95% confidential intervals are indicated by shaded area.

Table 1 shows the details of these species that belong to lysophosphatidylcholine (LPC), phosphatidylcholine (PC), phosphatidylinositol (PI), and sphingomyelin (SM) classes. Two phosphatidylcholines containing eicosatrienoic (20:3) and docosadienoic (22:2) acid, namely PC(20:0/22:2), and PC(20:3/24:0), had the highest VIP scores. In general, PC was down-regulated in patients of both types of psoriasis while two SM species, containing tetracosadienoic (24:2) and docosaenoic acid (22:1), respectively, were up-regulated. Other phospholipid species that were changed in the course of both forms of psoriasis belong to the PI class. PI species were down-regulated in both groups of patients with exception of PI(24:0/24:0), PI(24:0/24:1), and PI(18:0/22:0), which were highly up-regulated. Important to notice is that PI species containing arachidonic and linoleic acid, namely PI(16:0/20:4), PI(18:0/20:4), and PI(18:2/22:0) were significantly down-regulated in both groups of psoriatic patients in comparison to healthy subjects. Moreover, most of PI species were found to be more altered in PsA patients than those with Ps. LPC species with the score > 1, namely LPC(16:0) and LPC(18:0), were found to be highly up-regulated in psoriasis in comparison to healthy subjects. Hence, these two LPC species were mostly responsible for the differentiation of both types of psoriasis from healthy subjects (Table 1).

Table 1. Changes in mononuclear cells top 20 phospholipid species with VIP score greater than one comparing the healthy subjects (C; n = 10) to psoriasis vulgaris (n = 10) and psoriasis arthritis (n = 10) groups of patients; ns, not statistically significant.

m/z	RT	ID	Composition	VIP	Log2 (Fold-Change)					
					Control vs. Psoriasis Vulgaris	p Value	Control vs. Psoriatic Arthritis	p Value	Psoriasis Vulgaris vs. Psoriatic Arthritis	p Value
928.6940	18.31	PC(42:2)	PC(20:0/22:2)	1.97	0.63	2.34×10^{-5}	0.34	1.17×10^{-3}	0.29	ns
954.7113	18.12	PC(44:3)	PC(20:3/24:0)	1.89	0.54	3.76×10^{-5}	0.26	2.84×10^{-3}	0.29	ns
917.6085	3.47	PI(40:2)	PI(18:2/22:0)	1.57	0.68	1.13×10^{-5}	0.90	1.81×10^{-8}	-0.21	ns
915.5954	3.47	PI(40:3)	PI(18:0/22:3)	1.57	0.75	1.13×10^{-5}	0.97	3.91×10^{-8}	-0.21	ns
1033.7629	3.90	PI(48:0)	PI(24:0/24:0)	1.52	-1.06	5.81×10^{-4}	-0.85	2.06×10^{-3}	-0.21	ns
857.6755	18.16	SM(d41:2)	SM(d17:0/24:2)	1.51	-0.50	5.81×10^{-4}	-0.26	3.36×10^{-2}	-0.23	ns
868.6052	16.49	PC(38:4)	PC(18:0/20:4)	1.47	-0.181	2.00×10^{-3}	0.31	1.66×10^{-2}	0.26	ns
1031.7489	3.90	PI(48:1)	PI(24:0/24:1)	1.44	-1.64	1.03×10^{-3}	-1.43	1.93×10^{-3}	-0.2109	ns
857.5159	3.85	PI(36:4)	PI(16:0/20:4)	1.39	0.68	5.81×10^{-4}	0.89	1.26×10^{-5}	-0.21	ns
840.5732	16.71	PC(36:4)	PC(16:0/20:4)	1.39	0.56	3.51×10^{-3}	0.31	3.00×10^{-2}	0.25	ns
896.6372	16.37	PC(40:4)	PC(18:0/22:4)	1.38	0.42	4.04×10^{-3}	0.14	ns	0.27	ns
909.5490	3.84	PI(40:6)	PI(18:2/22:4)	1.38	0.61	3.33×10^{-4}	0.82	2.76×10^{-6}	-0.21	ns
792.5746	17.39	PC(32:0)	PC(16:0/16:0)	1.37	0.54	4.04×10^{-3}	0.28	ns	0.25	ns
921.6399	3.99	PI(40:0)	PI(18:0/22:0)	1.36	-1.89	1.63×10^{-3}	-1.68	3.02×10^{-3}	-0.21	ns
885.5472	3.83	PI(38:4)	PI(18:0/20:4)	1.35	0.57	2.61×10^{-4}	-0.26	ns	-0.21	ns
554.3463	20.37	LPC(16:0)		1.33	-1.77	5.81×10^{-4}	-2.6	3.53×10^{-6}	0.83	ns
582.3771	20.10	LPC(18:0)		1.31	-1.50	3.32×10^{-5}	-2.3	7.98×10^{-8}	0.83	ns
894.6222	16.40	PC(40:5)	PC(18:1/22:4)	1.30	0.50	4.72×10^{-3}	0.80	ns	0.26	ns
843.6591	18.25	SM(d40:2)	SM(d18:1/22:1)	1.26	-0.50	4.70×10^{-3}	-0.20	ns	-0.29	ns
911.5644	3.84	PI(40:5)	PI(18:1/20:4)	1.26	0.59	1.63×10^{-3}	0.24	4.78×10^{-5}	-0.21	ns

It is often assumed that the reduced level of PUFAs is related to their ROS-dependent and enzyme-dependent metabolism. Consequently, the elevated levels of lipid peroxidation products belonging to compounds generated during PUFAs' oxidative fragmentation, such as 4-HNE, as well as to compounds generated during PUFAs oxidative cyclisation, such as 8-iso prostaglandin F2α (8-isoPGF2α), was observed, in particular in patients with PsA (Figure 2).

Figure 2. The level of phospholipid oxidative modifications products and of 4-HNE-protein adducts in mononuclear cells of healthy peoples (n = 16) and patients with psoriasis vulgaris (n = 32) and psoriatic arthritis (n = 16). 8-isoPGF2α, F2α-8-isoprostaglandin; 4-HNE, 4-hydroxynonenal. Data points represent the mean ± SD; a, significantly different from healthy subject, $p < 0.05$; x, significantly different from patients with psoriasis vulgaris, $p < 0.05$.

That might indeed be that case with psoriatic patients because their observed decrease of PUFAs was associated by enhanced activities of the enzymes metabolizing lipids including phospholipases (PLA2 and PAF-AH), as well as of cyclooxygenase 1 (COX1) and cyclooxygenase2 (COX2), especially in Ps (Figure 3).

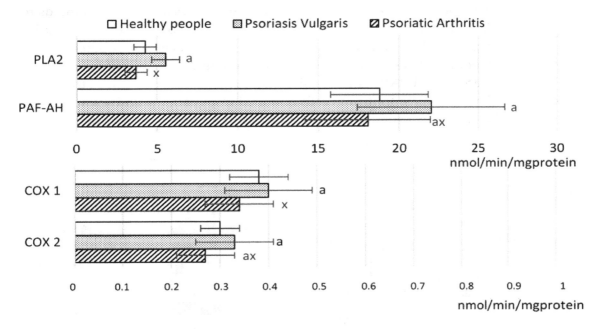

Figure 3. The activity of the enzymes involved in phospholipid metabolism in mononuclear cells of patients psoriasis vulgaris (n = 32) and psoriatic arthritis (n = 16) as well as healthy subjects (n = 16). PLA2, phosholipase A2; PAF-AF, platelet-activating factor acetylhydrolase; COX, cyclooxygenases. Data points represent the mean ± SD; a, significantly different from healthy subject, $p < 0.05$; x, significantly different from patients with psoriasis vulgaris, $p < 0.05$.

It is likely that increased activity of the above listed enzymes promoted generation of endocannabinoids. The levels of anandamide and LEA increased more in mononuclear cells of patients with PsA, while the concentration of 2-AG, 2-LG (2-linoleoylglycerol), and OEA (oleoylethanolamide) was higher in patients with Ps (Table 2). An elevated level of endocannabinoids was observed despite the increased activity of enzymes degrading them (FAAH—fatty acid amide hydrolase and MAGL—monoacylglycerol lipase), especially in mononuclear cells of patients with Ps (Table 2).

Table 2. The level of endocannabinoids and enzymes degrading them (FAAH and MAGL) in mononuclear cells of patients with psoriasis vulgaris (n = 32) and psoriatic arthritis (n = 16) Abbreviations: 2-AG, 2-arachidonoylglycerol; 2-LG, 2-linoleoylglycerol; AEA, anandamide; FAAH, fatty acid amide hydrolase; LEA, dihomo-γ-linolenoylethanolamine; MAGL, monoacylglycerol lipase; OEA, oleoylethanolamide. Data points represent the mean ± SD; a, significantly different from healthy subject, $p < 0.05$; x, significantly different from patients with Ps, $p < 0.05$.

Analyzed Parameters	Healthy Subjects	Psoriasis Vulgaris	Psoriatic Arthritis
AEA (pmol/mg protein)	0.17 ± 0.02	0.19 ± 0.03a	0.23 ± 0.04ax
2-AG (pmol/mg protein)	1.87 ± 0.18	3.24 ± 0.45a	2.78 ± 0.37ax
2-LG (pmol/mg protein)	5.59 ± 0.87	7.92 ± 0.99a	7.41 ± 0.93a
LEA (pmol/mg protein)	0.79 ± 0.08	0.94 ± 0.15a	1.17 ± 0.15ax
OEA (pmol/mg protein)	0.33 ± 0.05	0.47 ± 0.07a	0.36 ± 0.05a
FAAH (pmol/min/mg protein)	170 ± 16	219 ± 28a	242 ± 31ax
MAGL (pmol/min/mg protein)	55 ± 6	75 ± 10a	83 ± 14ax

Increased level of endocannabinoids resulted in enhanced expression of cannabinoids receptors (CB1 and CB2), as well as other receptors activated also by endocannabinoids (GPR55 and TRPV1) in Ps and decreased expression of these receptors in PsA (Figure 4). Products of phospholipid metabolism including endocannabinoids, but also fatty acids and eicosanoids, are ligands of nuclear peroxisome proliferator-activated receptors (PPARα, PPARγ, PPARδ). A significant increase in the expression of these receptors was observed in mononuclear cells obtained from patients with Ps, while it was only moderately raised in mononuclear cells of patients with PsA (Figure 4).

Figure 4. The expression of receptors involved in phospholipid metabolism in mononuclear cells of patients with psoriasis vulgaris (n = 16) and psoriatic arthritis (n = 8) and healthy peoples (n = 8). CB1, CB2, cannabinoid receptors; GRP55, G protein-coupled receptor 55; TRPV, the transient receptor potential cation channel subfamily V member 1; PPAR, peroxisome proliferator-activated receptor. Data points represent the mean ± SD; a, significantly different from healthy subjects, $p < 0.05$; x, significantly different from patients with psoriasis vulgaris, $p < 0.05$.

Increased activity of PLA2 lead to the enhanced release of arachidonic acid, which is further metabolized (mainly by cyclooxygenases and lipoxygenases) into another large group of active lipid mediators, notably eicosanoids (Figure 5) Among them, pro-inflammatory factors, such as 13-hydroxyoctadecadienoic acid (13-HODE) and leukotriene B$_4$ (LTB4) levels, were increased in both forms of the disease. In particular LTB4 level increased dramatically in psoriasis, especially in Ps. In addition, thromboxane B$_2$ (TxB2), (metabolite of pro-inflammatory thromboxane A$_2$ (TxA2) level was increased in Ps, which might be related to the activities of cyclooxygenases. The analysis of anti-inflammatory mediators revealed decreased levels of 15-deoxy-Δ12,14-prostaglandin J$_2$ (15-d-PGJ$_2$) in patients with Ps, while 15-hydroxyeicosatetraenoic acid (15-HETE) levels were slightly, but significantly, increased in Ps, and prostaglandin E1 (PGE$_1$) levels were increased both in Ps (four-fold) and in PsA (two-fold).

Since psoriasis is known to be associated with inflammation, basic pro-inflammatory and anti-inflammatory parameters were examined (Figure 6). The levels of pro-inflammatory cytokine IL-2 was increased above normal in mononuclear cells of both forms of psoriasis, while anti-inflammatory IL-10 levels were not changed in psoriatic patients.

Figure 5. The level of the eicosanoids in mononuclear cells of patients with psoriasis (n = 32), psoriatic arthritis (n = 16), as well as healthy subjects (n = 16). Data points represent the mean ± SD; a, significantly different from healthy subject, $p < 0.05$; x, significantly different from patients with psoriasis vulgaris. Prostaglandin E1 (PGE1), leukotriene B4 (LTB4), 13-hydroxyoctadecadienoic acid (13HODE), thromboxane B2 (TXB2). Surprisingly, some of major eicosanoids 15-deoxy-Δ12,14-prostaglandin J$_2$ (15-d-PGJ$_2$), 15-hydroxyeicosatetraenoic acid (15-HETE). Data points represent the mean ± SD; a, significantly different from healthy subject, $p < 0.05$; x, significantly different from patients with Ps, $p < 0.05$.

Figure 6. The expression of interleukins and pro-inflammatory mediators in mononuclear cells from patients with psoriasis vulgaris (n = 16), psoriatic arthritis (n = 8), and healthy subjects (n = 8). IL-interleukine. Data points represent the mean ± SD; a, significantly different from healthy subjects, $p < 0.05$.

3. Discussion

Psoriasis is a complex inflammatory disease associated with increased activation of lymphocytes [14], which leads to the generation of pro-inflammatory cytokines and to pro-oxidative processes causing oxidative stress [3]. The results of our study confirm the onset of oxidative stress in psoriasis, which is, in particular in PsA, manifested by changes in the metabolism of phospholipids in mononuclear cells, mainly containing lymphocytes, thus offering better understanding of the diseases, due to differentially expressed changes in lipid metabolism between Ps and PsA examined mononuclear cells.

The main source of ROS in cells are usually mitochondria whose respiratory chain may be disrupted by various factors, including phospholipids' metabolites, such as endocannabinoids, the levels of which were, in the current study, found to be increased in the mononuclear cells of psoriatic patients. It is known that the main endocannabinoids, AEA and 2-AG, may stimulate the function of mitochondria, including the production of hydrogen peroxide by enhanced entry of calcium ions into the cell [15]. In addition, activation of cannabinoid receptors (CB1), caused by endocannabinoids, which was, in our study, also found to be increased in mononuclear cells of psoriatic patients, may promote oxidative stress by enhanced inflammation, e.g., through NOS stimulation leading to increased generation of superoxide and nitric oxide [16]. In favor of this possibility are increased activities of cytosolic NADPH and xanthine oxidases in granulocytes and in plasma of patients with psoriasis, in particular if obtained from patients with PsA [4]. Such changes were accompanied by disturbances in the antioxidant system, which was spread in a stress-response manner lowering the level/activity of cellular antioxidants.

Similarly, redox imbalance and inflammation observed in psoriatic patients were, in the current study, associated with changes in ROS-dependent and enzyme-dependent phospholipid metabolism of mononuclear cells affecting especially PUFAs, which are lipid species the most sensitive to the ROS attack causing lipid peroxidation. Different phospholipid species, including phosphatidylcholines and phosphatidylinositols containing linoleic, arachidonic, eicosatetraenoic and docosadienoic acids, in particular, were down-regulated in mononuclear cells of psoriatic patients. Arachidonic acid and linoleic acid are the major PUFAs, which are oxidized in a ROS-dependent manner to biologically-active lipid mediators, including products of oxidative fragmentation (mainly α,β-unsaturated electrophilic aldehydes, with 4-HNE as the most important one) and products of oxidative cyclisation (mainly prostaglandin derivatives, such as 8-isoPGF2α) that further propagate oxidative damages altering functional activities of the immune-competent cells [17]. The mechanism of 8-isoPGF$_{2\alpha}$ action is based on TNFα activation [18]. So far, increased levels of 8-isoPGF$_{2\alpha}$ have been found in psoriatic patients' serum [19] as well as in the skin cells [20] being accompanied by elevated TNFα expression [21]. However, 4-HNE is a more potent biomarker of lipid peroxidation, which is involved in complex regulation of inflammatory and immunological responses [6]. The increased levels of the free 4-HNE were observed in our study especially in the mononuclear cells of PsA patients. Opposite to that, the levels of histidine-bound protein adducts of 4-HNE were higher in examined cells of patients with Ps indicating differential metabolic and scavenging pathways for this "second messenger of free radicals" in Ps and in PsA patients. It is known that unsaturated aldehydes, such as 4-HNE, have a strong affinity for covalently linking with nucleophilic amino and thiol groups of biomolecules, including proteins and glutathione (GSH) [17]. Since the thiol groups of protein cysteine residues act as redox switches controlling cell signaling and metabolism [22], versatile interactions of cysteine with signaling molecules, such as 4-HNE, can selectively modulate protein functions [23]. Complementary to that, modifications of protein residues, not only cysteine but also histidine or lysine, may lead to disturbances of biological functions of modified proteins and their translocation to the cell membrane and activation of protein G [24–26]. Our findings suggest that such protein adducts may participate in enhanced expression of protein G-coupled receptors (including cannabinoid receptors), as was observed in this study in mononuclear cells of psoriatic patients.

The cellular metabolism of phospholipids, independent of ROS, also includes enzymatic reactions leading to the generation of endocannabinoids dependent on the activity of phospholipases [27]. Despite the increased activity of endocannabinoid-metabolizing enzymes (FAAH and MAGL), endocannabinoid levels were elevated in our patients. The main endocannabinoids, anandamide and 2-arachidonoylglycerol (2-AG), participate in the modulation of inflammation and redox balance mainly through the activation of cannabinoid receptors [28]. Crosstalk between ROS and endocannabinoids has been proven in various diseases [27], but so far not in patients with psoriasis, as was done for the first time in the present study.

In addition, inflammation is associated with increased expression of lymphocyte receptors: GPR55 and TRPV1 [29,30]. According to in vitro studies endocannabinoids themselves may also act as anti-inflammatory agents by promoting the Th2 cell phenotype and further inhibit the production of pro-inflammatory cytokines by lymphocytes [31]. This may suggest that endocannabinoids are generated, among others, to alleviate the inflammatory aspects of psoriasis. In fact, in the case of Ps we observed a higher expression of endocannabinoid receptors but, surprisingly, in the case of PsA, the expression of these receptors has been reduced, suggesting no cellular response to the regulatory role of endocannabinoids. It is possible that the receptors or membrane protein G have been modified by 4-HNE, which can explain also less pronounced increase of the soluble 4-HNE-protein adducts in patients with PsA, who have otherwise higher levels of the free aldehyde than patients with Ps. In any case, the disrupted immunosuppressive effect of endocannabinoids in PsA may be an important factor differentiating the pathophysiology of both forms of psoriasis and may promote exacerbation of Ps into the form of PsA.

Enzymatic degradation of endocannabinoids, with COXs participation in particular, plays a critical role in the onset of the inflammatory cascade with the generation of different biologically-active compounds, including eicosanoids [32]. Among them are various bioactive agents, such as prostaglandins, thromboxanes, and leukotrienes, which can participate in the pathophysiology of psoriasis. Eicosanoids may have opposite inflammatory effects and, thus, modulate skin disorders. The results of this study revealed a significant increase in mononuclear cells of patients with psoriasis TxB2, a stable metabolite of TxA2, which plays a pro-inflammatory role in imiquimod-induced psoriatic dermatitis [33]. Additionally, elevated LTB4 levels may promote skin inflammation [34]. Inflammation may also be modified by 15d-PGJ$_2$, which is elevated in Ps, and which inhibits NFκB mediated metabolic pathways by inhibiting IκB kinase (IKK) activity [35].

Another mechanism of interactions redox biology-lipid metabolism in the mononuclear cells of psoriatic patients may be associated with the expression of nuclear receptors like peroxisome proliferator-activated receptors—PPARs [36], whose forms: PPARα, PPARγ, and PPARδ were enhanced in mononuclear cells of patients with psoriasis, particularly with Ps. Moreover, PUFAs, eicosanoids, and endocannabinoids may be ligands of PPARs, which in B and T lymphocytes serve as important regulators of the immune system as potential anti-inflammatory targets for PPAR ligands [37,38].

PPARα and PPARδ show antioxidant properties by suppressing enzymes involved in ROS/RNS generation [39], while enhanced activation of PPARα may also prevent NFκB–dependent inflammation [40]. The results obtained by the murine translation study indicated that PPARα activation may be one of the protective mechanisms against progression of skin inflammation [41]. Additionally, the PPARδ promotes synthesis of antioxidants, such as thioredoxin, superoxide dismutase, or heme oxygenase [42]. Thus, PPARδ enhanced expression seems to be an important antioxidative mechanism in patients with Ps. The significant decrease in their expression observed in PsA confirms that the lack of anti-stress protection against ROS leads to an increase the severity of this disease. In addition, increased PPARγ expression, as discovered in this study, may be involved in reduction of TNFα level, particularly in PsA [43].

4. Materials and Methods

4.1. Materials

Blood samples were collected from 32 patients with psoriasis vulgaris (Ps) (16 females, 16 men; mean age 38) and 16 patients with psoriatic arthritis (seven females, nine men; mean age 35).

Only patients with psoriasis vulgaris for at least six months and characterized by at least 10% of the total body surface affected by the disease were included in the study (the median of their psoriasis surface index and severity index (PASI) was 21, with a range of 15–25). Patients with psoriatic arthritis (PsA) were diagnosed on the basis of a questionnaire CASPAR (ClASsification criteria for Psoriatic Arthritis). All participants gave their informed consent for inclusion in the research. The research was carried out in accordance with the Helsinki Declaration, and the protocol was approved by the Local Bioethics Commission at the Medical University of Białystok (Poland), no. R-I-002/289/2017 (2017.09.28). People receiving topical or oral medications during the four weeks before the study and comorbidities/smoking or alcohol abuse were excluded from examinations.

Blood was collected into tubes with ethylenediaminetetraacetic acid as an anti-coagulant and butylhydroxytoluene as an antioxidant. Density gradient centrifugation (Gradisol L, 300 g, 25 min) was used to obtain mononuclear cells mainly containing lymphocytes fraction from blood. This fraction was washed in phosphate-buffered saline (PBS), then resuspended in PBS containing proteases inhibitors mix. Purity of the cells has been examined microscopically (Nikon Eclipse Ti, Nikon Instruments Inc., Melville, NY, USA). Isolated fractions were lysed by sonification on ice and stored at −80 °C before further analysis. All obtained parameters are expressed per mg of protein (protein levels were examined using Bradford method [44]).

4.2. Methods

4.2.1. Phospholipid Profile Estimation

Mononuclear cells from ten patients with Ps, ten patients with PsA (5f + 5m) and ten healthy subjects (5f + 5m) were used to estimate phospholipid profile of each group. Total lipids from all samples were extracted by the modified Bligh and Dyer method [45]. The total amount of phospholipids (PL) was calculated by using a phosphorus assay, performed according to Bartlett and Lewis [46]. Hydrophilic interaction chromatography liquid chromatography-mass spectrometry (HILIC-LC)-MS, performed on an Agilent 1290 ultra-performance liquid chromatography (UPLC) system coupled to an Agilent 6540 quadrupole time of flight mass spectrometer (Agilent Technologies, Palo Alto, CA, USA) was applied to obtain the phospholipid profile. An Ascentis Si HPLC Pore column (15 cm × 1.0 mm, 3 µm; Sigma Aldrich, St. Louis, MO, USA) was used for chromatographic separation in gradient mode. The method was described in details previously [47]. Internal standards PC 14:0/14:0, PI 16:0/16:0, and PE 14:0/14:0 (Avanti Polar Lipids, Alabaster, AL, USA) were used to confirm the ion variations observed in the MS spectra. Identification of each phospholipid species was performed according to the typical fragmentation pathways [48]. The area of each extracted ion chromatogram peak was normalized to the area of an internal standard to calculate relative abundance of each ion. Detailed description of the lipidomic methodology is provided in supplementary materials.

4.2.2. Determination of the Activity of Lipid Metabolizing Enzymes

Spectrophotometric method was used to assay phospholipase A2 (PLA2-EC.3.1.1.4) activity using PLA2 Assay Kit (no. 765021, Cayman Chemical Company, Ann Arbor, MI, USA) according to the kit instructions [49].

PAF acetylhydrolase (PAF-AH-EC.3.1.1.47) activity was measured spectrophotometrically using the Cayman's PAF Acetylhydrolase Assay Kit (no. 760901, Cayman Chemical Company, Ann Arbor, MI, USA) according to kit instructions [50].

Cyclooxygenase 1 and 2 (COX1/2-EC.1.14.99.1) activities were measured spectrophotometrically using a commercial assay kit (Cayman Chemical Company, Ann Arbor, MI, USA) [51]. For distinguishing COX1 activity from COX2 activity the specific COX1 inhibitor SC-560 was used [52].

4.2.3. 4-HNE Determination

Gas chromatography-mass spectrometry (GC/MS) using the selected ion monitoring (SIM) mode, as the O-PFB-oxime-TMS derivatives, using minor modifications of the method of Luo [53] was used to measure product of phospholipid fragmentation—4-HNE. Transitions of the precursor to the product ion were as follows: m/z 333.0 and 181.0 for 4-HNE-PFB-TMS and m/z 307 for IS (benzaldehyde-D_{6+}) derivative. (7890A GC-7000 quadrupole MS/MS, Agilent Technologies, Palo Alto, CA, USA).

4.2.4. 4-HNE-Protein Adducts Determination

The 4-HNE-protein adducts level was measured using ELISA method using anti-4-HNE-His murine monoclonal antibody (genuine anti-4-HNE-Hismurine monoclonal antibody, clone 4-HNE 1g4) and goat anti-mouse antibody (Dako, Carpinteria, CA, USA) as primary and secondary antibodies [54]. Results were shown as a percentage of the expression determined in control cells.

4.2.5. 8-isoPGF2α Determination

LC-MS/MS method of Coolen [55] was used to determination of phospholipid oxidative cyclisation product, 8-isoPGF2α, which was analyzed in negative-ion mode using MRM mode: m/z 353.2→193.1 (for 8-isoPGF2α) and 357.2→197.1 (for 8-isoPGF2α-d4 used as an internal standard) (LCMS 8060, Shimadzu, Kyoto, Japan).

4.2.6. Determination of Endocannabinoids and Enzymes Them Degradation

The LC-MS/MS method was used for the quantification of the endocannabinoids level [56]. Endocannabinoids were analyzed in positive-ion mode using MRM mode. Transitions of the precursors to the product ions were as follows: m/z 348.0→62.15 for AEA, m/z 379.0→269.35 for 2-AG, m/z 356.0→63.05 for AEA-d8, m/z 387.0→294.0 m/z for 2-AG-d8, m/z 430.0→66.0 for OEA-d4, m/z 324.0→62.0 for LEA, m/z 355.0→263.0 for 2-LG, 326.0→62.0 for OEA. (LCMS 8060, Shimadzu, Kyoto, Japan). Results were expressed as amount of cannabinoids per mg of protein. The Siegmund procedure [57] was used to determine FAAH (EC.3.5.1.99) activity, following the releasing of m-nitroaniline (m-NA) from decanoyl m-nitroaniline at 410 nm. Enzyme activity was expressed as the amount of enzyme metabolizing 1 pmol of substrat per minute per mg of protein. Releasing of 5′-thio-2-nitrobenzoic acid from arachidonoyl-1-thio-glycerol was used to spectrophotometric [340 nm] determination of MAGL (EC.3.1.1.23) activity [58]. Enzyme activity was expressed as the amount of enzyme metabolizing 1 pmol of substrate per minute per mg of protein.

4.2.7. Lipid Mediators Determination

Lipid mediators levels: TXB_2, PGE_1, 15d-PGJ_2, 13-HODE, LTB_4, and 15-HETE were estimated using ultra-performing liquid chromatography tandem mass spectrometry (LCMS 8060, Shimadzu, Kyoto, Japan) [59]. 15-HETE-d8, LTB_4-d4, PGF2α-d4 and PGD_2-d4 were used as internal standards for quantification. Lipid mediators were extracted using SPE and analyzed in negative-ion mode (MRM). The precursor to the product ion transition was as follows: m/z 369.3→169.1 for TXB_2, m/z 353.3→317.2 for PGE_1, 315.2→271.2 for 15-d-PGJ_2, m/z 295→277 for 13-HODE, and m/z 319→301.2 for 15-HETE.

4.2.8. Proteins Examination

Western blot analysis of protein expression was performed according to Eissa and Seada [60]. Samples were electrophoretically separated on 10% gels, transferred to 0.2 μm pore-sized nitrocellulose, and incubated overnight with primary antibodies against: GPR55, PPARα (host: rabbit) β-actin (host: mouse) that were purchased from Sigma-Aldrich, (St. Louis, MO, USA). Primary antibodies against: Il-10 (host mouse), CB1, CB2, TRPV1 (host rabbit) were purchased from Santa Cruz Biotechnology (Santa Cruz, CA, USA). Primary antibodies against PPARγ (host: rat) were purchased from Abcam (Cambridge, UK). Primary antibodies against PPARδ were purchased from Invitrogen (Carlsbad,

CA, USA). Primary antibodies against IL-2 (host: rat) were purchased from Thermo Fisher Scientific (Thermo Fisher Scientific, Waltham, MA, USA). Next membranes were incubated for 2 h with alkaline phosphatase secondary IgG antibody against corresponding primary antibody (Sigma-Aldrich, St. Louis, MO, USA). Protein bands were visualized using the BCIP/NBT Liquid substrate system (Sigma-Aldrich, St. Louis, MO, USA). To compare the proteins expression between samples, each band intensity was estimated using VersaDoc System and Quantity One software (Bio-Rad Laboratories Inc., Hercules, CA, USA). The results are expressed as a percentage of the expression determined in the control cells.

4.3. Statistical analysis

All data were expressed as mean ± SD. For data analysis program Statistica (Statistica 13.3, StatSoft Polska, Cracow, Poland) were used. These data were analyzed using one-way analysis of variance followed by a post hoc Tukey test. Values of $p < 0.05$ were considered significant.

5. Conclusions

In conclusion, the results of our research suggest that the development of both forms of psoriasis is strongly associated with oxidative stress resulting in altered lipid metabolism and cytokine production, leading to the development of pro-inflammatory preconditioning of the immune cells. In such a vicious circle, mononuclear cells additionally activate pro-inflammatory states and enhance pro-oxidative, stressful conditions. Thus, ROS and enzyme-dependent changes in mononuclear cell phospholipids can be considered as important processes associated with the pathophysiology of psoriasis. Moreover, the reduced expression of endocannabinoid receptors in PsA suggests the failure of the anti-inflammatory mechanism and may be an important factor leading to the transformation of Ps into a more severe form of PsA. Finally, we assume that monitoring the level of 4-HNE adducts can help predict the progression of Ps into PsA if done complementary to the other parameters of lipid metabolism and the levels of respective cytokines that should be analyzed in further studies.

Author Contributions: Conceptualization: E.S. and N.Z.; methodology: P.W.; software: W.L.; validation: W.L., P.W.; formal analysis: W.L.; investigation: M.B.; G.W.; resources: P.W.; data curation: A.W.; writing—original draft preparation: P.W.; writing—review and editing: E.S.; visualization: P.W.; supervision: N.Z.; project administration: E.S.; funding acquisition: E.S.

Abbreviations

2-AG	2-Arachidonylglycerol
2-LG	2-Linoleoylglycerol
4-HNE	4-Hydroxynonenal
4-ONE	4-Oxynonenal
8-isoPGF2α	8-iso prostaglandin F2α
13-HODE	13-hydroxyoctadecadienoic acid
15-HETE	15-Hydroxyeicosatetraenoic acid$_2$
15d-PGJ$_2$	15-deoxy-Δ12,14-prostaglandin J
AEA	Anandamide
AIDS	Acquired immunodeficiency syndrome
CB	Cannabinoid receptor
COX	Cyclooxygenase

EDTA	Ethylenediaminetetraacetic acid
ELISA	Enzyme-linked immunosorbent assay
ERK5	Extracellular-signal-regulated kinase 5
FAAH	Fatty acid amide hydrolase
GC	Gas chromatography
GPR55	G protein-coupled receptor 55
HILIC	Hydrophilic interaction chromatography
HPLC	High-performance liquid chromatography
IFNγ	Interferon γ
IKK	IκB kinase
IL	Interleukin
IMQ	Imiquimod
LC	Liquid chromatography
LEA	Dihomo-γ-linolenoylethanolamine
LOX	Lipoxygenases
LPC	Lysophosphatidylcholine
LTB$_4$	Leukotriene B4
MAGL	Monoacylglycerol lipase
MS	Mass spectrometry
NFκB	Nuclear factor kappa-light-chain-enhancer of activated B cells
NOX	NADPH oxidase
Ns	Not significant
OEA	Oleoylethanolamide
PAF-AH	Platelet-activating factor acetylhydrolase
PBS	Phosphate-buffered saline
PC	Phosphatidylcholine
PCA	Principal component analysis
PGE1	Prostaglandin E1
PI	Phosphatidylinositol
PLA2	Phospholipase A2
PLS-DA	partial least squares-discriminate analysis
PPAR	Peroxisome proliferator-activated receptor
Ps	Psoriasis vulgaris
PsA	Psoriatic arthritis
PUFAs	Polyunsaturated fatty acids
ROS	Reactive oxygen species
RT	Retention time
SIM	Selected ion monitoring
SLE	Systemic lupus erythematosus
SM	Sphingomyelin
Th	T helper lymphocytes
TNFα	Tumor necrosis factor α
TNFR	Tumor necrosis factor receptor
TRPV1	The transient receptor potential cation channel subfamily V member 1
TxA2	Thromboxane A2
TxB2	Thromboxane B2
UPLC	Ultra-performance liquid chromatography
VIP	variable importance in projection

References

1. Mease, P.J.; Armstrong, A.W. Managing Patients with Psoriatic Disease: The Diagnosis and Pharmacologic Treatment of Psoriatic Arthritis in Patients with Psoriasis. *Drugs* **2014**, *74*, 423–441. [CrossRef] [PubMed]

2. Hawkes, J.E.; Chan, T.C.; Krueger, J.G. Psoriasis pathogenesis and the development of novel targeted immune therapies. *J. Allergy Clin. Immunol.* **2017**, *140*, 645–653. [CrossRef] [PubMed]

3. Huang, N.; Perl, A. Metabolism as a Target for Modulation in Autoimmune Diseases. *Trends Immunol.* **2018**, *39*, 562–576. [CrossRef] [PubMed]

4. Ambrożewicz, E.; Wójcik, P.; Wroński, A.; Łuczaj, W.; Jastrząb, A.; Žarković, N.; Skrzydlewska, E. Pathophysiological Alterations of Redox Signaling and Endocannabinoid System in Granulocytes and Plasma of Psoriatic Patients. *Cells* **2018**, *7*, 159. [CrossRef] [PubMed]

5. Belikov, A.V.; Schraven, B.; Simeoni, L. T cells and reactive oxygen species. *J. Biomed. Sci.* **2015**, *22*. [CrossRef] [PubMed]

6. Łuczaj, W.; Gęgotek, A.; Skrzydlewska, E. Antioxidants and HNE in redox homeostasis. *Free Radic. Biol. Med.* **2017**, *111*, 87–101. [CrossRef] [PubMed]

7. Phillis, J.W.; O'Regan, M.H. The role of phospholipases, cyclooxygenases, and lipoxygenases in cerebral ischemic/traumatic injuries. *Crit. Rev. Neurobiol.* **2003**, *15*, 61–90. [CrossRef]

8. Barrie, N.; Manolios, N. The endocannabinoid system in pain and inflammation: Its relevance to rheumatic disease. *Eur. J. Rheumatol.* **2017**, *4*, 210–218. [CrossRef]

9. Navarini, L.; Bisogno, T.; Mozetic, P.; Piscitelli, F.; Margiotta, D.P.E.; Basta, F.; Afeltra, A.; Maccarrone, M. Endocannabinoid system in systemic lupus erythematosus: First evidence for a deranged 2-arachidonoylglycerol metabolism. *Int. J. Biochem. Cell Biol.* **2018**, *99*, 161–168. [CrossRef]

10. Mukhopadhyay, P.; Rajesh, M.; Bátkai, S.; Pan, H.; Mukhopadhyay, B.; Haskó, G.; Mackie, K.; Pacher, P. Opposing effects of cb1 and cb2 receptors on inflammation, oxidative stress, and cell death in nepropathy. *Faseb. J.* **2011**, *25*, 1087.

11. Siegmund, S.V.; Wojtalla, A.; Schlosser, M.; Schildberg, F.A.; Knolle, P.A.; Nüsing, R.M.; Zimmer, A.; Strassburg, C.P.; Singer, M.V. Cyclooxygenase-2 contributes to the selective induction of cell death by the endocannabinoid 2-arachidonoyl glycerol in hepatic stellate cells. *Biochem. Biophys. Res. Commun.* **2016**, *470*, 678–684. [CrossRef] [PubMed]

12. Meirer, K.; Steinhilber, D.; Proschak, E. Inhibitors of the Arachidonic Acid Cascade: Interfering with Multiple Pathways. *Basic Clin. Pharmacol. Toxicol.* **2014**, *114*, 83–91. [CrossRef] [PubMed]

13. Gachet, M.S.; Rhyn, P.; Bosch, O.G.; Quednow, B.B.; Gertsch, J. A quantitiative LC-MS/MS method for the measurement of arachidonic acid, prostanoids, endocannabinoids, N-acylethanolamines and steroids in human plasma. *J. Chromatogr. B Anal. Technol. Biomed. Life Sci.* **2015**, *976–977*, 6–18. [CrossRef] [PubMed]

14. Diani, M.; Altomare, G.; Reali, E. T cell responses in psoriasis and psoriatic arthritis. *Autoimmun. Rev.* **2015**, *14*, 286–292. [CrossRef] [PubMed]

15. Nunn, A.; Guy, G.; Bell, J.D. Endocannabinoids in neuroendopsychology: Multiphasic control of mitochondrial function. *Philos Trans. R Soc Lond B Biol Sci* **2012**, *367*, 3342–3352. [CrossRef] [PubMed]

16. Carney, S.T.; Lloyd, M.L.; MacKinnon, S.E.; Newton, D.C.; Jones, J.D.; Howlett, A.C.; Norford, D.C. Cannabinoid Regulation of Nitric Oxide Synthase I (nNOS) in Neuronal Cells. *J. Neuroimmune Pharm.* **2009**, *4*, 338–349. [CrossRef] [PubMed]

17. Csala, M.; Kardon, T.; Legeza, B.; Lizák, B.; Mandl, J.; Margittai, É.; Puskás, F.; Száraz, P.; Szelényi, P.; Bánhegyi, G. On the role of 4-hydroxynonenal in health and disease. *Biochim. Et Biophys. Acta (Bba)-Mol. Basis Dis.* **2015**, *1852*, 826–838. [CrossRef]

18. Timmermann, M.; Högger, P. Oxidative stress and 8-iso-prostaglandin F(2alpha) induce ectodomain shedding of CD163 and release of tumor necrosis factor-alpha from human monocytes. *Free Radic. Biol. Med.* **2005**, *39*, 98–107. [CrossRef]

19. Jiao, X.; Guo, Z.; Chen, T.; Zhang, Y.; Li, M. Determination of antioxidant capacity and 8-iso-prostaglandin F2α levels in patients with psoriasis and their significance. *Chin. J. Dermatol.* **2012**, *45*, 388–391.

20. Basu, S.; Whiteman, M.; Mattey, D.; Halliwell, B. Raised levels of F2-isoprostanes and prostaglandin F2α in different rheumatic diseases. *Ann. Rheum. Dis.* **2001**, *60*, 627–631. [CrossRef]

21. Man, X.-Y.; Zheng, M. Role of Angiogenic and Inflammatory Signal Pathways in Psoriasis. *J. Investig. Derm. Symp. Proc.* **2015**, *17*, 43–45. [CrossRef]

22. Miki, H.; Funato, Y. Regulation of intracellular signalling through cysteine oxidation by reactive oxygen species. *J. Biochem.* **2012**, *151*, 255–261. [CrossRef] [PubMed]

23. Castro, J.P.; Jung, T.; Grune, T.; Siems, W. 4-Hydroxynonenal (HNE) modified proteins in metabolic diseases. *Free Radic. Biol. Med.* **2017**, *111*, 309–315. [CrossRef] [PubMed]

24. Grabarczyk, D.B.; Chappell, P.E.; Eisel, B.; Johnson, S.; Lea, S.M.; Berks, B.C. Mechanism of Thiosulfate Oxidation in the SoxA Family of Cysteine-ligated Cytochromes. *J. Biol. Chem.* **2015**, *290*, 9209–9221. [CrossRef] [PubMed]

25. Agarwal, R.; MacMillan-Crow, L.A.; Rafferty, T.M.; Saba, H.; Roberts, D.W.; Fifer, E.K.; James, L.P.; Hinson, J.A. Acetaminophen-Induced Hepatotoxicity in Mice Occurs with Inhibition of Activity and Nitration of Mitochondrial Manganese Superoxide Dismutase. *J. Pharm. Exp.* **2011**, *337*, 110–118. [CrossRef] [PubMed]

26. Westcott, P.M.K.; To, M.D. The genetics and biology of KRAS in lung cancer. *Chin. J. Cancer* **2013**, *32*, 63–70. [CrossRef] [PubMed]

27. Turcotte, C.; Chouinard, F.; Lefebvre, J.S.; Flamand, N. Regulation of inflammation by cannabinoids, the endocannabinoids 2-arachidonoyl-glycerol and arachidonoyl-ethanolamide, and their metabolites. *J. Leukoc. Biol.* **2015**, *97*, 1049–1070. [CrossRef] [PubMed]

28. Jean-Gilles, L.; Braitch, M.; Latif, M.L.; Aram, J.; Fahey, A.J.; Edwards, L.J.; Robins, R.A.; Tanasescu, R.; Tighe, P.J.; Gran, B.; et al. Effects of pro-inflammatory cytokines on cannabinoid CB1 and CB2 receptors in immune cells. *Acta Physiol. (Oxf)* **2015**, *214*, 63–74. [CrossRef] [PubMed]

29. Włodarczyk, M.; Sobolewska-Włodarczyk, A.; Cygankiewicz, A.I.; Jacenik, D.; Krajewska, W.M.; Stec-Michalska, K.; Piechota-Polańczyk, A.; Wiśniewska-Jarosińska, M.; Fichna, J. G protein-coupled receptor 55 (GPR55) expresses differently in patients with Crohn's disease and ulcerative colitis. *Scand. J. Gastroenterol.* **2017**, *52*, 711–715. [CrossRef] [PubMed]

30. Gouin, O.; L'Herondelle, K.; Lebonvallet, N.; Le Gall-Ianotto, C.; Sakka, M.; Buhé, V.; Plée-Gautier, E.; Carré, J.-L.; Lefeuvre, L.; Misery, L.; et al. TRPV1 and TRPA1 in cutaneous neurogenic and chronic inflammation: Pro-inflammatory response induced by their activation and their sensitization. *Protein Cell* **2017**, *8*, 644–661. [CrossRef] [PubMed]

31. Klein, T.W.; Newton, C.; Larsen, K.; Chou, J.; Perkins, I.; Lu, L.; Nong, L.; Friedman, H. Cannabinoid receptors and T helper cells. *J. Neuroimmunol.* **2004**, *147*, 91–94. [CrossRef] [PubMed]

32. Camara-Lemarroy, C.R.; Gonzalez-Moreno, E.I.; Guzman-de la Garza, F.J.; Fernandez-Garza, N.E. Arachidonic Acid Derivatives and Their Role in Peripheral Nerve Degeneration and Regeneration. *Sci. World J.* **2012**, *2012*, 7. [CrossRef] [PubMed]

33. Tanada-Ueharaguchi, Y.; Honda, T.; Murata, T.; Arita, M.; Miyachi, Y.; Kabashima, K. Thromboxane A2 promotes the development of imiquimod-induced mouse psoriasis model via TP receptor. *J. Dermatol. Sci.* **2016**, *84*, e5. [CrossRef]

34. Del Prete, A.; Shao, W.-H.; Mitola, S.; Santoro, G.; Sozzani, S.; Haribabu, B. Regulation of dendritic cell migration and adaptive immune response by leukotriene B4 receptors: A role for LTB4 in up-regulation of CCR7 expression and function. *Blood* **2007**, *109*, 626–631. [CrossRef] [PubMed]

35. Paul, S.; Traver, M.K.; Kashyap, A.K.; Washington, M.A.; Latoche, J.R.; Schaefer, B.C. T cell receptor signals to NF-κB are transmitted by a cytosolic p62-Bcl10-Malt1-IKK signalosome. *Sci. Signal.* **2014**, *7*, ra45. [CrossRef] [PubMed]

36. Ament, Z.; Masoodi, M.; Griffin, J.L. Applications of metabolomics for understanding the action of peroxisome proliferator-activated receptors (PPARs) in diabetes, obesity and cancer. *Genome Med.* **2012**, *4*, 32. [CrossRef] [PubMed]

37. O'Sullivan, S.E. Cannabinoids go nuclear: Evidence for activation of peroxisome proliferator-activated receptors. *Br. J. Pharm.* **2007**, *152*, 576–582. [CrossRef] [PubMed]

38. Xu, Z.; Wang, G.; Zhu, Y.; Liu, R.; Song, J.; Ni, Y.; Sun, H.; Yang, B.; Hou, M.; Chen, L.; et al. PPAR-γ agonist ameliorates liver pathology accompanied by increasing regulatory B and T cells in high-fat-diet mice. *Obesity* **2017**, *25*, 581–590. [CrossRef]

39. Aleshin, S.; Reiser, G. Role of the peroxisome proliferator-activated receptors (PPAR)-α, β/δ and γ triad in regulation of reactive oxygen species signaling in brain. *Biol. Chem.* **2013**, *394*, 1553–1570. [CrossRef]

40. Contreras, A.V.; Torres, N.; Tovar, A.R. PPAR-α as a Key Nutritional and Environmental Sensor for Metabolic Adaptation. *Adv. Nutr.* **2013**, *4*, 439–452. [CrossRef]

41. Kim, M.-S.; Pyun, H.-B.; Hwang, J.-K. Panduratin A, an activator of PPAR-α/δ, suppresses the development of oxazolone-induced atopic dermatitis-like symptoms in hairless mice. *Life Sci.* **2014**, *100*, 45–54. [CrossRef] [PubMed]

42. Kim, H.J.; Ham, S.A.; Paek, K.S.; Hwang, J.S.; Jung, S.Y.; Kim, M.Y.; Jin, H.; Kang, E.S.; Woo, I.S.; Kim, H.J.; et al. Transcriptional up-regulation of antioxidant genes by PPARδ inhibits angiotensin II-induced premature senescence in vascular smooth muscle cells. *Biochem. Biophys. Res. Commun.* **2011**, *406*, 564–569. [CrossRef] [PubMed]

43. Marx, N.; Kehrle, B.; Kohlhammer, K.; Grüb, M.; Koenig, W.; Hombach, V.; Libby, P.; Plutzky, J. PPAR Activators as Antiinflammatory Mediators in Human T Lymphocytes. *Circ. Res.* **2002**, *90*, 703–710. [CrossRef] [PubMed]

44. Bradford, M.M. A rapid and sensitive method for the quantitation of microgram quantities of protein utilizing the principle of protein-dye binding. *Anal. Biochem.* **1976**, *72*, 248–254. [CrossRef]

45. Bligh, E.G.; Dyer, W.J. A Rapid Method of Total Lipid Extraction and Purification. *Can. J. Biochem. Physiol.* **1959**, *37*, 911–917. [CrossRef] [PubMed]

46. Bartlett, E.M.; Lewis, D.H. Spectrophotometric determination of phosphate esters in the presence and absence of orthophosphate. *Anal. Biochem.* **1970**, *36*, 159–167. [CrossRef]

47. Łuczaj, W.; Domingues, P.; Domingues, M.R.; Pancewicz, S.; Skrzydlewska, E. Phospholipidomic Analysis Reveals Changes in Sphingomyelin and Lysophosphatidylcholine Profiles in Plasma from Patients with Neuroborreliosis. *Lipids* **2017**, *52*, 93–98. [CrossRef] [PubMed]

48. Pulfer, M.; Murphy, R.C. Electrospray mass spectrometry of phospholipids. *Mass Spectrom. Rev.* **2003**, *22*, 332–364. [CrossRef] [PubMed]

49. Reynolds, L.J.; Hughes, L.L.; Yu, L.; Dennis, E.A. 1-Hexadecyl-2-arachidonoylthio-2-deoxy-sn-glycero-3-phosphorylcholine as a substrate for the microtiterplate assay of human cytosolic phospholipase A2. *Anal. Biochem.* **1994**, *217*, 25–32. [CrossRef] [PubMed]

50. Aarsman, A.J.; Neys, F.W.; Van den Bosch, H. Catabolism of platelet-activating factor and its acyl analog. Differentiation of the activities of lysophospholipase and platelet-activating-factor acetylhydrolase. *Eur. J. Biochem.* **1991**, *200*, 187–193. [CrossRef]

51. Kulmacz, R.J.; Lands, W.E. Requirements for hydroperoxide by the cyclooxygenase and peroxidase activities of prostaglandin H synthase. *Prostaglandins* **1983**, *25*, 531–540. [CrossRef]

52. Smith, C.J.; Zhang, Y.; Koboldt, C.M.; Muhammad, J.; Zweifel, B.S.; Shaffer, A.; Talley, J.J.; Masferrer, J.L.; Seibert, K.; Isakson, P.C. Pharmacological analysis of cyclooxygenase-1 in inflammation. *PNAS* **1998**, *95*, 13313–13318. [CrossRef] [PubMed]

53. Luo, X.P.; Yazdanpanah, M.; Bhooi, N.; Lehotay, D.C. Determination of aldehydes and other lipid peroxidation products in biological samples by gas chromatography-mass spectrometry. *Anal. Biochem.* **1995**, *228*, 294–298. [CrossRef]

54. Weber, D.; Milkovic, L.; Bennett, S.J.; Griffiths, H.R.; Zarkovic, N.; Grune, T. Measurement of HNE-protein adducts in human plasma and serum by ELISA—Comparison of two primary antibodies. *Redox Biol.* **2013**, *1*, 226–233. [CrossRef] [PubMed]

55. Coolen, S.A.J.; van Buuren, B.; Duchateau, G.; Upritchard, J.; Verhagen, H. Kinetics of biomarkers: Biological and technical validity of isoprostanes in plasma. *Amino Acids* **2005**, *29*, 429–436. [CrossRef] [PubMed]

56. Gouveia-Figueira, S.; Nording, M.L. Development and validation of a sensitive UPLC-ESI-MS/MS method for the simultaneous quantification of 15 endocannabinoids and related compounds in milk and other biofluids. *Anal. Chem.* **2014**, *86*, 1186–1195. [CrossRef] [PubMed]

57. Siegmund, S.V.; Seki, E.; Osawa, Y.; Uchinami, H.; Cravatt, B.F.; Schwabe, R.F. Fatty acid amide hydrolase determines anandamide-induced cell death in the liver. *J. Biol. Chem.* **2006**, *281*, 10431–10438. [CrossRef]

58. Ulloa, N.M.; Deutsch, D.G. Assessment of a Spectrophotometric Assay for Monoacylglycerol Lipase Activity. *AAPS J.* **2010**, *12*, 197–201. [CrossRef]

59. Watkins, B.A.; Kim, J.; Kenny, A.; Pedersen, T.L.; Pappan, K.L.; Newman, J.W. Circulating levels of endocannabinoids and oxylipins altered by dietary lipids in older women are likely associated with previously identified gene targets. *Biochim. et Biophys. Acta (BBA)-Mol. Cell Biol. Lipids* **2016**, *1861*, 1693–1704. [CrossRef]

60. Eissa, S.; Seada, L.S. Quantitation of bcl-2 protein in bladder cancer tissue by enzyme immunoassay: Comparison with Western blot and immunohistochemistry. *Clin. Chem.* **1998**, *44*, 1423–1429.

4

Immunological Memory of Psoriatic Lesions

Agnieszka Owczarczyk-Saczonek [1,*], **Magdalena Krajewska-Włodarczyk** [2,3], **Marta Kasprowicz-Furmańczyk** [1] **and Waldemar Placek** [1]

[1]   Department of Dermatology, Sexually Transmitted Diseases and Clinical Immunology, The University of Warmia and Mazury, Al. Wojska Polskiego 30, 10-229 Olsztyn, Poland; martak03@wp.pl (M.K.-F.); w.placek@wp.pl (W.P.)

[2]   Department of Rheumatology, Municipal Hospital in Olsztyn, 10-229 Olsztyn, Poland; magdalenakw@op.pl

[3]   Department of Internal Medicine, School of Medicine, Collegium Medicum, University of Warmia and Mazury, 10-900 Olsztyn, Poland

*   Correspondence: aganek@wp.pl

Abstract: The natural course of psoriasis is the appearance of new lesions in the place of previous ones, which disappeared after a successful therapy. Recent studies of psoriasis etiopathogenesis showed that after psoriatic plaques have disappeared, in healthy skin we can still find a trace of inflammation in the form of tissue resident memory cells (TRM). They are originally responsible for protection against viral and bacterial infections in non-lymphatic tissues. In psoriatic inflammation, they are characterized by heterogeneity depending on their origin. CD8+ T cells TRM are abundantly present in psoriatic epidermis, while CD4+ TRM preferentially populate the dermis. In psoriasis, epidermal CD8+ TRM cells express CLA, CCR6, CD103 and IL-23R antigen and produce IL-17A during ex vivo stimulation. However, CD4+ CD103+ TRM can also colonize the epidermis and produce IL-22 during stimulation. Besides T cells, Th22 and epidermal DCs proved that epidermal cells in healed skin were still present and functioning after several years of disease remission. It explains the clinical phenomenon of the tendency of psoriatic lesions to relapse in the same location and it allows to develop new therapeutic strategies in the future.

Keywords: psoriasis; tissue resident memory cells; IL-17

1. Introduction

The natural course of psoriasis is the long-term persistence of lesions in the same anatomical regions and the appearance of new ones in places where they have resolved after successful therapy. The appearance of new lesions in the place of previous ones, which disappeared after a successful therapy, evokes feelings of depression, hopelessness and depression in patients and induces conviction in the lack of effective therapies. Recent studies of psoriasis etiopathogenesis showed that after psoriatic plaques have disappeared, in healthy skin we can still find a trace of inflammation in the form of tissue resident memory cells (TRM). They are able to initiate an inflammatory cascade and cause a relapse in the same location. In psoriasis, even during remission, they become a source of important inflammatory cytokines IL-17A and IL-22 [1–4]. T cell-associated gene (*LCK* and *TRCB1*) and inflammatory gene (*IL17*, *IL22* and *IFN-γ*) activity remains increased in the skin after psoriasis lesions, at least three months after the onset of the treatment with TNF-α inhibitors [5,6]. However, not only TRMs are responsible for clinical relapses at the same location (Figure 1) (Table 1). This article is a review of current knowledge about the "immune memory" of psoriatic lesions.

Figure 1. The relapse of psoriatic lesions in the same localization despite efficient treatment.

Table 1. The Cells Responsible for the "memory" of Psoriatic Lesions.

Type of Cells		Psoriasis Lesions	Resolved Psoriasis Skin
TRM	**CD4+**	A few in dermis CD103- and a low number in epidermis CD103+	A few
	CD8+	A lot of in epidermis CD103+: CD8+CD49a+ producing perforin, IFN-γ CD8+CD49a- producing IL-17 IL-22, IFN-γ, a few in dermis CD103- and a low number CD103+	A few in epidermis
Dendritic Cells	**LC**	In epidermis producing a lot of IL-23	In epidermis producing IL-23
	eDC	In epidermis producing of IL-1β, IL-23, TNFα	Absent

2. Tissue Resident Memory Cells (TRM)

TRM cells are transcriptionally, phenotypically and functionally different from traditional central memory cells (TCM) and effector memory T cells (TEM). They recirculate among blood, T cell zones of secondary lymphoid organs, lymph and non-lymphoid tissues, such as the skin, where they act as alarm sensors or cytotoxic killers. They are characterized by heterogeneity depending on their origin [5,7–11].

They are originally responsible for protection against viral and bacterial infections in non-lymphatic tissues. The protective activity of TRM has been confirmed in HSV infection, vaccinia pox, lymphocytic choriomeningitis virus (LCMV), influenza, listeriosis, malaria, as well as in some types of cancer. The vaccination task is, among others, the education of TRM to react very quickly against an infection [9]. TRM cells are locally found in many tissues providing a rapid in situ response to infectious agents more effectively than T cells of effector memory. They also secrete granzyme B, which helps to reduce the spread of pathogens at the site of infection. They can activate the innate and adaptive mechanisms of the immune response [2,10,12–15]. TRM acts as a bridge between the adaptive and innate immune systems. Because many viruses have tissue tropism, TRM also provides protective immune responses for tissue that it has previously encountered. Since, HSV-specific TRMs have been found in the skin, rotavirus-specific TRMs in the intestines and flu-specific TRMs in the lungs [16,17]. However, in addition to their protective functions, there is more and more evidence of their involvement in the pathogenesis of autoimmune disorders such as psoriasis, vitiligo, autoimmune hepatitis, rheumatoid arthritis and lymphomas [11].

The main surface markers of human TRM cells are CD49a, CD69 and CD103. The CD103 marker (integrin αE subunit) is only expressed on CD8+ TRM cells, not CD4+ TRM. Its expression is most prominent on epidermal CD4+ and CD8+ TRM cells because it enables TRM binding to E-cadherin, which is widely expressed by epithelial cells [8,13,18]. The CD69 marker plays a key role in distinguishing T cells in tissues from those in circulation and it is responsible for the colonization of these cells in tissues, preventing them from recirculating. CD69 binds and inhibits the expression of the cell surface of sphingosine-1-phosphate receptor (S1PR1). The transcription factor KLF2 promotes the expression of S1PR1, thereby CD69 and may allow recirculation of TRM in unusual situations [19]. S1PR1 reacts to the S1P ligand, which is released by endothelial cells in the blood and lymph, allowing TRM cells to leave the tissues for circulation. This situation is observed, among others, after exposure to an allergen resulting in formation of secondary TRM cells [19]. However, the latest findings indicate that the importance of CD69 for TRM residence may depend on the tissue in which they are located (essential for TRM in the kidneys, no relevance in the gut) [18]. However, expression levels may vary between T cells in different tissues. Another marker that can be used to differentiate two subsets of TRM cells is CD49a—the α-subunit of the α1β1 integrin receptor (also known as very late antigen VLA-1). It determines a subset of CD8+ TRM cells that are localized in the epidermis. These cells produce IFN-γ and acquire high cytotoxic capacity upon IL-15 stimulation [20]. CD8+ CD49a+ TRM cells produce perforin and IFN-γ, which is a key cytokine in fighting viral infections. CD8+ CD49-TRM cells produce IL-17 [20,21]. TRM also expresses the Program Cell Death Protein-1 (PD-1) and T-cell immunoglobulin mucin receptor 3 (TIM3), which are the surface proteins that suppress T cell activity. Their expression occurs in inflamed tissues. In such situations, TRMs have an anti-inflammatory effect, which indicates the ambiguous nature of these cells [22,23].

In healthy individuals, CD8$^+$CD103$^+$CD49a$^-$TRM cells were present in both dermis and epidermis, whereas CD8$^+$CD103$^+$CD49a$^+$TRM cells were localized in the epidermis. Epidermal CD8$^+$CD103$^+$CD49a$^-$TRM cells were predominant IL-17 producers, whereas CD8$^+$CD103$^+$CD49a$^+$TRM cells excelled at IFN-γ production and rapidly gained a cytotoxic capacity following IL-15 stimulation [21].

TRM cells develop from circulating effector T cell precursors in response to an antigen. CD103 plays a major role in their formation, and the expression of this integrin depends on the TGF-β cytokine. CD8+ T effector cells, which do not produce TGF-β, have no expression of CD103 and they do not differentiate into TRM cells. The homeostatic IL-15 cytokine, pro-inflammatory cytokines (IL-12 and IL-18) and barrier cytokines, such as IL-33, which support TRM cell formation and survival, play an important role in the development of TRM cells [7,8].

The second type of TRM are CD4+ cells, which are less-known ones, and are located near the vessels in the dermis; they do not express CD103 and have a high proliferative capacity. They are responsible for defense against *Leishmania* and *Candida albicans* in the gut, lungs and reproductive system [24].

3. Tissue Resident Memory Cells in Psoriasis

CD4+ T cells with the Th1 and Th17 phenotype have long been considered the main pathogenic subpopulations of T cells. LL37 (antimicrobial peptide derived from keratinocytes) and ADAMTSL5 (protein produced by melanocytes) in the pathogenesis of the disease has been more appreciated. The abovementioned proteins are considered as autoantigens in psoriasis. Similarly, CD4 T-cells recognize LL37 as an autoantigen and they correlate with PASI [25,26]. CD8+ T cells with resident memory tissue phenotype (TRM) are abundantly present in psoriatic epidermis, while CD4+ TRM preferentially populate the dermis. The differences in colonization result from the expression of CD69, which blocks the sphingosine-1-phosphate receptor (S1P1), a receptor normally allowing lymph entry. In addition, a significant proportion of skin TRM expresses CD103, the αEβ7 integrin chain, which interacts with E-cadherin expressed by keratinocytes (Figure 2). The signal required for their residence is TGF-β via TGF-βRII [9]. Hair follicles through IL-15 and IL-7 production are also important in their recruitment [27]. In addition to cytokines, lipids available in the skin are essential to maintain TRM [10,17]

Figure 2. The receptors and secretory activity of tissue resident memory (TRM) CD8+ [5,22]

TRMs have been described in unchanged, healed skin in places of recurrent psoriasis, which indicates their role in the disease's local memory [28]. Recirculation of memory T cells between the skin and circulation is a newly recognized immunological mechanism that plays an important role in the initiation of psoriasiform response [3,29,30] (Figure 3). Their particular pathogenicity is determined by the fact that they have the ability to produce IL-17 and IL-22, pro-inflammatory, key cytokines involved in this process [23,29].

Figure 3. The role of TRM in psoriatic inflammation.

The first study that highlighted the role of resident skin T cells in psoriasis was the experiment of Boyman et al. [31]. They implanted unchanged human psoriatic skin to immunodeficient mice (AGR129 mice, deficient in type I and II interferon receptors and the recombination activating gene 2). The reproduction of resident human T cells and the formation of psoriatic lesions were observed within eight weeks. They showed the CD8+ phenotype with TNF-α susceptibility and were located mainly in the epidermis and the dermal–epidermal junction [31].

Diani et al. [1] analyzed the phenotype of circulating T cells in patients with psoriasis with the assessment of gene expression in psoriatic skin. It was found that circulating CCR6+ CD4+ TEM (effector memory cells) and T effector cells significantly correlated with the severity of skin lesions and inflammation (CRP) while the percentage of CXCR3+ CD4+ TEM cells correlated negatively. In addition, CLA+ CD4+ TCM cells expressing CCR6+ or CCR4+ CXCR3+ negatively correlated with the severity of psoriasis. CLA expression is associated with the recruitment of CD4+ T cells into the skin, mainly when expressed on TCM cells, in particular on CD4+ TCM with the CCR4+ and CCR6+ phenotype [1,26]. In an earlier study, Bose et al. [32] proved that inhibition of the CCR7/CCL19 axis was critical for remission of psoriasis induced by TNF inhibitors [3]. In psoriasis, circulating CCR4 + CD4+ T cells significantly correlate with disease severity (PASI), and a strong negative correlation has been found for CCR5+ CD4+ T cells [32]. A subset of T effector CCR4+ CD8+ CD103+ cells also positively correlates with both systemic inflammation (CRP) and the severity of skin lesions [4,33]. It was also found that the fraction of IL-17 secreting CD4+ T-lymphocytes and probably γδ T-lymphocytes may play a role in the formation of a self-sustaining inflammatory loop [1].

Lymphocytes CD4+ Th producing pro-inflammatory cytokines, such as IL-17A, IL-22 and IFN-γ, are considered to be the main pathogenic T cell subpopulation, whereas CD8+, present in healthy skin as memory T cells, have a similar pro-inflammatory cytokine profile. They are in large quantities in the psoriatic epidermis and can recognize peptide antigens presented on MHC class I molecules like HLA-Cw6 [29]. Blockade of β1-integrin hinders entry of T cells into the epidermis, which prevents the development of disease eruptions on the murine AGR model of psoriasis [34]. Di Meglio et al. [29] showed that the accumulation of epidermal CD8+ cells induces both hyperproliferation of keratinocytes and papillomatosis (increase in CD8 + a parallel to the intensity of Ki67 staining in keratinocytes) [29]. CD8+ T cells isolated from psoriasis patients produce psoriasis-related cytokines. After treatment they remain in the skin as TRM and LL-37-specific CD8 + T cells, expressing integrin α1β1 [29].

In the study of Kurihara et al. [13], biopsies from psoriatic lesions were examined. The number of CD8+CD103+ TRM cells in the epidermis correlated with the thickness of the epidermis ($p = 0.016$), suggesting their role in the formation of psoriatic lesions [13]. They were mostly CD8+ CD69+ T cells, expressing skin colonization antigens, and the count of CD4+ CD103+ TRM was low. Some CD8+ CD103+ T cells produced IFN-γ, IL-17A or IL-22. In addition, CD8+ CD103+ TRM cells more frequently produced IL-17A than CD8+ CD103- and effector cells CD8+ CD103 or CD4+ CD103+. Interestingly, the number of CD8+ CD103+ IL-17A + TRM cells in patients treated with biological or systemic therapy was higher [13]. In contrast, in the dermis of the psoriatic plaques, TRM cells show lower expression of CD103, as demonstrated by Cheuk et al. [5]. In the first stage of psoriatic inflammation, in the skin without lesions yet, epidermal TRM cells expressing CCR6 cooperate with CCL20 expressing keratinocytes [35,36].

In turn, Vo et al. [36] evaluated the phenotypic features of TRM in non-lesional, lesional psoriasis and healthy skin. Immunofluorescence study showed that CD103+ CD8 TRM, both in non-lesional and lesional were dominant in the epidermis compared to the skin of healthy volunteers. In addition, IL-17A production was higher in patients with longer disease duration [36].

The optimal treatment time needed to completely silence TRM, which could ensure that there is no recurrence of lesions at the location is unknown [37]. Therefore, psoriatic lesions preferentially recur in previously affected areas of the skin, and pathogenic TRM cells exposed to IL-17A and IL-22 accumulate in resolved lesions [5,35]. In the study of Gallais Serezal et al. [38], tissue responses after T cell stimulation in healthy and psoriatic lesions were analyzed. An increase in the number of epidermal IL-17 and IL-22—producing skin-resident T CCR6 + cells—may be a genetically predisposed reaction to microbial stimulation in never-lesional skin in patients with psoriasis. The consequence is an increase in IFN-g production and stimulation of keratinocytes that release INF-a, which stimulates psoriatic inflammation.

At the same time psoriasis plaques showed IL-17-induced response patterns, indicating a relapse. The proportional amount of induced IFN-γ, IL-10e and IL-17A correlated with relapse time in patients after discontinuation of the treatment [38].

For the complete remission of the disease, full TRM suppression is required. Unfortunately, TRM cells are long-lived, and resistant to damaging factors and apoptosis. This explains the frequent relapses at the same location for psoriasis. Even after the clinical lesions have resolved, they are capable of producing IL-17A, and effective therapy only suppresses their activity [3,37]. Furthermore, CD8+ TRM cells accumulate in untreated psoriasis localizations, probably in correlation with disease duration [4,11]. An interesting issue is the explanation of the longevity of memory cells. One of the reasons is its resistance to apoptosis. The heterodimeric marker molecule CD8+ ($\alpha E\beta 7$) consists of CD103 and $\beta 7$ subunits and plays a key role in the stability of CD8+ TRM cells by increasing the level of the Bcl-2 molecule with anti-apoptotic activity [8,13]. In contrast, TRM can produce granzyme B (serine protease), which can induce cellular apoptosis [23]. Moreover, IL-15 probably plays an important role in TRM cell survival [24].

What is surprising, the effector T cells use glycolysis energy, which is less efficient in generating ATP, but faster. TCM, on the other hand, use endogenously synthesized fatty acids, glucose catabolism and oxidative phosphorylation to support their long-term survival and function [17,39]. TCMs use extracellular glucose from the blood to synthesize fatty acids in the endoplasmic reticulum, using lysosomal acid lipase, which is important in the hydrolysis of cholesteryl esters and triglycerides in LDL molecules to cholesterol and free fatty acids (FFA). Thanks to such mechanisms, they can be long-lived and able to react quickly to antigen [17]. Cui et al. additionally showed that IL-7, a cytokine critical for TCM differentiation and survival, induced glycerol transport and triacylglycerol synthesis via enhanced gene expression of glycerol channel aquaporin 9, thus providing substrates for mitochondria via fatty acid oxidation (FAO) [17,40].

Unfortunately, there is currently no detailed data on the metabolic properties of TRM. However, it is known that CD8+ TRM develop a transcriptional program with overexpression of FABP4 (adipocyte-FABP), FABP5 (epidermal-FABP), CD36 (a lipid scavenger receptor) and lipoprotein lipase (cleaves triglycerides to yield FFA and diacylglycerol). Such activity of genes responsible for the activity of these molecules is not found in naive T cells, TCM or effector memory cells [17].

The study by Pan et al. [17] showed that mouse CD8 + TRM cells generated by skin viral infection show different expression level of genes of proteins mediating the intracellular uptake and transport of lipids, including fatty acid-binding protein—FABP4 (adipocyte-FABP) and FABP5 (epidermal-FABP). These are molecules facilitating exogenous FFAs acquisition and metabolism [17]. CD8 + TRM upregulated the gene expression of FABP4/FABP5 in a peroxisome proliferator-activated receptor gamma (PPAR-γ)—dependent manner [17,41]. T-specific deficiency of these molecules has been shown to impair the uptake of exogenous FFA by CD8+ TRM cells, which significantly reduces their long-term survival in vivo, but does not affect the survival of TCM in lymph nodes. In addition, CD8+ TRM skin cells lacking FABP4/FABP5 were less effective in protecting mice against cutaneous viral infection [41]. It is interesting whether in patients with psoriasis the described situation will be similar to the one in healthy individuals. No studies have been published on this subject yet.

In vitro, CD8+ TRM cells showed increased oxidative metabolism of mitochondria in the presence of exogenous FFA in normal and psoriatic skin. These results suggest that FABP4 and FABP5 play a key role in the maintenance, longevity and function of CD8+ TRM cells, and suggest that CD8+ TRM cells use exogenous FFA and their oxidative metabolism to survive in tissue. It has been shown that the lack of FABP4 and FABP5 does not affect CD8+ T cell proliferation or skin recruitment, but they are necessary for their long-term survival in the skin [41]. Perhaps the blockade of PPAR-γ functions will allow the development of strategies for the treatment of psoriatic lesions.

Oxidative stress plays an important role in psoriatic inflammation. In the study of Esmaeili et al. [42], the redox status of TRM CD4+ and its correlation with IL-17 response were assessed. The increased intracellular ROS production in memory CD4+ T cells in psoriasis patients decreased catalase gene expression compared to healthy ones, but no differences in intracellular glutathione levels and plasma total antioxidant capacity were revealed. However, the above disorders did not affect the IL-17 response in memory T cells [42].

4. Tissue Resident Memory Cells in Psoriatic Arthritis (PsA)

Recently, data has shown that TRM cells are responsible for the development of synovitis in PsA. However, they were not observed in rheumatoid arthritis [23].

The latest study on psoriatic arthritis (PsA) and other spondyloarthritides (SpA) assessed the molecular profile, phenotype and function of synovial Tc17 cells (IL-17A + CD8 + T cells) to clarify their role in pathogenesis. It turned out that, as in psoriasis, they were mainly TCRαβ +, and their number was increased in synovial fluid vs. peripheral blood in patients with PsA or other SpA. In addition, synovial TA17 PsA cells had the characteristics of Th17 (RORC/IL23R/CCR6/CD161) and Tc1 cells (A/B granzyme). The synovial marker Tc17 was CXCR6, and elevated levels of CXCR6 CXCL16 ligand in PsA were found in synovial fluid, which could contribute to their retention in the joints [43]. However, there are many doubts if TRMs are responsible for the initiation of inflammation and whether it is the same phenotype that persists after the treatment [23].

A new theory has emerged that TRMs involved in synovitis migrate from the skin and gut. Although TRMs do not circulate in the blood, they can sometimes be activated so that they travel within the lymphatic system [23,44,45]. A study by Guggino et al. [45], assessing TRM cells in peripheral blood, gut and synovium in patients with SpA, showed that the expression of α4β7 may support the recirculation of these cells from the gut and peripheral blood to foci of inflammation in the joints. Although this study applies to the entire group of patients with ankylosing spondylitis, probably patients with PSA were also included. Unfortunately, PSA patients were not analyzed separately and there is no research on these patients.

5. The Role of Memory γδ T Cells

Matos et al. found that TRM in psoriasis patients had specific properties that TRM did not have in healthy skin. These pathogenic clones preferentially had Vβ and Vα in the TCR region. Researchers identified 15 TCRβ and 4 TCRα antigen receptor sequences in patients with psoriasis that were not seen in the skin of healthy patients or atopic dermatitis patients. In addition, they observed a reduced amount of γδ T cells in psoriasis compared to αβ T cells. It has been proven that IL-17- and IL-22-producing T-cell clones with IL-17- and IL-22-specific antigen receptors still exist in the skin after the active psoriatic lesions have resolved. Therefore, for full disease remission, suppression of these resident T lymphocyte populations is required [3].

However, in psoriasis a reduced amount of γδ T cells was observed compared to αβ T cells [3]. In contrast, γδ T lymphocytes, considered innate immune cells that can also give rise to TRM populations, are far less known. Recently it has been shown in a mouse model that they can produce IL-17A and IL-17F in the skin in response to imiquimod. Each subsequent test with imiquimod resulted in an ever stronger proliferation of γδ T cells compared to the skin of mice after the first provocation [46].

6. Th22 and Tc17 Lymphocytes

In active psoriasis, we observe increased expression of IL17A, IL22 and IFN-γ in the effector T CD4+ and CD8+ cells of the epidermis in the immediate vicinity of keratinocytes, whereas cutaneous T cells show less activity of these genes. Cheuk et al. [5] proved that Th22 epidermal cells in healed skin were still present and functioning after several years of disease remission. After their stimulation, an increase in local IL-22, IL-17A and IFN-γ production by CD4+ T cells was observed. The percentage of IL-22-producing CD4+ epidermal cells did not correlate with the number of years of treatment, which indicates a preserved effector function even after 6 years of the treatment [5]. It has been shown that CD4+ epidermal T cells produced mainly IL-22, which activates keratinocytes leading to acanthosis. In contrast, epidermal CD8+ T cells mainly produced IL-17A, which drives the production of pro-inflammatory cytokines and chemokines by keratinocytes and is involved in the recruitment of neutrophils [5].

Studies have also shown that there are T-cells producing both IL-22 and IL-17 in the epidermis, which are present in lesions and healed skin in patients receiving nb-UVB therapy, and are practically absent in patients treated with biological drugs. Perhaps this type of T cell is more pathogenic [5]. It is known that effective nb-UVB therapy induces T cell apoptosis in the skin, but highly active effector lymphocytes can be constantly recruited from circulation [5].

Of note, active effector T cells involved in the inflammatory process may develop into long-lived epidermal TRM cells as the disease subsides [5,7,8].

7. Epidermal Langerhans Cells (LCs)

Psoriatic lesions' "memory" may also be affected by Langerhans cells dysfunction. In normal skin, epidermal Langerhans cells (eLC) are located in the epidermis and separated from dendritic skin cells (DC) by the basal membrane. Compared with cutaneous DC, LCs express fewer Toll-like receptors (TLRs), indicating an impaired ability to respond to TLR signaling, probably to maintain a state of tolerance to commensal [47]. In active psoriasis, under the influence of IL-23 and IL-17, inflammatory DCs penetrate both to the epidermis and dermis. In inflammatory DC epidermal expression of CCR2+ (eDC) occurs only in psoriasis and is phenotypically different from normal DCs'. Their number is higher than eLC and they show high expression of genes involved in the recruitment of neutrophils, keratinocytes and T lymphocytes. On the other hand, colonization of epidermis by eLC, under the influence of TLR-4 and TLR-7/8 activation, produce large amounts of IL-23, and eDCs secrete IL-1β together with IL-23 and TNF-α. After the psoriasis eruption, eDCs are absent in unchanged skin, while eLC retain high IL-23A expression and continue to respond to TLR stimulation, producing IL-23 [47,48]. Although eDCs are 3–10 times more numerous than eLC and drive the psoriatic condition, they also have the ability to produce anti-inflammatory IL-10 [48].

In individuals with early type of psoriasis (under 40 years of age) LCs do not show the ability to migrate under the influence of stimuli (chemical allergens, IL-1b and TNF-α). It is probably a phenomenon caused by the influence of the psoriatic environment rather than their defect [49,50]. Their ability to migrate is restored under the influence of treatment (among others anti-TNF, anti-IL-12/23, fumaric acid esters and UVB), except for therapies directed mainly towards T cells (ciclosporin A, MTX) [50–52]. Therefore, the observed rapid relapses after discontinuation of ciclosporin A may be explained by the role of LC in the rapid initiation of the inflammation in the same location (effect on TRM expressing IL-23R), which thus affects the memory of psoriatic eruptions [48].

8. Clinical Significance of the Memory of Psoriasis Lesions

Psoriatic lesions are characterized by the presence of massive inflammatory infiltrates (lymphocytes, neutrophils), proliferation and disturbance of epidermal differentiation (parakeratosis) as well as the formation of new blood vessels. Despite being such large structures, their resolution leaves no scars. This is quite unusual, especially comparing to other conditions in which neutrophils (pyoderma gangrenosum) are involved, where scars are present [12]. However, after discontinuation of treatment, a rapid recurrence of lesions is usually observed (90% in the same location) [24]. The understanding of the psoriasis context and the role of TRM can explain the key issues associated with this disease:

- the role in resistance to treatment and reactivation of changes in the same location [24];
- the role in the Koebner isomorphic symptom [24];

- the decision about adequate treatment time to limit lesions relapse and withdraw and reduce the amount of TRM.

The clinical characteristics of recurrence of psoriatic lesions mirrors the biology of TRMs. Since TRM does not work, inflammatory lesions induced by TRM are usually well demarcated with clear margins. The relapse of lesions can be fast because they occur in TRM skin and cooperate with local dendritic cells [12,52]. In understanding the abovementioned mechanisms, one stands a chance to provide more effective treatment and thus long-lasting remissions in psoriasis patients.

9. Conclusions

The discovery of TRM cells in psoriasis allows a better understanding of the complicated relationships between mediators and cells of the innate and adaptive immune system, keratinocytes and endothelial cells. It explains the clinical phenomenon of the tendency of psoriatic lesions to relapse in the same location and it allows to develop new therapeutic strategies in the future.

Author Contributions: A.O.-S. and W.P. conceived and designed manuscript; A.O.-S., M.K.-W., M.K.-F. analyzed the data; A.O.-S., M.K.-W., M.K.-F. contributed materials; A.O.-S. wrote the paper. All authors have read and agreed to the published version of the manuscript.

References

1. Diani, M.; Altomare, G.; Reali, E. T helper cell subsets in clinical manifestations of psoriasis. *J. Immunol. Res.* **2016**, *2016*, 1–7. [CrossRef]
2. Eberle, F.C.; Brück, J.; Holstein, J.; Hirahara, K.; Ghoreshi, K. Recent advances in understanding psoriasis. *F1000 Res.* **2016**, *5*, 770. [CrossRef]
3. Matos, T.; O'Malley, J.T.; Lowry, E.L.; Hamm, D.; Kirsch, I.R.; Robins, H.S.; Kupper, T.S.; Krueger, J.G.; Clark, R.A. Clinically resolved psoriatic lesions contain psoriasis-specific IL-17–producing αβ T cell clones. *J. Clin. Invest.* **2017**, *127*, 4031–4041. [CrossRef]
4. Watanabe, R. Protective and pathogenic roles of resident memory T cells in human skin disorders. *J. Dermatol. Sci.* **2019**, *95*, 2–7. [CrossRef]
5. Cheuk, S.; Wikén, M.; Blomqvist, L.; Nylén, S.; Talme, T.; Ståhle, M.; Eidsmo, L. Epidermal Th22 and Tc17 cells form a localized disease memory in clinically healed psoriasis. *J. Immunol.* **2014**, *192*, 3111–3120. [CrossRef]
6. Suarez-Farinas, M.; Fuentes-Duculan, J.; Lowes, M.A.; Krueger, J.G. Resolved psoriasis lesions retain expression of a subset of disease-related genes. *J. Investig. Dermatol.* **2011**, *131*, 391–400. [CrossRef]
7. Casey, K.A.; Fraser, K.A.; Schenkelm, J.M.; Moran, A.; Abt, M.C.; Beura, L.K.; Lucas, P.J.; Artis, D.; Wherry, E.J.; Hogquist, K.; et al. Antigen-independent differentiation and maintenance of effector-like resident memory T cells in tissues. *J. Immunol.* **2012**, *188*, 4866–4875. [CrossRef]
8. Mackay, L.K.; Rahimpour, A.; Ma, J.Z.; Collins, N.; Stock, A.T.; Hafon, M.L.; Vega-Ramos, J.; Lauzurica, P.; Mueller, S.N.; Stefanovic, T.; et al. The developmental pathway for CD103(+)CD8+ tissue-resident memory T cells of skin. *Nat. Immunol.* **2013**, *14*, 1294–1301. [CrossRef]
9. Milner, J.J.; Goldrath, A.W. Transcriptional programming of tissue-resident memory CD8+ T cells. *Curr. Opin. Immunol.* **2018**, *51*, 162–169. [CrossRef]
10. Patra, V.; Laoubi, L.; Nicolas, J.F.; Vocanson, M.; Wolf, P. A perspective on the interplay of ultraviolet-radiation, skin microbiome and skin resident memory TCRαβ+ cells. *Front. Med. (Lausanne)* **2018**, *5*, 166. [CrossRef]
11. Wu, H.; Liao, W.; Li, Q.; Long, H.; Yin, H.; Zhao, M.; Chan, V.; Lau, C.S.; Lu, Q. Pathogenic role of tissue-resident memory T cells in autoimmune diseases. *Autoimmun. Rev.* **2018**, *17*, 906–911. [CrossRef]
12. Clark, R.A. Resident memory T cells in human health and diseases. *Sci. Transl. Med.* **2015**, *7*, 269rv1. [CrossRef]
13. Kurihara, K.; Fujiyama, T.; Phadungsaksawasdi, P.; Ito, T.; Tokura, Y. Significance of IL-17A-producing CD8+CD103+ skin resident memory T cells in psoriasis lesion and their possible relationship to clinical course. *J. Dermatol. Sci.* **2019**, *95*, 21–27. [CrossRef]

14. Rosato, P.C.; Beura, L.K.; Masopust, D. Tissue resident memory T cells and viral immunity. *Curr. Opin. Virol.* **2017**, *22*, 44–50. [CrossRef]

15. Shin, H.; Iwasaki, A. Tissue-resident memory T cells. *Immunol. Rev.* **2013**, *255*, 165–181. [CrossRef]

16. Khan, A.A.; Srivastava, R.; Chentoufi, A.A.; Kritzer, E.; Chilukuri, S.; Garg, S.; Yu, D.C.; Vahed, H.; Huang, L.; Syed, S.A.; et al. Bolstering the number and function of HSV-1-specific CD8(+) effector memory T cells and tissue-resident memory T cells in latently infected trigeminal ganglia reduces recurrent ocular herpes infection and disease. *J. Immunol.* **2017**, *199*, 186–203. [CrossRef]

17. Pan, Y.; Kupper, T.S. Metabolic reprogramming and longevity of tissue-resident memory T cells. *Front. Immunol.* **2018**, *9*, 1347. [CrossRef]

18. Walsh, D.A.; Borges da Silva, H.; Beura, L.K.; Peng, C.; Hamilton, S.E.; Masopust, D.; Jameson, S.C. The functional requirement for CD69 in establishment of resident memory CD8^{+} T cells varies with tissue location. *J. Immunol.* **2019**, *203*, 946–955. [CrossRef]

19. Behr, F.M.; Chuwonpad, A.; Stark, R.; van Gisbergen, K. Armed and ready: Transcriptional regulation of Tissue-Resident Memory CD8 T cells. *Front. Immunol.* **2018**, *9*, 1770. [CrossRef]

20. Schenkel, J.M.; Masopust, D. Tissue-resident memory T cells. *Immunity* **2014**, *41*, 886–897. [CrossRef]

21. Cheuk, S.; Schlums, H.; Gallais Sérézal, I.; Martini, E.; Chiang, S.C.; Marquardt, N.; Gibbs, A.; Detlofsson, E.; Introini, A.; Forkel, M.; et al. CD49a expression defines tissue-resident CD8^{+} T cells poised for cytotoxic function in human skin. *Immunity* **2017**, *46*, 287–300. [CrossRef] [PubMed]

22. Petrelli, A.; van Wijk, F. CD8(+) T cells in human autoimmune arthritis: The unusual suspects. *Nat. Rev. Rheumatol.* **2016**, *12*, 421–428. [CrossRef] [PubMed]

23. Ritchlin, C. Tissue-resident T cells: Sequestered immune sensors and effectors of inflammation in spondyloarthritis. *Arthritis Rheumatol.* **2019**, *17*. [CrossRef]

24. Chen, L.; Shen, Z. Tissue-resident memory T cells and their biological characteristics in the recurrence of inflammatory skin disorders. *Cell. Mol. Immunol.* **2019**, *8*. [CrossRef]

25. Lande, R.; Botti, E.; Jandus, C.; Dojcinovic, D.; Fanelli, G.; Conrad, C.; Chamilos, G.; Feldmeyer, L.; Marinari, B.; Chon, S.; et al. The antimicrobial peptide LL37 is a T-cell autoantigen in psoriasis. *Nat. Commun.* **2014**, *5*, 5621. [CrossRef]

26. Arakawa, A.; Siewert, K.; Stöhr, J.; Besgen, P.; Kim, S.M.; Rühl, G.; Nickel, J.; Vollmer, S.; Thomas, P.; Krebs, S.; et al. Melanocyte antigen triggers autoimmunity in human psoriasis. *J. Exp. Med.* **2015**, *212*, 2203–2212. [CrossRef]

27. Adachi, T.; Kobayashi, T.; Sugihara, E.; Yamada, T.; Ikuta, K.; Pittaluga, S.; Saya, H.; Amagai, M.; Nagao, K. Hair follicle-derived IL-7 and IL-15 mediate skin-resident memory T cell homeostasis and lymphoma. *Nat. Med.* **2015**, *21*, 1272–1279. [CrossRef]

28. Diani, M.; Galasso, M.; Cozzi, C.; Sgambelluri, F.; Altomare, A.; Cigni, C.; Frigerio, E.; Drago, L.; Volinia, S.; Granucci, F.; et al. Blood to skin recirculation of CD4+ memory T cells associates with cutaneous and systemic manifestations of psoriatic disease. *Clin. Immunol.* **2017**, *180*, 84–94. [CrossRef]

29. Di Meglio, P.; Villanova, F.; Navarini, A.A.; Mylonas, A.; Tosi, I.; Nestle, F.O.; Conrad, C. Targeting CD8(+) T cells prevents psoriasis development. *J. Allergy Clin. Immunol.* **2016**, *138*, 274–276. [CrossRef]

30. Farber, D.L.; Yudanin, N.A.; Restifo, N.P. Human memory T cells: Generation, compartmentalization and homeostasis. *Nat. Rev. Immunol.* **2014**, *14*, 24–35. [CrossRef]

31. Boyman, O.; Hefti, H.P.; Conrad, C.; Nickoloff, B.J.; Suter, M.; Nestle, F.O. Spontaneous development of psoriasis in a new animal model shows an essential role for resident T cells and tumor necrosis factor-alpha. *J. Exp. Med.* **2004**, *199*, 731–736. [CrossRef] [PubMed]

32. Bosè, F.; Petti, L.; Diani, M.; Moscheni, C.; Molteni, S.; Altomare, A.; Rossi, R.L.; Talarico, D.; Fontana, R.; Russo, V.; et al. Inhibition of CCR7/CCL19 axis in lesional skin is a critical event for clinical remission induced by TNF blockade in patients with psoriasis. *Am. J. Pathol.* **2013**, *183*, 413–421. [CrossRef] [PubMed]

33. Sgambelluri, F.; Diani, M.; Altomare, A.; Frigerio, E.; Drago, L.; Granucci, F.; Banfi, G.; Altomare, G.; Reali, E. A role for CCR5(+)CD4 T cells in cutaneous psoriasis and for CD103(+) CCR4(+) CD8 Teff cells in the associated systemic inflammation. *J. Autoimmun.* **2016**, *70*, 80–90. [CrossRef] [PubMed]

34. Conrad, C.; Boyman, O.; Tonel, G.; Tun-Kyi, A.; Laggner, U.; de Fougerolles, A.; Kotelianski, V.; Gardner, H.; Nestle, F.O. Alpha1beta1 integrin is crucial for accumulation of epidermal T cells and the development of psoriasis. *Nat. Med.* **2007**, *13*, 836–842. [CrossRef] [PubMed]

35. Gallais Sérézal, I.; Classon, C.; Cheuk, S.; Barrientos-Somarribas, M.; Wadman, E.; Martini, E.; Chang, D.; Xu Landén, N.; Ehrström, M.; Nylén, S.; et al. Resident T cells in resolved psoriasis steer tissue responses that stratify clinical outcome. *J. Invest. Dermatol.* **2018**, *138*, 1754–1763. [CrossRef] [PubMed]

36. Vo, S.; Watanabe, R.; Koguchi-Yoshioka, H.; Matsumura, Y.; Ishitsuka, Y.; Nakamura, Y.; Okiyama, N.; Fujisawa, Y.; Fujimoto, M. CD8 resident memory T cells with interleukin 17A producing potential are accumulated in disease-naïve nonlesional sites of psoriasis possibly in correlation with disease duration. *Br. J. Dermatol.* **2019**, *181*, 410–412. [CrossRef]

37. Campbell, J.J.; Clark, R.A.; Watanabe, R.; Kupper, T.S. Sezary syndrome and mycosis fungoides arise from distinct T-cell subsets: A biologic rationale for their distinct clinical behaviors. *Blood* **2010**, *116*, 767–771. [CrossRef]

38. Gallais Sérézal, I.; Hoffer, E.; Ignatov, B.; Martini, E.; Zitti, B.; Ehrström, M.; Eidsmo, L. A skewed pool of resident T cells triggers psoriasis-associated tissue responses in never-lesional skin from patients with psoriasis. *J. Allergy Clin. Immunol.* **2019**, *143*, 1444–1454. [CrossRef]

39. Pearce, E.L.; Walsh, M.C.; Cejas, P.J.; Harms, G.M.; Shen, H.; Wang, L.S.; Jones, R.G.; Choi, Y. Enhancing CD8 T-cell memory by modulating fatty acid metabolism. *Nature* **2009**, *460*, 103–107. [CrossRef]

40. Cui, G.; Staron, M.M.; Gray, S.M.; Ho, P.C.; Amezquita, R.A.; Wu, J.; Kaech, S.M. IL-7-induced glycerol transport and TAG synthesis promotes memory CD8+ T cell longevity. *Cell* **2015**, *161*, 750–761. [CrossRef]

41. Pan, Y.; Tian, T.; Park, C.O.; Lofftus, S.Y.; Mei, S.; Liu, X.; Luo, C.; O'Malley, J.T.; Gehad, A.; Teague, J.E.; et al. Survival of tissue-resident memory T cells requires exogenous lipid uptake and metabolism. *Nature* **2017**, *9*, 252–256. [CrossRef] [PubMed]

42. Esmaeili, B.; Mansouri, P.; Doustimotlagh, A.H.; Izad, M. Redox imbalance and IL-17 responses in memory CD4$^+$ T cells from patients with psoriasis. *Scand. J. Immunol.* **2019**, *89*, e12730. [CrossRef] [PubMed]

43. Steel, K.J.A.; Srenathan, U.; Ridley, M.; Durham, L.E.; Wu, S.Y.; Ryan, S.E.; Hughes, C.D.; Chan, E.; Kirkham, B.W.; Taams, L.S. Synovial IL-17A+ CD8+ T cells display a polyfunctional, pro-inflammatory and tissue-resident memory phenotype and function in psoriatic arthritis. *Arthritis Rheumatol.* **2019**, *2*. [CrossRef] [PubMed]

44. Beura, L.K.; Wijeyesinghe, S.; Thompson, E.A.; Macchietto, M.G.; Rosato, P.C.; Pierson, M.J.; Schenkel, J.M.; Mitchell, J.S.; Vezys, V.; Fife, B.T.; et al. T cells in nonlymphoid tissues give rise to lymph-node-resident memory T Cells. *Immunity* **2018**, *48*, 327–338e5. [CrossRef] [PubMed]

45. Guggino, G.; Rizzo, A.; Mauro, D.; Macaluso, F.; Ciccia, F. Gut-derived CD8$^+$ tissue-resident memory T cells are expanded in the peripheral blood and synovia of SpA patients. *Ann. Rheum. Dis.* **2019**, *18*. [CrossRef]

46. Lalor, S.J.; McLoughlin, R.M. Memory γδ T cells-newly appreciated protagonists in infection and immunity. *Trends Immunol.* **2016**, *37*, 690–702. [CrossRef] [PubMed]

47. Eidsmo, L.; Martini, E. Human langerhans cells with pro-inflammatory features relocate within psoriasis lesions. *Front. Immunol.* **2018**, *22*, 300. [CrossRef]

48. Martini, E.; Wikén, M.; Cheuk, S.; Gallais Sérézal, I.; Baharom, F.; Ståhle, M.; Smed Sörensen, A.; Eidsmo, L. Dynamic changes in resident and infiltrating epidermal dendritic cells in active and resolved psoriasis. *J. Invest. Dermatol.* **2017**, *137*, 865–873. [CrossRef]

49. Cumberbatch, M.; Singh, M.; Dearman, R.J.; Young, H.S.; Kimber, I.; Griffiths, C.E. Impaired Langerhans cell migration in psoriasis. *J. Exp. Med.* **2006**, *203*, 953–960. [CrossRef]

50. Shaw, F.L.; Mellody, K.T.; Ogden, S.; Dearman, R.J.; Kimber, I.; Griffiths, C. Treatment-related restoration of Langerhans cell migration in psoriasis. *J. Investig. Dermatol.* **2014**, *134*, 268–271. [CrossRef]

51. Mohammed, J.; Beura, L.K.; Bobr, A.; Astry, B.; Chicoine, B.; Kashem, S.W.; Welty, N.E.; Igyártó, B.Z.; Wijeyesinghe, S.; Thompson, E.A.; et al. Stromal cells control the epithelial residence of DCs and memory T cells by regulated activation of TGF-beta. *Nat. Immunol.* **2016**, *17*, 414–421. [CrossRef] [PubMed]

52. Clark, R.A. Gone but not forgotten: Lesional memory in psoriatic skin. *J. Invest. Dermatol.* **2011**, *131*, 283–285. [CrossRef] [PubMed]

5

The Roles of Lipoprotein in Psoriasis

Chun-Ming Shih [1,2,3,†]**, Chang-Cyuan Chen** [4,†]**, Chen-Kuo Chu** [5,†]**, Kuo-Hsien Wang** [6]**, Chun-Yao Huang** [1,2,3] **and Ai-Wei Lee** [2,3,4,*]

[1] Department of Internal Medicine, School of Medicine, College of Medicine, Taipei Medical University, Taipei 11031, Taiwan; cmshih53@tmu.edu.tw (C.-M.S.); cyhuang@tmu.edu.tw (C.-Y.H.)
[2] Cardiovascular Research Center, Taipei Medical University Hospital, Taipei 11031, Taiwan
[3] Taipei Heart Institute, Taipei Medical University, Taipei 11031, Taiwan
[4] Department of Anatomy and Cell Biology, School of Medicine, College of Medicine, Taipei Medical University, Taipei 11031, Taiwan; chance03070307@gmail.com
[5] Department of Emergency Medicine, Taichung Veterans General Hospital, Taichung 40705, Taiwan; drckchu@gmail.com
[6] Department of Dermatology, Taipei Medical University Hospital, Taipei 11031, Taiwan; khwang40@gmail.com
* Correspondence: ammielee@tmu.edu.tw
† These authors contributed equally to this work.

Abstract: The association between psoriasis and cardiovascular disease risk has been supported by recent epidemiological data. Patients with psoriasis have an increased adjusted relative risk for myocardial infarction. As such, the cardiovascular risk conferred by severe psoriasis may be comparable to what is seen with other well-established risk factors, such as diabetes mellitus. Previous studies demonstrated that low-density lipoprotein (LDL) plays critical roles during atherogenesis. It may be caused by the accumulation of macrophages and lipoprotein in the vessel wall. Oxidized LDL (ox-LDL) stimulates the expression of adhesion molecules, such as ICAM-1 and VCAM-1, on endothelial cells and increases the attachment of mononuclear cells and the endothelium. Even though previous evidence demonstrated that psoriasis patients have tortuous and dilated blood vessels in the dermis, which results in the leakage of ox-LDL, the leaked ox-LDL may increase the expression of adhesion molecules and cytokines, and disturb the static balance of osmosis. Therefore, exploration of the relationship between hyperlipidemia and psoriasis may be another novel treatment option for psoriasis and may represent the most promising strategy.

Keywords: lipid; psoriasis; inflammation

1. Introduction

Psoriasis is a chronic inflammatory disease related to many diseases, especially cardiovascular disease. Among these diseases, atherosclerosis plays the most important role [1]. Atherosclerosis is caused by inflammation and an imbalance of the lipid metabolism. Psoriasis and atherosclerosis not only share the same cytokines involved in the immunological mechanism, such as interleukin (IL)-17, but also have common angiogenic factors and oxidative pathways [2]. In addition, both of them have similar lipid profiles, including decreased high-density lipoprotein (HDL) levels and/or increased low-density lipoprotein (LDL) levels [3]. In the pathological process of atherosclerosis, the accumulation of cholesterol triggers the production of pro-inflammatory cytokines, such as tumor necrosis factor alpha (TNFα), and also leads to the aggregation of monocytes and differentiation into foam cells [4]. TNFα eventually induces an inflammatory cascade in blood vessels [5]. In chronic inflammation, TNFα may also influence the lipid profile, such as LDL-C levels, via a decreased concentration of apolipoproteins. Moreover, TNFα lowers the quality of lipoprotein by inducing the production of

LDL and oxLDL and reducing the level of HDL-C at the same time [6]. Oxidized LDL (oxLDL) not only exacerbates inflammation but also promotes cholesterol accumulation in lysosomes, which eventually leads to cell death [7]. On the other hand, HDL has a reverse cholesterol transport (RCT) function, anti-oxidative capacity, and anti-inflammatory properties by regulating dendritic cells' (DCs) differentiation [8], and reducing T cell activation and IL-12 production [9]. However, these properties are reduced during chronic inflammation, such as psoriasis [10]. Previous studies have clarified the immunological pathway of psoriasis; however, the mechanism between psoriasis and an abnormal lipid profile remains unknown. Thus, identification of the relationship between hyperlipidemia and psoriasis is of paramount importance to develop a new therapeutic prospect for psoriasis.

2. Psoriasis

2.1. The Etiology of Psoriasis

Psoriasis is a chronic inflammatory skin disease related to immune inheritance. However, to date, the true cause of the disease remains unclear. According to epidemiological statistics, approximately 1%–3% of people worldwide develop psoriasis every year [11]. Psoriasis has long been considered a skin disease. However, according to recent research findings, psoriasis is actually a multisystem disease. It may be related to the occurrence and course of other diseases, including rheumatological (psoriatic arthritis (PsA)), cardiovascular and psychiatric complications [12,13], as well as cardiometabolic diseases, such as obesity, hypertension, and dyslipidemia [14]. At present, comorbid cardiovascular diseases are the main cause of death in patients with psoriasis [15]. The risk of suffering myocardial infarction in patients with severe psoriasis is seven times that in individuals with corresponding age, sex, body mass index (BMI), and cardiovascular risk factors, and the risk of cardiovascular mortality increases by 57% in patients with severe psoriasis [16]. In addition, patients with psoriasis are at a higher risk for cardiovascular diseases. Psoriasis is also related to accelerated atherosclerosis. It has been found that all T cells involved in the pathogenesis of psoriasis are also involved in atherosclerosis [17]. Clinically, psoriasis is divided into many categories, and psoriasis vulgaris (PV) accounts for approximately 90%. Psoriasis often causes symptoms, such as desquamation, skin redness, and itching. In addition to affecting appearance, psoriasis causes great psychological pressure and social distress to patients, thus reducing quality of life [18].

2.2. The Molecular Mechanism of Psoriasis

Previous studies have shown that CD4+ helper T cells may differentiate into regulatory T cells and effector T cells (including T-helper cell type 1 (Th1) cells, T-helper cell type 2 (Th2) cells, T-helper cell type 17 (Th17) cells, follicular helper T (Tfh) cells, and regulatory T cells (Tregs)), which are subsequently activated. Before the discovery of other cell lineages, Th1 and Th2 cells were considered to be the only T cells that differentiated from progenitor CD4+ helper T cells [19]. However, a new CD4+ helper T cell subset was discovered, named Th17 cells [20]. Th17 cells produce interleukin 17 (IL-17). Among all Th cell subsets, IL-17-producing T cells play an important role in autoimmune diseases, including multiple sclerosis, psoriasis, inflammatory bowel diseases, and steroid-resistant asthma [21]. At present, psoriasis is generally considered to be derived from the chronic activation of the IL-23/Th17 cell signaling axis, in which dominant T cell subsets are Th1 and Th17 cells. The cytokines released by Th1 and Th17 cells facilitate immune cell aggregation, promote keratinocyte proliferation, and increase the inflammatory response [22]. More precisely, CD4+ and CD8+ T cells with an IL-17-secretory phenotype are most important because they produce pro-inflammatory cytokines IL-17, IL-22, and tumor necrosis factor alpha (TNFα) [23]. The pathogenic mechanism of psoriasis is divided into the primary initiation phase and the chronic inflammatory phase. In the primary initiation phase, the pathogenic inflammatory response is initiated. The subsequent chronic inflammatory phase is continued by feedback loops and amplification signals. During the development of psoriasis, T cell predominance shifts from Th1 predominance in the initiation phase to Th17 predominance in the chronic inflammatory phase [24]. External stimuli, such as trauma, infection, or drug administration, cause the release of self-nucleotides. Self-nucleotides then bind to antimicrobial peptides (AMPs) released by keratinocytes, forming complexes [19]. AMPs are positively charged proteins and members of the innate immune system and include cathelicidin antimicrobial peptide (CAMP), pro-inflammatory cytokines and chemokines (for example, TNF, IL-17, IL-22, and CC-chemokine ligand 20 (CCL20), among numerous others), and angiogenic factors [24]. Among the AMPs, CAMP is not produced when keratinocytes are healthy. However, CAMP is upregulated when epidermal cells are destroyed. In psoriasis lesions, the increase in CAMP production initiates pathogenic interferon (IFN) signaling cascades and the activation of DCs, resulting in uncontrolled inflammatory reactions [25]. The complexes of self-nucleotides and AMPs then bind to the receptors on antigen-presenting cells, such as toll-like receptor 7 (TLR7) and TLR9 on the surface of plasmacytoid dendritic cells (pDCs). pDCs are a member of the innate immune system circulating in the blood. After antigen presentation, pDCs promote the activation and clonal expansion of antigen-specific CD8+ T cells, and such processes occur in the dermis (activation of memory resident T cells) and local lymph nodes (activation of naive T cells). In addition, in the initiation phase of psoriasis, pDCs release the inflammatory mediators IFNα and IFNβ, thereby stimulating the secretion of pro-inflammatory mediators (such as IL-12, IL-23, and TNF) by myeloid DCs. Subsequently, the activated CD8+ T cells migrate to the epidermal layer and encounter class I major histocompatibility complex (MHC) receptors on the surface of keratinocytes (or melanocytes), triggering the local release of soluble factors, including cytokines, chemokines, and innate immune mediators, to increase local inflammation and stimulate keratinocyte proliferation [24]. In addition to being a skin barrier, keratinocytes release inflammatory cytokines, such as TNF; express IL-17 receptors; and participate in the initiation and amplification of psoriasis [26]. The IL-17 family consists of 6 members, IL-17A to IL-17F, among which IL-17A is the most studied member while IL-17E (also known as IL-25) is an inhibitor of IL-17 [27]. In addition to IL-17A, Th17 cells also release various inflammatory cytokines, including IL-17F, IL-21, IL-22, and granulocyte macrophage colony-stimulating factor (GM-CSF). Therefore, targeting the Th17 cell subset is more therapeutically effective than targeting a single cytokine [21]. Innate immunity mediators stimulate the activation of T cell populations, such as Th1, Th17, and Th22 cells, and then release additional cytokines and chemokines. In particular, IL-1 allows Th17 cells to respond to IL-23 [24]. Th17 cells then release IL-17, IL-22, TNF-α, and other cytokines [28], and participate in the macrophage-dependent and -independent stimulation of DCs, thereby enhancing the immune response [29]. They may participate in the production of angiogenic inflammatory mediators, including monocyte chemoattractant protein (MCP-1), nitric oxide, and vascular endothelial growth factor [30]. The expression of vascular endothelial growth factor receptors on epidermal cells induces cardiovascular endothelial hyperplasia and the expression of adhesion molecules in the vascular endothelium, thereby aggregating immune cells. Angiogenic factors induce tortuous characteristics in papillary dermal vessels at the sites of psoriasis lesions, manifesting as the Auspitz sign. In addition, IL-17 acts on the IL-17 receptor on keratinocytes to stimulate the production of TNF and CCL20 (a chemotactic for T cells and DCs208) by keratinocytes [24]. IL-17 and TNF and/or other pro-inflammatory cytokines stimulate the activation of defensins and chemokines to promote host defense and the accumulation of other immune cells [31]. IL-22 is related to the pathological characteristics of psoriasis, including epidermal hyperplasia, acanthosis, and parakeratosis. Important transcription factors in psoriasis include cyclic AMP, the Janus kinase (JAK) signal transducer and activator of transcription (STAT) family, and nuclear factor-κB (NF-κB). Activation of these transcription factors results in the production of other factors, such as TNF and IL-17, as well as downstream amplification loops. Notably, although IL-17 is a signature cytokine of TH17 cells, other innate and acquired immune cells also produce IL-17, including CD8+ T cells, γδ T cells, innate lymphoid cells, and natural killer (NK) T cells [32]. Compared with a healthy control group, patients with psoriasis display higher serum concentrations of IL-17. However, the paradigm of Th17 cells as the main cellular source of IL-17 is no longer fully valid [33].

Recent studies have noted that the innate immune system, including neutrophils, mast cells, $\gamma\delta$ T cells, and innate lymphoid cells, is the most important source of IL-17 in patients with psoriasis [34].

3. The Relationships among Psoriasis, Cardiovascular Diseases, and Dyslipidemia

3.1. Normal Function of Fat and Cholesterol in Skin Cells

The stratum corneum is the outermost layer of the epidermis, and is a barrier protecting humans from the external environment. In addition to protecting humans against external harm, the stratum corneum prevents water loss from the body [35]. The structure of the stratum corneum is often described as bricks and mortar [36]. The bricks are fully differentiated keratinocytes, mostly consisting of keratin filaments and filaggrin [37]. The mortar refers to intracellular lipids, which consist of ceramides (CERs), free fatty acids (FFAs), and cholesterol. These lipids are arranged into a lamellar structure, and CERs account for 50%. CERs are the main polar lipids in the stratum corneum, and their basic composition is a sphingoid base connected to fatty acids by amide bonds. However, the composition of CERs varies appreciably in the human body. CERs are divided into 12 categories according to the head group composition or fatty acid esterification [38]. CERs play an important role in skin barriers, cell adhesion, and epidermal differentiation. In addition, CERs act as second messengers in stress-induced apoptosis [39]. CERs induce the apoptosis of tumor cells and reduce the resistance of tumor cells to chemotherapy drugs [40]. In psoriasis, the barrier function of the skin and water loss by the epidermis are mainly related to an abnormal composition ratio of CERs [41]. However, the total amount of CERs does not differ significantly between patients with psoriasis and healthy individuals [42]. Studies have shown that prosaposin, a precursor of saposin, and its mRNA were decreased in patients with psoriasis [43]. Saposins are a class of nonenzymatic proteins involved in the hydrolysis of sphingolipids, including the postsecretory glucosyl-CERs in the stratum corneum [44]. Sphingomyelinase is also significantly downregulated in the stratum corneum of patients with psoriasis. The reduction in the enzymes involved in CER production and metabolism may lead to decreases in ceramide 1 and other CERs at the sites of psoriasis lesions [41] as well as decreases in long-chain CERs containing ester-linked fatty acids and CERs containing phytosphingosine, thereby altering CER composition and increasing transepidermal water loss. In addition, the proportion of the three major intracellular lipids varies in the stratum corneum. At the sites of psoriasis lesions, the FFA content is significantly reduced while the cholesterol content is slightly increased [42]. Cholesterol constitutes approximately 25% of animal cell membranes and maintains cell integrity and fluidity. Moreover, the dynamic arrangement of cholesterol enhances the coating ability of the cell membrane, allowing the cell membrane to increase fluidity at low temperatures and increase stability at high temperatures [45]. For circulating low-density lipoprotein (LDL), cholesterol is transported via LDL receptor (LDL-R)-mediated endocytosis of holo-particles. Cholesteryl esters (CEs) delivered by the endocytosed LDL are hydrolyzed by lysosomal acid lipase in the lysosomes. The released unesterified (free) cholesterol is transported to the endoplasmic reticulum (ER), in which the cholesterol is re-esterified to form CEs. The CEs are stored in cytoplasmic lipid droplets (LDs) or are transported to the cell membrane or mitochondria. HDL binds to scavenger receptor class B type 1 (SR-B1) on the cell surface, and CEs are selectively transported into the cells without the internalization of the whole lipoprotein molecule. Subsequently, the CEs are hydrolyzed into free cholesterol by hormone-sensitive lipase (HSL). This mechanism is used by steroidogenic cells that rely on cholesterol as a precursor. Large amounts of CE-rich LDs are found in steroidogenic cells, in which the CEs are hydrolyzed into cholesterol by HSL to supply the steroidogenic cells [46]. Each has a unique receptor specificity and mechanism of transporting cholesterol. SR-B1 is a lipoprotein receptor [47] and plays an important role in cholesterol efflux and steroid hormone production [48]. In addition, SR-B1 has an RCT function and determines HDL-C levels through selectively transporting HDL-CEs to the liver, where the HDL-CEs are converted to bile acids, or through biliary cholesterol secretion [49]. Various mouse model studies have shown that SR-B1-null mice exhibit an increase in the amount and size of HDL-CE, which is accompanied by a reduced level of cholesterol in secreted bile and accelerated atherosclerosis. In contrast, SR-B1-overexpressing mice exhibit decreased levels of HDL-CE, a reduced degree of atherosclerosis, and a reduced extent of atherosclerosis in the liver [49]. Binding of HDL to SR-B1 increases anti-inflammatory cytokines, such as IL-10 and transforming growth factor-beta (TGF-β), by initiating Akt and reducing NF-κB activation, thereby regulating the inflammatory response of macrophages. SR-B1 in macrophages also regulates efferocytosis or the removal of apoptotic cells through the Src/phosphoinositide 3-kinase (PI3K)/Akt/Rac1 signaling pathway, thereby enhancing survival and the anti-inflammatory response of phagocytes. In endothelial cells, SR-B1 participates in the translocation of HDL from the apical to basolateral side, which further promotes the removal of cholesterol from intimal macrophages and lymphatic vessels [50].

3.2. The Correlation Between Psoriasis and Atherosclerosis

Patients with psoriasis are at a high risk for the incidence of cardiovascular disease and myocardial infarction [51]. Compared with the general population, the risk factors for cardiovascular diseases in patients with psoriasis have a high incidence, such as diabetes, hypertension, obesity, and hyperlipidemia [51]. Psoriasis is highly correlated with cardiovascular diseases, and hyperlipidemia-induced atherosclerosis is the predominant disease [1]. A large amount of evidence indicates that psoriasis is related to severe atherosclerosis and cardiovascular diseases while inflammation plays an important role in psoriasis and atherosclerosis [1]. Atherosclerosis and psoriasis have very similar immune response profiles. In addition, atherosclerosis and psoriasis share the same immunological pathways (including DCs, Th1 cells, Th17 cells, and Tregs) as well as angiogenic factors and oxidative mechanisms [2]. A number of studies show that patients with psoriasis exhibit decreased HDL levels and/or increased low-density lipoprotein (LDL), very-low-density lipoprotein (VLDL), and triglyceride (TG) levels [3].

3.3. The Relationship Between Psoriasis and Blood Lipids

Obesity is related to many immune diseases, including cardiovascular diseases, arteriosclerosis, and psoriasis [52]. However, in mouse models, both obese and lean mice develop severe psoriasiform skin inflammation after being fed a high-fat diet (HFD). Such a phenomenon is related to FFAs but is not related to the fat mass extension, blood glucose levels, and adipose tissue-derived mediators. The increase in FFAs leads to an immune response and insulin resistance, which alters the homeostasis and function of immune cells. HFD also increases the level of saturated fatty acids (SFAs). SFAs stimulate myeloid cells to produce TLR-like stimuli, which induce a pro-immune response, thus resulting in keratinocyte activation. Therefore, decreasing the SFA content in food reduces psoriasiform inflammation. HFD-induced obesity does not directly alter the proinflammatory status of skin and immune cells. However, it renders the skin and immune cells more susceptible to proinflammatory stimuli, such as imiquimod (IMQ), thereby enhancing the immune response [53]. Certain studies failed to establish a correlation between psoriasis and lipid serum levels [54], including a large population-based cross-sectional study conducted in the UK [55].

3.4. The Relationships among Oxidized LDL (oxLDL), the Inflammatory Response, and Psoriasis

The accumulation of excessive cholesterol in blood vessel walls could promote the dysfunction and activation of epidermal cells, which induces an inflammatory response and eventually leads to the production of pro-inflammatory cytokines and reactive oxygen species, the overexpression of adhesion molecules and chemokines, and a reduction in nitric oxide levels [4]. The above processes lead to the aggregation and invasion of monocytes and the differentiation of monocytes into macrophages. After receiving modified LDL via scavenger receptors, macrophages are converted to foam cells. In addition, TNFα triggers endothelial dysfunction and induces an inflammatory cascade in the blood vessel wall, ultimately resulting in vascular sclerosis [5]. Although elevated TNFα exerts a protective effect during acute immunity, the maintenance of a high concentration of TNFα during chronic inflammation may alter lipid and carbohydrate metabolism. In fact, TNFα decreases the concentration of LDL-C through diminishing the secretion of apolipoproteins and reducing cholesterol catabolism and excretion, thereby interfering with cholesterol metabolism. In addition, TNFα promotes the production of pro-atherogenic small dense LDL and oxLDL to alter the quality of lipoproteins. TNFα also reduces HDL-C levels and changes HDL composition [6]. Patients with chronic inflammatory responses experience qualitative and quantitative changes in lipid and lipoprotein profiles, including decreases in cholesterol, HDL-C, and apolipoprotein A-1, and increases in small dense LDL, lipoprotein(a) [Lp(a)], and TG. In addition to TNFα, IL-6 and IL-1ß also alter lipid metabolism, including increasing VLDL and reducing TG-rich lipoprotein clearance. An increase in serum TG levels enhances the expression of cholesteryl ester transfer protein (CETP), which transfers TG from VLDL/LDL to LDL/HDL. These TG-enriched particles become the substrate for hepatic lipase and lipoprotein lipase, resulting in the production of small dense LDL and HDL as the final products. Small dense LDL more readily enters into the arteries [9] and is more susceptible to oxidation. As a result, the antioxidant and anti-inflammatory activities of small dense HDL become limited [56]. LDL levels and composition are also altered due to inflammation. First, the increase in LDLR expression reduces LDL-C levels and thus promotes the intracellular accumulation of cholesterol. Second, circulating LDL is more prone to oxidation. Therefore, patients with chronic inflammatory diseases have high plasma levels of oxLDL. oxLDL is more atherogenic and can enhance the inflammatory response. Moreover, oxLDL promotes the accumulation of cholesterol and the formation of cholesterol crystals in lysosomes, which causes lysosomal disruption and leads to increased cellular toxicity [7].

3.5. The Relationships among HDL, the Inflammatory Response, and Psoriasis

HDL has RCT, anti-inflammatory, and antioxidant functions, which are related to the prevention of cardiovascular diseases [57]. In addition, HDL has anti-apoptotic and anti-thrombotic activities. The protective effect of HDL is mostly due to its role in RCT. RCT refers to the process of cholesterol transport from the peripheral tissues to the liver, where the cholesterol is secreted, converted into bile acid, or synthesized into sterol hormones [58]. The first step in RCT is the removal of excess cholesterol from macrophage foam cells at sclerotic sites via HDL or macrophage-derived apolipoproteins [59]. Cholesterol efflux can be achieved through a number of ways, including (a) unidirectional efflux to lipid-free apolipoproteins, particularly apoA-1, mediated by ATP-binding cassette A1 (ABCA1); (b) unidirectional efflux to mature HDL particles mediated by ABCG1; and (c) efflux to mature HDL particles via passive diffusion facilitated by SR-B1 [60]. Once cholesterol is transferred to the cytoplasm, SR-B1 delivers the macrophage-derived (HDL) cholesterol to the liver for bile acid production. The next step is biliary secretion or transport to steroidogenic tissues, especially the adrenal gland and ovary, for steroid production and storage. HDL terminates lipid peroxidation chain reactions via apolipoproteins (such as apoA) and enzymes (paraoxonase (PON1), lecithin-cholesterol acyltransferase (LCAT), and platelet activating factor-acetyl hydrolase), thereby exhibiting an antioxidant function [61]. HDL not only inhibits monocyte transmigration and the expression of adhesion molecules in endothelial cells but also plays an immunomodulating role in the innate and acquired immune systems. HDL regulates DCs, monocytes, macrophages, T cells, and B cells mainly through modification of the cholesterol content of lipid rafts [62]. The anti-inflammatory properties of HDL are achieved through apoA-1, a major HDL-associated protein. apoA-1 stimulates the production of IL-10 and prostaglandin E2 (PGE2), thereby inhibiting the differentiation and functions of DCs [63], and reducing T cell activation and IL-12 production [8]. During a chronic inflammatory response, the antioxidative and anti-inflammatory properties of HDL are reduced. In addition, RCT and the ability to resist LDL oxidation are affected. The decrease in the antioxidative property is due to proteome alterations, including decreased activity of HDL-associated enzymes and the accumulation of complement (C3), ceruloplasmin, and serum amyloid A (SAA) [58]. The reduced anti-inflammatory property may be related to decreased apoA-1 and apoM levels. In addition, enhancement of the pro-inflammatory mechanism is due to the impaired cellular efflux of lipids to HDL, which initiates intracellular STAT3 signaling and induces vascular inflammation. In addition to low plasma levels of HDL [9], HDL proteomic and lipid composition are altered in psoriasis [15,16], which leads to a decrease in the cholesterol efflux capacity [12,15] and a reduction in the anti-inflammatory and antioxidant capacities of HDL. Moreover, other properties of HDL are also altered, such as the anti-LDL oxidation capability, inhibition of TNF-α-induced monocyte adhesion to epidermal cells, prevention of the ox-LDL-induced monocyte migration, and protection of epidermal cells from TNF-α-induced apoptosis [14]. Patients with psoriasis exhibit low PON-1 activity, which is negatively correlated with psoriasis area and severity index (PASI) scores [58]. Conversely, anti-psoriatic therapy restores the composition and function of HDL [64]. HDL-associated proteins also undergo changes, among which apoA-1 and apoM are significantly reduced. In contrast, the levels of acute-phase proteins, such as SAA, prothrombin, α-1-antitrypsin, and α-1-acid glycoprotein 1, are significantly increased. The cholesterol efflux capacity is related to decreased apoA-1, phosphatidylcholine, and sphingomyelin in HDL. Under chronic inflammatory conditions, such as psoriasis, the changes in protein structure and the appearance of neo-epitopes may lead to autoantibody production and HDL dysfunction and are even related to cardiovascular diseases [10]. Therefore, these antibodies may serve as new biomarkers for autoimmune diseases in cardiovascular diseases. High titers of autoantibodies against HDL (aHDL) and apoA-I are present in chronic inflammatory diseases, which is related to high cardiovascular risk. aHDL and aapoA-I are also found in patients with psoriasis. These antibodies are correlated with the severity of diseases and may be related to the development of vascular sclerosis.

4. Conclusions

Psoriasis affects at least 125 million people across the world. Additional development and evaluation of the relationship between the lipid profile and psoriasis to explore treatment efficacy is required. In chronic inflammation, TNFα may influence the lipid profile, such as LDL-C levels, via decreased concentrations of apolipoproteins. Moreover, TNFα lowers the quality of lipoprotein by inducing the production of LDL and oxLDL but reducing the level of HDL-C at the same time. Oxidized LDL (oxLDL) not only exacerbates inflammation but also promotes cholesterol accumulation in lysosomes, which eventually leads to cell death. On the other hand, HDL has a reverse cholesterol transport (RCT) function, anti-oxidative capacity, and anti-inflammatory properties by regulating dendritic cells' (DCs) differentiation and reducing T cell activation and cytokine production. However, these properties are reduced during chronic inflammation, such as psoriasis. Thus, identification of the relationship between hyperlipidemia and psoriasis is of paramount importance to develop a new therapeutic prospect for psoriasis (Figure 1).

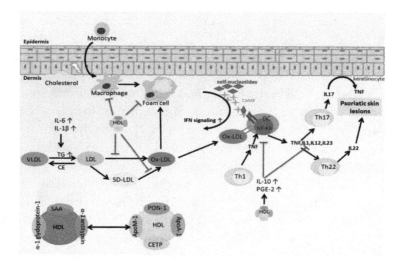

Figure 1. Immune cells and lipoprotein-associated cytokines implicated in psoriasis pathogenesis. Characteristic markers and cytokines related to the interleukin (IL)-17/IL-23 immune signature of T cells, lipoprotein, dendritic cells (DCs), and associated immune cells in psoriatic skin inflammation.

Author Contributions: Conceptualization, methodology, A.-W.L. and K.-H.W.; writing—original draft preparation, C.-C.C.; writing—review and editing, C.-M.S., C.-Y.H. and C.-K.C. All authors have read and agreed to the published version of the manuscript.

Acknowledgments: This work was supported by grants from National Science Council (MOST 108-2320-B-038-046) in Taiwan.

Abbreviations

apoA-I	Apolipoprotein A1
ABCA1	ATP-binding cassette A1
aHDL	autoantibodies against HDL
AMP	Antimicrobial peptide
apo	apolipoprotein
BMI	Body mass index
C3	Complement 3
CAMP	Cathelicidin antimicrobial peptide
CCL20	C-C motif chemokine ligand 20
CD	Cluster of differentiation
CE	Cholesteryl ester
CER	Ceramide
CETP	Cholesteryl ester transfer protein
DC	Dendritic cell
ER	Endoplasmic reticulum
FFA	Free fatty acid
GM-CSF	Granulocyte macrophage colony stimulating factor
HDL	High density lipoprotein
HDL-C	High-density lipoprotein cholesterol
HDL-CE	High density lipoprotein cholesteryl ester
HFD	High fat diet
HSL	Hormone-sensitive lipase
ICAM-1	Intercellular Adhesion Molecule 1
IFN	Interferon
IL	Interleukin
IMQ	Imiquimod
JAK	Janus kinase
LCAT	Lecithin-cholesterol acyltransferase
LD	Lipid droplet
LDL	Low density lipoprotein
LDL-R	Low density lipoprotein receptor
Lp(a)	Lipoprotein(a)
MCP-1	Monocyte chemoattractant protein 1
MHC	Major histocompatibility complex
NF-κB	Nuclear factor-κB
NK	Natural killer
ox-LDL	Oxidized LDL
pDC	Plasmacytoid dendritic cell
PI3K	Phosphoinositide 3 kinase
PON	Paraoxonase
PsA	Psoriatic arthritis
PV	Psoriasis vulgaris
RCT	Reverse cholesterol transport
SAA	Serum amyloid A
SFA	Saturated fatty acid
SR-B1	Scavenger receptor class B type 1

STAT	Signal transducer and activator of transcription
Th	T helper cell
Tfh	T follicular helper cells
TG	Triglyceride
TGF-β	Transforming growth factor beta
TLR	Toll-like receptor
TNF	Tumor necrosis factor
Treg	Regulatory T cell
VCAM-1	Vascular cell adhesion molecule 1
VLDL	Very-low-density lipoprotein

References

1. Ghazizadeh, R.; Tosa, M.; Ghazizadeh, M. Clinical improvement in psoriasis with treatment of associated hyperlipidemia. *Am. J. Med. Sci.* **2011**, *341*, 394–398. [CrossRef]

2. Harrington, C.L.; Dey, A.K.; Yunus, R.; Joshi, A.A.; Mehta, N.N. Psoriasis as a human model of disease to study inflammatory atherogenesis. *Am. J. Physiol. Heart Circ. Physiol.* **2017**, *312*, H867–H873. [CrossRef]

3. Kimball, A.B.; Szapary, P.; Mrowietz, U.; Reich, K.; Langley, R.G.; You, Y.; Hsu, M.C.; Yeilding, N.; Rader, D.J.; Mehta, N.N. Underdiagnosis and undertreatment of cardiovascular risk factors in patients with moderate to severe psoriasis. *J. Am. Acad Derm.* **2012**, *67*, 76–85. [CrossRef]

4. Gimbrone, M.A., Jr.; Garcia-Cardena, G. Endothelial Cell Dysfunction and the Pathobiology of Atherosclerosis. *Circ. Res.* **2016**, *118*, 620–636. [CrossRef] [PubMed]

5. Sorci-Thomas, M.G.; Thomas, M.J. Microdomains, Inflammation, and Atherosclerosis. *Circ. Res.* **2016**, *118*, 679–691. [CrossRef] [PubMed]

6. Amezaga Urruela, M.; Suarez-Almazor, M.E. Lipid paradox in rheumatoid arthritis: Changes with rheumatoid arthritis therapies. *Curr. Rheumatol. Rep.* **2012**, *14*, 428–437. [CrossRef] [PubMed]

7. Favari, E.; Thomas, M.J.; Sorci-Thomas, M.G. High-Density Lipoprotein Functionality as a New Pharmacological Target on Cardiovascular Disease: Unifying Mechanism That Explains High-Density Lipoprotein Protection Toward the Progression of Atherosclerosis. *J. Cardiovasc. Pharm.* **2018**, *71*, 325–331. [CrossRef]

8. Wang, S.H.; Yuan, S.G.; Peng, D.Q.; Zhao, S.P. HDL and ApoA-I inhibit antigen presentation-mediated T cell activation by disrupting lipid rafts in antigen presenting cells. *Atherosclerosis* **2012**, *225*, 105–114. [CrossRef]

9. Whetzel, A.M.; Sturek, J.M.; Nagelin, M.H.; Bolick, D.T.; Gebre, A.K.; Parks, J.S.; Bruce, A.C.; Skaflen, M.D.; Hedrick, C.C. ABCG1 deficiency in mice promotes endothelial activation and monocyte-endothelial interactions. *Arter. Thromb Vasc. Biol.* **2010**, *30*, 809–817. [CrossRef]

10. Batuca, J.R.; Ames, P.R.; Amaral, M.; Favas, C.; Isenberg, D.A.; Delgado Alves, J. Anti-atherogenic and anti-inflammatory properties of high-density lipoprotein are affected by specific antibodies in systemic lupus erythematosus. *Rheumatol. (Oxf.)* **2009**, *48*, 26–31. [CrossRef]

11. Spah, F. Inflammation in atherosclerosis and psoriasis: Common pathogenic mechanisms and the potential for an integrated treatment approach. *Br. J. Derm.* **2008**, *159*, 10–17. [CrossRef] [PubMed]

12. Gelfand, J.M.; Feldman, S.R.; Stern, R.S.; Thomas, J.; Rolstad, T.; Margolis, D.J. Determinants of quality of life in patients with psoriasis: A study from the US population. *J. Am. Acad Derm.* **2004**, *51*, 704–708. [CrossRef] [PubMed]

13. Kim, N.; Thrash, B.; Menter, A. Comorbidities in psoriasis patients. *Semin Cutan Med. Surg.* **2010**, *29*, 10–15. [CrossRef] [PubMed]

14. Langan, S.M.; Seminara, N.M.; Shin, D.B.; Troxel, A.B.; Kimmel, S.E.; Mehta, N.N.; Margolis, D.J.; Gelfand, J.M. Prevalence of metabolic syndrome in patients with psoriasis: A population-based study in the United Kingdom. *J. Invest. Derm.* **2012**, *132*, 556–562. [CrossRef]

15. Yeung, H.; Takeshita, J.; Mehta, N.N.; Kimmel, S.E.; Ogdie, A.; Margolis, D.J.; Shin, D.B.; Attor, R.; Troxel, A.B.; Gelfand, J.M. Psoriasis severity and the prevalence of major medical comorbidity: A population-based study. *Jama Derm.* **2013**, *149*, 1173–1179. [CrossRef]

16. Gelfand, J.M.; Neimann, A.L.; Shin, D.B.; Wang, X.; Margolis, D.J.; Troxel, A.B. Risk of myocardial infarction in patients with psoriasis. *JAMA* **2006**, *296*, 1735–1741. [CrossRef]

17. Hansson, G.K.; Hermansson, A. The immune system in atherosclerosis. *Nat. Immunol.* **2011**, *12*, 204–212. [CrossRef]

18. Parisi, R.; Symmons, D.P.; Griffiths, C.E.; Ashcroft, D.M.; Identification and Management of Psoriasis and Associated ComorbidiTy (IMPACT) project team. Global epidemiology of psoriasis: A systematic review of incidence and prevalence. *J. Invest. Derm.* **2013**, *133*, 377–385. [CrossRef]

19. Zhu, J.; Yamane, H.; Paul, W.E. Differentiation of effector CD4 T cell populations (*). *Annu Rev. Immunol.* **2010**, *28*, 445–489. [CrossRef]

20. Harrington, L.E.; Hatton, R.D.; Mangan, P.R.; Turner, H.; Murphy, T.L.; Murphy, K.M.; Weaver, C.T. Interleukin 17-producing CD4+ effector T cells develop via a lineage distinct from the T helper type 1 and 2 lineages. *Nat. Immunol.* **2005**, *6*, 1123–1132. [CrossRef]

21. Yang, J.; Sundrud, M.S.; Skepner, J.; Yamagata, T. Targeting Th17 cells in autoimmune diseases. *Trends Pharm. Sci.* **2014**, *35*, 493–500. [CrossRef] [PubMed]

22. Furue, M.; Tsuji, G.; Chiba, T.; Kadono, T. Cardiovascular and Metabolic Diseases Comorbid with Psoriasis: Beyond the Skin. *Intern. Med.* **2017**, *56*, 1613–1619. [CrossRef] [PubMed]

23. Karczewski, J.; Dobrowolska, A.; Rychlewska-Hanczewska, A.; Adamski, Z. New insights into the role of T cells in pathogenesis of psoriasis and psoriatic arthritis. *Autoimmunity* **2016**, *49*, 435–450. [CrossRef]

24. Greb, J.E.; Goldminz, A.M.; Elder, J.T.; Lebwohl, M.G.; Gladman, D.D.; Wu, J.J.; Mehta, N.N.; Finlay, A.Y.; Gottlieb, A.B. Psoriasis. *Nat. Rev. Dis. Primers* **2016**, *2*, 16082. [CrossRef]

25. Lande, R.; Gregorio, J.; Facchinetti, V.; Chatterjee, B.; Wang, Y.H.; Homey, B.; Cao, W.; Wang, Y.H.; Su, B.; Nestle, F.O.; et al. Plasmacytoid dendritic cells sense self-DNA coupled with antimicrobial peptide. *Nature* **2007**, *449*, 564–569. [CrossRef] [PubMed]

26. Chiricozzi, A.; Nograles, K.E.; Johnson-Huang, L.M.; Fuentes-Duculan, J.; Cardinale, I.; Bonifacio, K.M.; Gulati, N.; Mitsui, H.; Guttman-Yassky, E.; Suarez-Farinas, M.; et al. IL-17 induces an expanded range of downstream genes in reconstituted human epidermis model. *PLoS ONE* **2014**, *9*, e90284. [CrossRef]

27. Lavocat, F.; Ndongo-Thiam, N.; Miossec, P. Interleukin-25 Produced by Synoviocytes Has Anti-inflammatory Effects by Acting As a Receptor Antagonist for Interleukin-17A Function. *Front. Immunol.* **2017**, *8*, 647. [CrossRef]

28. Chiricozzi, A.; Guttman-Yassky, E.; Suarez-Farinas, M.; Nograles, K.E.; Tian, S.; Cardinale, I.; Chimenti, S.; Krueger, J.G. Integrative responses to IL-17 and TNF-alpha in human keratinocytes account for key inflammatory pathogenic circuits in psoriasis. *J. Invest. Derm.* **2011**, *131*, 677–687. [CrossRef]

29. Nestle, F.O.; Kaplan, D.H.; Barker, J. Psoriasis. *N. Engl. J. Med.* **2009**, *361*, 496–509. [CrossRef]

30. Takahashi, H.; Numasaki, M.; Lotze, M.T.; Sasaki, H. Interleukin-17 enhances bFGF-, HGF- and VEGF-induced growth of vascular endothelial cells. *Immunol. Lett.* **2005**, *98*, 189–193. [CrossRef]

31. Leonardi, C.; Matheson, R.; Zachariae, C.; Cameron, G.; Li, L.; Edson-Heredia, E.; Braun, D.; Banerjee, S. Anti-interleukin-17 monoclonal antibody ixekizumab in chronic plaque psoriasis. *N. Engl. J. Med.* **2012**, *366*, 1190–1199. [CrossRef] [PubMed]

32. Gaffen, S.L.; Jain, R.; Garg, A.V.; Cua, D.J. The IL-23-IL-17 immune axis: From mechanisms to therapeutic testing. *Nat. Rev. Immunol.* **2014**, *14*, 585–600. [CrossRef] [PubMed]

33. Keijsers, R.R.; Joosten, I.; van Erp, P.E.; Koenen, H.J.; van de Kerkhof, P.C. Cellular sources of IL-17 in psoriasis: A paradigm shift? *Exp. Derm.* **2014**, *23*, 799–803. [CrossRef] [PubMed]

34. Zheng, Y.; Wang, Z.; Deng, L.; Zhang, G.; Yuan, X.; Huang, L.; Xu, W.; Shen, L. Modulation of STAT3 and STAT5 activity rectifies the imbalance of Th17 and Treg cells in patients with acute coronary syndrome. *Clin. Immunol.* **2015**, *157*, 65–77. [CrossRef]

35. Del Rosso, J.Q.; Levin, J. Clinical relevance of maintaining the structural and functional integrity of the stratum corneum: Why is it important to you? *J. Drugs Derm.* **2011**, *10*, s5–s12.

36. Harding, C.R. The stratum corneum: Structure and function in health and disease. *Dermatol. Ther.* **2004**, *17*, 6–15. [CrossRef]

37. Proksch, E.; Brandner, J.M.; Jensen, J.M. The skin: An indispensable barrier. *Exp. Derm.* **2008**, *17*, 1063–1072. [CrossRef]

38. van Smeden, J.; Hoppel, L.; van der Heijden, R.; Hankemeier, T.; Vreeken, R.J.; Bouwstra, J.A. LC/MS analysis of stratum corneum lipids: Ceramide profiling and discovery. *J. Lipid Res.* **2011**, *52*, 1211–1221. [CrossRef]

39. Komatsu, M.; Takahashi, T.; Abe, T.; Takahashi, I.; Ida, H.; Takada, G. Evidence for the association of ultraviolet-C and H(2)O(2)-induced apoptosis with acid sphingomyelinase activation. *Biochim. Biophys. Acta* **2001**, *1533*, 47–54. [CrossRef]

40. Charles, A.G.; Han, T.Y.; Liu, Y.Y.; Hansen, N.; Giuliano, A.E.; Cabot, M.C. Taxol-induced ceramide generation and apoptosis in human breast cancer cells. *Cancer Chemother Pharm.* **2001**, *47*, 444–450. [CrossRef]

41. Motta, S.; Monti, M.; Sesana, S.; Mellesi, L.; Ghidoni, R.; Caputo, R. Abnormality of water barrier function in psoriasis. Role of ceramide fractions. *Arch. Derm.* **1994**, *130*, 452–456. [CrossRef]

42. Motta, S.; Monti, M.; Sesana, S.; Caputo, R.; Carelli, S.; Ghidoni, R. Ceramide composition of the psoriatic scale. *Biochim. Biophys. Acta* **1993**, *1182*, 147–151. [CrossRef]

43. Alessandrini, F.; Stachowitz, S.; Ring, J.; Behrendt, H. The level of prosaposin is decreased in the skin of patients with psoriasis vulgaris. *J. Invest. Derm.* **2001**, *116*, 394–400. [CrossRef]

44. Nemes, Z.; Marekov, L.N.; Fesus, L.; Steinert, P.M. A novel function for transglutaminase 1: Attachment of long-chain omega-hydroxyceramides to involucrin by ester bond formation. *Proc. Natl. Acad. Sci. USA* **1999**, *96*, 8402–8407. [CrossRef]

45. Incardona, J.P.; Eaton, S. Cholesterol in signal transduction. *Curr. Opin. Cell Biol.* **2000**, *12*, 193–203. [CrossRef]

46. Kraemer, F.B.; Shen, W.J.; Harada, K.; Patel, S.; Osuga, J.; Ishibashi, S.; Azhar, S. Hormone-sensitive lipase is required for high-density lipoprotein cholesteryl ester-supported adrenal steroidogenesis. *Mol. Endocrinol.* **2004**, *18*, 549–557. [CrossRef]

47. Shen, W.J.; Azhar, S.; Kraemer, F.B. Lipid droplets and steroidogenic cells. *Exp. Cell Res.* **2016**, *340*, 209–214. [CrossRef]

48. Shen, W.J.; Hu, J.; Hu, Z.; Kraemer, F.B.; Azhar, S. Scavenger receptor class B type I (SR-BI): A versatile receptor with multiple functions and actions. *Metabolism* **2014**, *63*, 875–886. [CrossRef]

49. Ueda, Y.; Royer, L.; Gong, E.; Zhang, J.; Cooper, P.N.; Francone, O.; Rubin, E.M. Lower plasma levels and accelerated clearance of high density lipoprotein (HDL) and non-HDL cholesterol in scavenger receptor class B type I transgenic mice. *J. Biol. Chem.* **1999**, *274*, 7165–7171. [CrossRef]

50. Lim, H.Y.; Thiam, C.H.; Yeo, K.P.; Bisoendial, R.; Hii, C.S.; McGrath, K.C.; Tan, K.W.; Heather, A.; Alexander, J.S.; Angeli, V. Lymphatic vessels are essential for the removal of cholesterol from peripheral tissues by SR-BI-mediated transport of HDL. *Cell Metab.* **2013**, *17*, 671–684. [CrossRef]

51. Kaye, J.A.; Li, L.; Jick, S.S. Incidence of risk factors for myocardial infarction and other vascular diseases in patients with psoriasis. *Br. J. Derm.* **2008**, *159*, 895–902. [CrossRef] [PubMed]

52. Kanneganti, T.D.; Dixit, V.D. Immunological complications of obesity. *Nat. Immunol.* **2012**, *13*, 707–712. [CrossRef] [PubMed]

53. Herbert, D.; Franz, S.; Popkova, Y.; Anderegg, U.; Schiller, J.; Schwede, K.; Lorz, A.; Simon, J.C.; Saalbach, A. High-Fat Diet Exacerbates Early Psoriatic Skin Inflammation Independent of Obesity: Saturated Fatty Acids as Key Players. *J. Invest. Derm.* **2018**, *138*, 1999–2009. [CrossRef]

54. Farshchian, M.; Zamanian, A.; Farshchian, M.; Monsef, A.R.; Mahjub, H. Serum lipid level in Iranian patients with psoriasis. *J. Eur. Acad. Derm. Venereol.* **2007**, *21*, 802–805. [CrossRef] [PubMed]

55. Neimann, A.L.; Shin, D.B.; Wang, X.; Margolis, D.J.; Troxel, A.B.; Gelfand, J.M. Prevalence of cardiovascular risk factors in patients with psoriasis. *J. Am. Acad. Derm.* **2006**, *55*, 829–835. [CrossRef] [PubMed]

56. Catapano, A.L.; Pirillo, A.; Norata, G.D. Vascular inflammation and low-density lipoproteins: Is cholesterol the link? A lesson from the clinical trials. *Br. J. Pharm.* **2017**, *174*, 3973–3985. [CrossRef] [PubMed]

57. Paiva-Lopes, M.J.; Delgado Alves, J. Psoriasis-associated vascular disease: The role of HDL. *J. Biomed. Sci.* **2017**, *24*, 73. [CrossRef]

58. Goren, A.; Ozsolak, F.; Shoresh, N.; Ku, M.; Adli, M.; Hart, C.; Gymrek, M.; Zuk, O.; Regev, A.; Milos, P.M.; et al. Chromatin profiling by directly sequencing small quantities of immunoprecipitated DNA. *Nat. Methods* **2010**, *7*, 47–49. [CrossRef]

59. Ono, K. Current concept of reverse cholesterol transport and novel strategy for atheroprotection. *J. Cardiol.* **2012**, *60*, 339–343. [CrossRef]

60. Phillips, M.C. Molecular mechanisms of cellular cholesterol efflux. *J. Biol. Chem.* **2014**, *289*, 24020–24029. [CrossRef]

61. Rosenson, R.S.; Brewer, H.B., Jr.; Ansell, B.; Barter, P.; Chapman, M.J.; Heinecke, J.W.; Kontush, A.; Tall, A.R.; Webb, N.R. Translation of high-density lipoprotein function into clinical practice: Current prospects and future challenges. *Circulation* **2013**, *128*, 1256–1267. [CrossRef]

62. Barter, P.J.; Nicholls, S.; Rye, K.A.; Anantharamaiah, G.M.; Navab, M.; Fogelman, A.M. Antiinflammatory properties of HDL. *Circ. Res.* **2004**, *95*, 764–772. [CrossRef] [PubMed]

63. Kim, K.D.; Lim, H.Y.; Lee, H.G.; Yoon, D.Y.; Choe, Y.K.; Choi, I.; Paik, S.G.; Kim, Y.S.; Yang, Y.; Lim, J.S. Apolipoprotein A-I induces IL-10 and PGE2 production in human monocytes and inhibits dendritic cell differentiation and maturation. *Biochem. Biophys. Res. Commun.* **2005**, *338*, 1126–1136. [CrossRef] [PubMed]

64. Marsche, G.; Saemann, M.D.; Heinemann, A.; Holzer, M. Inflammation alters HDL composition and function: Implications for HDL-raising therapies. *Pharmacol. Ther.* **2013**, *137*, 341–351. [CrossRef] [PubMed]

6

Interleukin-17A and Keratinocytes in Psoriasis

Masutaka Furue [1,2,3,*], Kazuhisa Furue [1], Gaku Tsuji [1,2] and Takeshi Nakahara [1,3]

[1] Department of Dermatology, Graduate School of Medical Sciences, Kyushu University, Maidashi 3-1-1, Higashiku, Fukuoka 812-8582, Japan; ffff5113@gmail.com (K.F.); gakku@dermatol.med.kyushu-u.ac.jp (G.T.); nakahara@dermatol.med.kyushu-u.ac.jp (T.N.)

[2] Research and Clinical Center for Yusho and Dioxin, Kyushu University, Maidashi 3-1-1, Higashiku, Fukuoka 812-8582, Japan

[3] Division of Skin Surface Sensing, Graduate School of Medical Sciences, Kyushu University, Maidashi 3-1-1, Higashiku, Fukuoka 812-8582, Japan

* Correspondence: furue@dermatol.med.kyushu-u.ac.jp

Abstract: The excellent clinical efficacy of anti-interleukin 17A (IL-17A) biologics on psoriasis indicates a crucial pathogenic role of IL-17A in this autoinflammatory skin disease. IL-17A accelerates the proliferation of epidermal keratinocytes. Keratinocytes produce a myriad of antimicrobial peptides and chemokines, such as CXCL1, CXCL2, CXCL8, and CCL20. Antimicrobial peptides enhance skin inflammation. IL-17A is capable of upregulating the production of these chemokines and antimicrobial peptides in keratinocytes. CXCL1, CXCL2, and CXCL8 recruit neutrophils and CCL20 chemoattracts IL-17A-producing CCR6$^+$ immune cells, which further contributes to forming an IL-17A-rich milieu. This feed-forward pathogenic process results in characteristic histopathological features, such as epidermal hyperproliferation, intraepidermal neutrophilic microabscess, and dermal CCR6$^+$ cell infiltration. In this review, we focus on IL-17A and keratinocyte interaction regarding psoriasis pathogenesis.

Keywords: psoriasis; keratinocytes; interleukin-17A; Th17; ILC3; CCL20; CXCL1; CXCL8; Koebner phenomenon; antimicrobial peptides

1. Introduction

Psoriasis is an immune-mediated chronic skin disease characterized by epidermal hyperproliferation, an intraepidermal accumulation of neutrophils, and dermal inflammatory cell infiltrates that are composed of dendritic cells and T cells [1]. It has an estimated global prevalence of 2–4% [1,2]. Males are twice as likely as females to be affected [3,4]. As desquamative erythema can affect any skin site, psoriasis profoundly impairs the patients' quality of life, treatment satisfaction and adherence, and socioeconomic stability [5–7]. The skin lesion usually appears on the sites with frequent trauma such as elbows and knees [8,9]. This injury-induced development of psoriasis is called Koebner phenomenon [8,9]. Environmental factors, such as smoking, also trigger or exacerbate psoriatic lesions [10,11]. Genetic factors are critically involved in the development of psoriasis [12,13]. In addition to skin eruption, approximately 30% of patients with psoriasis manifest psoriatic arthritis [14–19]. Psoriasis is also significantly comorbid with other autoimmune diseases, such as bullous pemphigoid [20–24]. Psoriasis is frequently associated with cardiovascular diseases, metabolic diseases, and renal disorders [25–36]. Cancer risk is slightly higher in patients with psoriasis [37]. The topical application of steroids and vitamin D3 analogues inhibits psoriatic inflammation and normalizes epidermal differentiation [38,39]. Systemic treatments, such as methotrexate, cyclosporine, phototherapy, and the phosphodiesterase 4 inhibitor apremilast, are useful for patients with extensive lesions [40–45].

That the tumor necrosis factor-α (TNF-α) and IL-23/IL-17A axes appear to be major drivers in the pathogenesis of psoriasis is underscored by the excellent response of psoriasis to biologics targeting

TNF-α, IL-23, and IL-17A, although a difference exists in their efficacy [46–61]. Anti-TNF-α/IL-23/IL-17A biologics successfully improve psoriatic arthritis [18,56,62–64]. Reductions in comorbid cardiovascular events and systemic inflammation have been reported in patients with psoriasis treated with anti-TNF/IL23/IL17 biologics [65,66].

As the clinical response to anti-IL-23/IL-17A biologics seems better than that to anti-TNF-α biologics in psoriasis, the IL-23/IL-17A axis likely plays a more crucial role than the TNF-α axis in the development of psoriasis [67–71]. Under the regulation of IL-23p19, IL-17A-producing CD4$^+$ helper T (Th17) cells create a self-amplifying, feed-forward inflammatory response that is markedly augmented in the presence of TNF-α [68,72,73]. In addition, Th17 cells produce high amounts of TNF-α [74,75]. Therefore, IL-17A inhibition by the anti-IL-17A biologic results in early clinical, histopathologic, and molecular resolution of psoriasis [69].

In addition, various murine psoriasis models stress a pivotal role of the IL-23/IL-17A axis in experimental psoriasis [76–80]. Multiple animal studies have indicated that the interaction between IL-17A and keratinocyte is the key issue in the development of psoriasis [76–79]. In parallel, the importance of IL-17A and keratinocyte interaction is reinforced in patients with psoriasis who are successfully treated with the anti-IL-17A biologic [69]. In this review, we will focus on the multifaceted biological response in keratinocytes stimulated by IL-17A with regard to psoriatic pathogenesis.

2. IL-17A Signaling System

The IL-17 family plays a critical role in the immune response in infectious, inflammatory, autoimmune, and neoplastic disorders [81,82]. The IL-17 family and its receptors are evolutionarily ancient, and they are present in species as early as lamprey and sea urchins [83,84]. IL-17 family members comprise IL-17A, IL-17B, IL-17C, IL-17D, IL-17E, IL-17F, and IL-17AF [81,82]. IL-17AF is a hybrid heterodimer of IL-17A and IL-17F. IL-17E is also called IL-25 and is related to the type 2 immune response and allergies [81,82,85]. Among IL-17 family members, IL-17A has been the most strongly implicated in human health and disease. IL-17A is produced from hematopoietic cells, including Th17, CD8+ cytotoxic T cell (Tc17), γδ T cell, natural killer cell, group 3 innate lymphoid cell (ILC3), and "natural" Th17 cell [86–89], but IL-17B, IL-17C, and IL-25 are preferentially produced from nonhematopoietic cells, including keratinocytes [81,82,90]. Both hematopoietic cells and keratinocytes produce IL-17F [81,82,90]. Keratinocyte-derived IL-17C is capable of stimulating Th17 cells to secrete more IL-17A [91].

The IL-17 receptor (IL-17R) is composed of five members: IL-17RA, IL-17RB, IL-17RC, IL-17RD, and IL-17RE [81,82,90]. IL-17A, IL-17F, and IL-17AF all share the same IL-17R comprising IL-17RA and IL-17RC heterodimers [81,82,90]. IL-17C binds to IL-17RA and IL-17RE heterodimers [92]. IL-25 ligates IL-17RA and IL-17RB [81,82,90]. A recent study showed that IL-17A also activates IL-17RA and IL-17RD heterodimers [93] (Figure 1). IL-17B binds IL-17RB, but another heterodimeric IL-17R member remains unidentified [82]. Keratinocytes express both IL-17RA/IL-17RC and IL-17RA/IL-17RD, and the binding of IL-17A induces the transcription of differential gene sets [93]. Initial subcellular events in the ligation of IL-17RA/RC by IL-17A are the recruitment and activation of ACT1 encoded by the *TRAF3IP2* gene, TRAF6 and CARMA2 complexes, and the downstream activation of nuclear factor kappa-light-chain-enhancer of activated B cells (NF-κB) and MAPKs [93–97]. The ligation of IL-17RA/IL-17RC by IL-17A induces the activation of NF-κB, ERK, p38 MAPK, and JNK, while that of IL-17RA/IL-17-RD mainly activates p38 MAPK and JNK and barely affects NF-κB and ERK [93]. In addition, IL-17RA physically and functionally interacts with and transactivates epidermal growth factor (EGFR) [98]. IL-17RD potentially interacts with and transactivates fibroblast growth factor 2 receptor [82,99].

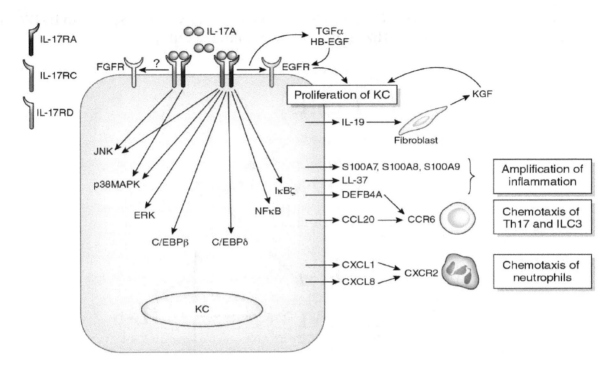

Figure 1. Simplified effects of anti-interleukin 17A (IL-17A) on keratinocyte (KC) with regard to psoriasis pathogenesis. IL-17A homodimers bind to IL-17 receptor A (IL-17RA) and IL-17RC or IL-17RA and IL-17RD heterodimers. The ligation of IL-17RA/IL-17RC activates epidermal growth factor receptor (EGFR) directly or by transforming growth factor-α (TGF-α) and heparin-binding EGF-like growth factor (HB-EGF) and promotes keratinocyte proliferation. The ligation of IL-17RA/IL-17RC activates various signal transduction molecules, including ERK, p38 MAPK, JNK, nuclear factor kappa-light-chain-enhancer of activated B cells (NFκB), IκBζ, C/CAAT-enhancer-binding protein β (C/EBPβ), and C/EBPδ. In contrast, the ligation of IL-17RA/IL-17RD preferentially activates JNK and p38 MAPK pathways. IL-17RA/IL-17RD is estimated to transactivate fibroblast growth factor receptor (FGFR); however, this is not conclusive. IL-17RA/IL-17RC signaling stimulates KCs to produce IL-19, which induces the production of keratinocyte growth factor (KGF) from fibroblasts. KGF also enhances the proliferation of KCs. IL-17A also induces the production of antimicrobial peptides, including S100A7, S100A8, S100A9, LL-37, and defensin β 4A (DEFB4A). These antimicrobial peptides amplify the local inflammatory process. Chemokines, such as CCL20, CXCL1, and CXCL8, are also produced from keratinocytes by IL-17RA/IL-17RC ligation. CCL20 is a key chemokine for the recruitment of CCR6[+] Th17 cells and group 3 innate lymphoid cells (ILC3). These CCR6[+] cells produce large amounts of IL-17A. DEFB4A also exhibits a chemotactic activity by binding to CCR6. CXCL1 and CXCL2 are potent chemoattractants for CXCR2[+] neutrophils. Therefore, IL-17A is associated with all of the histopathologic features of psoriasis.

In addition to the above-mentioned signaling cascades, IL-17A activates various other signal molecules including signal transducer and activator of transcription 3 (STAT3) in keratinocytes [100]. STAT3 is a very crucial signaling molecule in the development of psoriasis because transgenic mice with keratinocytes expressing a constitutively active Stat3 (K5.Stat3C mice) develop a skin phenotype either spontaneously, or in response to wounding, that closely resembles psoriasis [101]. Moreover, a STAT3 inhibitor STA-21 inhibits the generation of skin lesion in these psoriatic mice [102]. IL-17A is known to activate STAT3 via receptor-interacting protein 4 (RIP4) activation and upregulates the CCL20 expression [103]. IL-17A also upregulates keratin 17 expression via STAT1 and STAT3 activation [104]. IL-6 and IL-22 also play a synergistic role in development of psoriasis with IL-17A [68]. Notably, both IL-6 and IL-22 are potent STAT3 activators [105]. In accordance, biological or natural molecules such as indirubin and its derivatives useful for inactivating STAT3 exhibit therapeutic potential for psoriasis [106] (Figure 2). It reveals that IL-17 and IL-22 promote keratinocyte stemness and potentiate its regeneration [107]. IL-6 is produced from keratinocytes in response to IL-17A [108]. IL-22 is produced from Th17/22 cells, Th22 cells, and other immune cells [109,110].

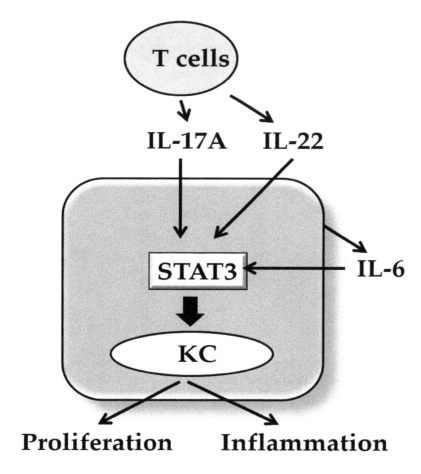

Figure 2. Pivotal role of signal transducer and activator of transcription 3 (STAT3) in psoriasis. The activation of STAT3 promotes keratinocyte (KC) proliferation and inflammatory response. IL-17A and IL-22 induce the STAT3 activation. IL-6 produced from KC also induces STAT3 activation.

In humans, impairment of the IL-17 signal causes infectious diseases, especially by *Candida albicans*, which is a ubiquitous fungus and commensal yeast of the intestines and skin [96]. Notably, deficiency of the *IL17RA, IL17RC, IL17F*, or *TRAF3IP2* genes is implicated in chronic mucocutaneous candidiasis disease (CMCD), which is characterized by recurrent or persistent infection affecting the nails, skin, and oral and genital mucosae caused by the *Candida* species, often *C. albicans* [96,111–113]. Impairment of the IL-17 signal is evident in other immunocompromised inborn errors, including autosomal-dominant hyper IgE syndrome, autosomal dominant *STAT1* gain-of-function, autosomal-recessive autoimmune polyendocrinopathy-candidiasis-ectodermal dystrophy (APECED), autosomal-recessive *CARD9* deficiency, *IL12RB1* deficiency, *IL12B* deficiency, and *RORC* deficiency [96]. However, these inborn errors seem to exhibit more complicated immune defects beyond IL-17 dysfunction and manifest CMCD together with other types of infection, including *Mycobacterium, Staphylococcus*, and viral disorders [96]. Of note, mice lacking *Traf3ip2* (*Act1*) or *Il17ra* manifest similar clinical phenotype as human CMCD patients lacking *IL17RA* or *IL17RC* [114–117]. A recent murine study by Sparber et al. also indicates that Malassezia infection selectively triggers the IL-17A-induced immune response [118]. These findings indicate a crucial role of IL-17A in anti-fungal immunity in humans and mice.

Mice overexpressing IL-17A in keratinocytes (K14-IL-17A$^{ind/+}$ mice) exhibit severe psoriasiform skin inflammation and vascular dysfunction in conjunction with infiltration of the vasculature by inflammatory myeloid cells [108]. The K14-IL-17A$^{ind/+}$ mice acquire the highest local and systemic IL-17A levels and exhibit a particularly severe psoriasis-like skin phenotype [108].

Homozygous CD11c-IL-17A$^{ind/ind}$ mice and heterozygous CD11c-IL-17A $^{ind/+}$ mice show a delayed onset of moderate to severe psoriasis-like skin disease associated with reduced amounts of cutaneous IL-17A compared with K14-IL-17A$^{ind/+}$ mice. In agreement with elevated skin and a stepwise increase in systemic IL-17A [119], homozygous CD11c-IL-17A $^{ind/ind}$ mice develop earlier and more severe skin lesions, as well as more pronounced vascular inflammation and dysfunction than heterozygous CD11c-IL-17A $^{ind/+}$ mice [76,119]. These experimental models indicate that IL-17A induces psoriasis-like lesions in a dose-dependent manner, irrespective of its cellular source [76,119].

3. IL-17A and Psoriasis

In the early 2000s, IL-23 was found to induce the production of IL-17A by activated CD4$^+$ T cells, which were later named Th17 cells [74,120]. These cells express RORγt (*RORC*) as the master transcription factor [121] and promoted the anti-infectious defense in the mucosa and skin [96], whereas excessive exposure to IL-23 induces their transformation into autoimmune or autoinflammatory immune cells [122,123]. Accordingly, the intradermal injection of IL-23 induces murine psoriasis-like dermatitis with epidermal acanthosis, neutrophil recruitment, and the infiltration of IL-17-producing T cells [78,79,124].

Psoriasis is one of the most typical IL-23/IL-17A-driven human diseases [68,72,73]. Th17 cells, Tc17 cells, IL-17-producing γδ T cells, and ILC3 can all be found in psoriatic skin [89,125,126]. IL-23 is composed of IL-23p40 and IL-23p19 subunits, and the expression of both is upregulated in the lesional skin compared to the nonlesional skin in psoriasis [127]. Dermal dendritic cells and monocytes are major sources of IL-23 production [128]. However, immunohistological staining also proves that IL23p40 and IL23p19 are expressed in normal and psoriatic keratinocytes [127–129]. Moreover, the epidermal expression of IL-23p40 and IL-23p19 is stronger in psoriasis lesions than in healthy controls [127–129]. Murine keratinocytes also produce biologically active IL-23 [130]. IL-23 can promote keratinocyte growth and histological acanthosis via the JAK2/AKT/STAT3/LMO4 signaling pathway [131]. LIM-domain only protein 4 (LMO4) is a LIM-domain protein that regulates keratinocyte proliferation and differentiation during embryogenesis [131]. In addition, TNF-α is an active stimulator of IL-23 production from keratinocytes in mice and possibly in humans [131]. In parallel, the anti-IL-23p40 antibody (Ustekinumab) [132,133] and anti-IL-23p19 antibodies (guselkumab, risankizumab, and tildrakizumab) [133–135] exhibit a high efficacy to psoriasis with a superiority of risankizumab over ustekinumab [133], and guselkumab over the anti-TNF-α antibody adalimumab [134].

The expression of *IL17A*, *IL17F*, and *IL17C* is upregulated in psoriatic lesional skin [136–138]. The intradermal injection of IL17C induces epidermal thickening and neutrophil infiltration [139]. As significant efficacy of the anti-IL17C antibody has recently been noted in murine psoriasis and atopic dermatitis [140], its human use has been suggested [141]. However, IL-17A is believed to be the most pathogenic IL-17 family member in psoriasis [68,69,72,73,142]. The lesional skin of psoriasis harbors IL-17A-producing immune cells [89,143], and transcriptomic analysis indicates a clear predominance of IL-17A signals [69,142]. Subsets of IL-17A-producing T cells are reactive to autoantigens, such as LL-37 (cathelicidin), a disintegrin and metalloprotease domain containing thrombospondin type 1 motif-like 5 (ADAMTSL5), keratin 17, and neolipid antigens generated by phospholipase A2 group IV D (PLA2G4D) [20,125,126,144–147]. IL-17A-dominant immune activation is also detected in the nonlesional skin of psoriasis [148].

There are three commercially available anti-IL17A biologics: secukinumab (fully human IgG1κ anti-IL17A antibody), ixekizumab (fully human IgG4 anti-IL17A antibody), and brodalumab (fully human IgG2 anti-IL17RA antibody). The severity of psoriatic skin lesions is generally evaluated by the Psoriasis Area and Severity Index (PASI) [149]. The efficacy of a therapeutic agent is assessed by the rate of responders who achieve 75%, 90%, and 100% reduction of PASI, namely, PASI75, PASI90, and PASI100, respectively. All three anti-IL-17A biologics exbibit remarkable therapeutic efficacy for psoriasis. The PASI90 scores of secukinumab, ixekizumab, and brodalumab are reported to be as high as 60% to 70% at 12 weeks post treatment [150–152].

Regarding histology, the psoriatic epidermis is acanthotic and the proliferating capacity of keratinocyte is increased as determined by Ki67 positivity and cytokeratin 16 expression [68,153,154]. In accordance with the accumulation of neutrophils in psoriasis, the gene expression of neutrophilic cytochemokines CXCL1, CXCL2, CXCL8, and IL-36 is upregulated in the lesional skin of psoriasis [68,155–157]. Psoriatic keratinocytes produce a large amount of CCL20 [158,159], which is a potent chemoattractant for CCR6+ IL-17A-producing Th17 [89,143,160], ILC3 [161,162], Tc17 [163,164], and γδ T cells [78,165]. Interestingly, IL-17A actively upregulates the production of these key cytochemokines as well as proliferative capacity in keratinocytes.

4. IL-17A and Keratinocyte Proliferation/Differentiation

Psoriatic keratinocytes simultaneously exhibit increased proliferation (Ki67+ or cytokeratin 16+ cell number) and differentiation [involucrin (IVL)+ cell number] [69,166–168]. Accordingly, IL17A is an active promoter of keratinocyte proliferation and differentiation [168–171]. In psoriasis patients, the neutralization of IL-17A by ixekizumab [168] or secukinumab [69] significantly decreases histological acanthosis, the number of Ki-67+-proliferating keratinocytes, and epidermal cytokeratin 16 expression. In the murine imiquimod-induced psoriasis model, topical imiquimod induces epidermal thickening that is significantly alleviated in *Traf3ip2* (*Act1*)-deficient mice in which IL-17 signaling is blocked [170]. The molecular mechanisms of the IL-17A-mediated acceleration of keratinocyte proliferation and differentiation are not yet fully understood.

IL-17A alone is likely to be insufficient to evoke a significant inflammatory response and may cooperatively or synergistically accelerate the proinflammatory cascade in combination with other cytokines, such as TNF-α, IL-23, IL-1β, IL-6, IL-22 and transforming growth factor-β (TGF-β) [68,172]. Transcriptomic analysis reveals a clear additive or synergistic gene regulation by IL-17A and TNF-α in human keratinocytes [173]. This gene regulation is likely attributable to two sets of transcription factors: NF-κB and the C/CAAT-enhancer-binding proteins (C/EBP), C/EBPβ, or C/EBPδ [169,173,174]. TNF-α is a strong inducer of active NF-κB, while IL-17A activates C/EBPβ or C/EBPδ and to a lesser extent NF-κB [169,173,174]. Therefore, the IL-17A blockade reduces the expression of these responsive genes to a greater extent than TNF-α inhibition [168].

The C/EBP family members are highly expressed transcription factors in epidermal keratinocytes and sebocytes in mice and humans and accelerate their differentiation [175]. The expression of C/EBPβ protein is located in the upper spinous layer and is strongly upregulated in the lesional skin of psoriasis [169]. Together with the elevated gene expression of *CEBPB*, the expression of keratinocyte-terminal differentiation genes, such as *IVL*, *FLG2*, and *TGM1*, is upregulated in the lesional skin of psoriasis [169]. In the promoter region of the *IVL* gene, there is a binding site for C/EBP, and the C/EBP transcription factor is necessary for the appropriate and continuous production of IVL protein [176]. These results suggest that IL-17A accelerates keratinocyte differentiation by increasing C/EBPβ protein in keratinocytes [168,169,173].

Regarding keratinocyte proliferation, IL-17A stimulates keratinocytes to produce IL-19 [173,177]. The combination of IL-17 and TNF-α results in the synergistic expression of IL-19 in keratinocytes. IL-17 alone promotes IL-19 expression by approximately 1.79-fold, and TNF-α alone slightly reduces IL-19 expression, whereas a combination of IL-17 and TNF-α promotes expression by 54.6-fold [173,177]. IL-19 itself promotes keratinocyte migration but not proliferation [178]. However, it activates fibroblasts to produce keratinocyte growth factor, which upregulates keratinocyte proliferation [178]. Additionally, the upregulation of cell cycle-related genes, such as CCNE1, CDCA5, and CDCA25A, suggests a direct contribution of IL-17 to epidermal KC proliferation [169]. The expression of cytokeratin 16 is upregulated in the lesional epidermis of psoriasis patients and in keratinocytes incubated with IL-17A [69,168,179]. The expression of cytokeratin 16 increases the proliferative capacity of keratinocytes via EGFR phosphorylation [180].

Other studies also underpin a possibility that IL-17A activates EGFR [98,181,182]. Chen et al. have demonstrated that IL-17A transactivates EGFR in keratinocyte stem cells [98]. IL-17A accelerates the enzymatic cleavage of amphiregulin, which activates EGFR in airway epithelial cells [181]. In the lesional skin of psoriasis, the expression of EGFR ligands, such as heparin-binding EGF, transforming growth factor-α, and amphiregulin, is overexpressed [183]. Consistent with these notions, the inhibition of EGFR by erlotinib or cetuximab successfully improves severe psoriasis [184–187]. These studies suggest that EGFR activation may partly explain the IL-17A-mediated upregulation of keratinocyte proliferation.

5. IL-17A and Cyto/Chemokines in Keratinocytes

In keratinocytes, IL-17A upregulates the expression of various psoriasis-related cyto/chemokines and antimicrobial peptides, such as CXCL1, CXCL8, IL-36G, CCL20, IL-19, IL-17C, S100A7, S100A8, S100A9, LL-37, and defensin β 4A (DEFB4A) [157,169,173,188–190]. The expression of these molecules is upregulated in the lesional skin of psoriasis and is downregulated to normal levels by biologics targeting TNF-α [128] or IL-17A [69,168]. Some are upregulated even in the nonlesional skin of patients with psoriasis [148]. The IL-17A-induced upregulation of these molecules is further amplified in the presence of TNF-α and IL-19 [173,177].

CXCL1 and CXCL8 are potent chemoattractants for neutrophils [191–193]. IL-36G induces CXCL1 and CXCL8 expression in an autocrine fashion in keratinocytes and recruits neutrophils [194]. Full-length IL-36G is cleaved by cathepsin G released from infiltrated neutrophils, and the cleaved IL-36G exhibits a more potent functional activity than the full-length one [192,195,196]. Moreover, IL-17A upregulates IL-36G production more potently in human psoriasis-derived keratinocytes than in healthy keratinocytes [197]. Therefore, the IL-17A, IL-36G, CXCL1/CXCL8, and neutrophils form a feed-forward vicious cycle, and an intraepidermal neutrophilic microabscess (Munro's microabscess or Kogoj's spongiform pustule) may develop [156,198,199]. The pathogenic significance of IL-36 is stressed more in pustular rather than plaque psoriasis [156,198,199]. In parallel, inhibition of the IL-36 pathway is efficacious for the treatment of pustular psoriasis [200].

While most chemokines redundantly bind to multiple receptors, CCL20 has only one known receptor, CCR6 [191]. CCR6 is expressed on dendritic cells [159] and IL-17-producing immune cells, including Th17 [89,143,201], ILC3 [161,162], Tc17 [163,164], and $\gamma\delta$ T cells [78,165]. CCR6 is now considered a representative marker for Th17 cells [202,203]. The human psoriatic epidermis expresses abundant CCL20 with the dermal infiltration of CCR6$^+$ dendritic cells and skin-homing T cells [143,158,159]. Although dermal dendritic cells and T cells express CCL20 in the psoriatic dermis [159], the expression of CCL20 is largely confined to the psoriatic epidermis, suggesting that epidermal keratinocytes are the major source of CCL20 production in psoriatic lesions [158,159]. CCL20 is constitutively expressed in cultured keratinocytes [201,204], and its production is upregulated by TNF-α and IL-17A [182,204]. Scratch injury upregulates the gene expression of *CCL20*, *CXCL8*, and *IL36G*, which may be related to the scratch-induced Koebner phenomenon frequently observed in patients with psoriasis [201]. Preclinical studies have revealed that the humanized anti-CCR6 antibody efficiently inhibits the cutaneous infiltration of CCR6$^+$ T cells in human and murine models [205,206]. The development of small molecule inhibitors against CCR6 is also ongoing [207,208]. Targeting the CCL20/CCR6 axis may be a potential therapeutic strategy for the treatment of psoriasis.

6. IL-17A and Anti-Microbial Peptides in Keratinocytes

S100A7, S100A8, S100A9, LL-37, and DEFB4A are anti-microbial peptides, and their expression is upregulated by IL-17A in keratinocytes [189,209,210]. S100A7 (psoriasin) has a multifaceted role in keratinocyte pathophysiology, including wound healing, keratinocyte differentiation, nucleocytoplasmic transport, and chemotaxis for CD4$^+$ T cells, neutrophils, and monocytes [211]. The production of S100A7 is augmented in the presence of IL-19 [212], IL-36G [188], and TNF-α [213]. S100A8, S100A9, and S100A12 are alternatively known as calgranulin A, B, and C, respectively, and exhibit antimicrobial activity [214]. All are elevated in psoriatic plaque and decreased by treatment with anti-IL-17A antibody secukinumab [69,168,215]. The S100 family members primarily form homodimers or higher-order oligomers, but S100A8 and S100A9 uniquely form heterodimeric complexes, which are known as calprotectin [214]. The chelation of Zn^{2+} and Mn^{2+} by extracellular S100A8/A9 is a proposed mechanism of antimicrobial activity [214]. S100A12 also has a chemotactic activity for mast cells and monocytes [216]. Pure human S100A8/A9 has broad spectrum antimicrobial activities against microorganisms, including *Capnocytophaga sputigena*, *C. albicans*, *Escherichia coli*, *Staphylococcus aureus*, *S. epidermis*, *Borrelia burgdorferi*, and *Listeria monocytogenes*, in vitro, and S100A12 has antimicrobial activity against filarial parasites [214]. The receptor for advanced glycation end-products (RAGE) may serve as a common receptor for S100 proteins, including S100A7, S100A8, S100A9, and S100A12 [214]. S100A8/S100A9 augments the production of CXCL1, CXCL2, CXCL3, CXCL8, CCL20, IL-6, and TNF-α in keratinocytes [217], and it enhances keratinocyte proliferation [217]. The transcriptional co-activator IκBζ, encoded by the *NFKBIZ* gene, plays a critical role in IL-17A-, IL-17F-, and IL-17A/F-mediated signaling, such as the gene expression of *S100A7* and *CCL20* [218–220].

LL-37 is an antimicrobial peptide of human cathelicidin that is produced when keratinocytes are injured by a broad range of bacteria, viruses, and fungi [221,222]. In addition to antimicrobial peptide activity, LL-37 exhibits "alarmin" function, affects adenosine triphosphate-receptor P2X7 and Toll-like receptor (TLR) signaling, and EGFR transactivation or intracellular $Ca2+$ mobilization [223–225]. The released LL-37 binds to the infiltrated neutrophils [221]. Neutrophils are a rich source of extracellular DNA due to their neutrophil extracellular traps [226]. Upon stimulation with complexes of host DNA and LL-37, plasmacytoid dendritic cells produce large amounts of IFN-α [227]. Notably, LL-37 induced the proliferation of circulating CD3+ T cells in 24 out of 52 patients with psoriasis (46%) [144]; therefore, LL-37 is effective for autoantigens. In total, 50 LL-37-reactive CD3+ T cells, including both CD4+ and CD8+ T cells, express the skin-homing receptor cutaneous lymphocyte antigen [144]. LL-37 peptides bind to HLA-DR in dendritic cells and are presented to CD4+ T cells, while LL-37 peptides and the HLA-C*0602 complex activate CD8+ T cells [144,228]. The majority of LL-37-reactive CD3+ T cells produce IL-17, and the capacity of their IL-17 production is associated with disease severity [144]. Interestingly, the LL-37-specific IL-17-producing T cells are exclusively CD4+, whereas the LL-37-specific CD8+ T cells do not produce IL-17 [144]. A recent study by Takahashi et al. revealed that LL-37 can bind to self-RNA and stimulate macrophages to produce IL-6 via a scavenger receptor [229].

DEFB4A is highly expressed in psoriasis plaques and is the most psoriasis-specific antimicrobial peptide [230,231]. In contrast, DEFB4A is expressed at negligible or low levels in normal skin and skin lesions of eczema [230–232]. The expression of DEFB4A is upregulated by IL-17A and synergistically by IL-17A and TNF-α [215,220]. The serum levels of DEFB4A are highly specific biomarkers for disease activity in patients with psoriasis [215]. The number of neutrophil extracellular traps increase in psoriasis and upregulate the expression of DEFB4A [226]. Notably, DEFB4A is a functional (non-chemokine) ligand for CCR6 and feasibly attracts Th17 cells [233,234].

Although the biological implications of increased antimicrobial peptides in psoriasis remain obscure, they are intimately associated with IL-17A-rich milieu. Therefore, the upregulated expression of these antimicrobial peptides is rapidly normalized by the neutralization of IL-17A by ixekizumab [168] or secukinumab [69].

7. Conclusions

IL-17A is a multifunctional cytokine produced from adaptive and innate immune cells, such as Th17 and ILC3s. It orchestrates and promotes the peripheral tissue defense system against microbial insult, especially fungal infection. Psoriasis is a major inflammatory skin disease in which the interaction between IL-17A and epidermal keratinocytes plays a critical pathogenic role. IL-17A stimulates the proliferation of keratinocytes. Keratinocytes also produce a variety of antimicrobial peptides and cytochemokines in response to IL-17A. The antimicrobial peptides further exacerbate skin inflammation. CCL20 produced from IL-17A-stimulated keratinocytes recruits IL-17A-producing Th17 cells and ILC3s and accelerates the feed-forward vicious cycle, which causes fully developed psoriasis. This pathogenetic scheme has been verified with a high clinical efficacy of anti-IL-17A biologics. Therefore, psoriasis is considered an excellent human model of how IL-17A works with target peripheral tissues, and it provides in-depth insight into human autoinflammatory diseases.

Author Contributions: M.F. wrote the first draft. K.F., G.T. and T.N. reviewed the draft. M.F. finalized the article. All authors have read and agreed to the published version of the manuscript.

References

1. Boehncke, W.H.; Schön, M.P. Psoriasis. *Lancet* **2015**, *386*, 983–994. [CrossRef]
2. Michalek, I.M.; Loring, B.; John, S.M. A systematic review of worldwide epidemiology of psoriasis. *J. Eur. Acad. Dermatol. Venereol.* **2017**, *31*, 205–212. [CrossRef] [PubMed]
3. Ito, T.; Takahashi, H.; Kawada, A.; Iizuka, H.; Nakagawa, H. Epidemiological survey from 2009 to 2012 of psoriatic patients in Japanese Society for Psoriasis Research. *J. Dermatol.* **2018**, *45*, 293–301. [CrossRef] [PubMed]
4. Ogawa, E.; Okuyama, R.; Seki, T.; Kobayashi, A.; Oiso, N.; Muto, M.; Nakagawa, H.; Kawada, A. Epidemiological survey of patients with psoriasis in Matsumoto city, Nagano Prefecture, Japan. *J. Dermatol.* **2018**, *45*, 314–317. [CrossRef] [PubMed]
5. Ichiyama, S.; Ito, M.; Funasaka, Y.; Abe, M.; Nishida, E.; Muramatsu, S.; Nishihara, H.; Kato, H.; Morita, A.; Imafuku, S.; et al. Assessment of medication adherence and treatment satisfaction in Japanese patients with psoriasis of various severities. *J. Dermatol.* **2018**, *45*, 727–731. [CrossRef]
6. Souza, C.S.; de Castro, C.C.S.; Carneiro, F.R.O.; Pinto, J.M.N.; Fabricio, L.H.Z.; Azulay-Abulafia, L.; Romiti, R.; Cestari, T.F.; Suzuki, C.E.; Biegun, P.M.; et al. Metabolic syndrome and psoriatic arthritis among patients with psoriasis vulgaris: Quality of life and prevalence. *J. Dermatol.* **2019**, *46*, 3–10. [CrossRef]
7. Takahashi, H.; Satoh, K.; Takagi, A.; Iizuka, H. Cost-efficacy and pharmacoeconomics of psoriatic patients in Japan: Analysis from a single outpatient clinic. *J. Dermatol.* **2019**, *46*, 478–481. [CrossRef]
8. Miller, R.A. The Koebner phenomenon. *Int. J. Dermatol.* **1982**, *21*, 192–197. [CrossRef]
9. Weiss, G.; Shemer, A.; Trau, H. The Koebner phenomenon: Review of the literature. *J. Eur. Acad. Dermatol. Venereol.* **2002**, *16*, 241–248. [CrossRef]
10. Dai, Y.X.; Wang, S.C.; Chou, Y.J.; Chang, Y.T.; Chen, T.J.; Li, C.P.; Wu, C.Y. Smoking, but not alcohol, is associated with risk of psoriasis in a Taiwanese population-based cohort study. *J. Am. Acad. Dermatol.* **2019**, *80*, 727–734. [CrossRef]
11. Kamiya, K.; Kishimoto, M.; Sugai, J.; Komine, M.; Ohtsuki, M. Risk factors for the development of psoriasis. *Int. J. Mol. Sci.* **2019**, *20*, 4347. [CrossRef] [PubMed]
12. O'Rielly, D.D.; Jani, M.; Rahman, P.; Elder, J.T. The Genetics of Psoriasis and Psoriatic Arthritis. *J. Rheumatol Suppl.* **2019**, *95*, 46–50. [PubMed]
13. Elder, J.T. Expanded genome-wide association study meta-analysis of psoriasis expands the catalog of common psoriasis-associated variants. *J. Investig. Dermatol. Symp. Proc.* **2018**, *19*, S77–S78. [CrossRef] [PubMed]
14. Diani, M.; Perego, S.; Sansoni, V.; Bertino, L.; Gomarasca, M.; Faraldi, M.; Pigatto, P.D.M.; Damiani, G.; Banfi, G.; Altomare, G.; et al. Differences in osteoimmunological biomarkers predictive of psoriatic arthritis among a large Italian cohort of psoriatic patients. *Int. J. Mol. Sci.* **2019**, *20*, 5617. [CrossRef] [PubMed]
15. Mease, P.J.; Palmer, J.B.; Hur, P.; Strober, B.E.; Lebwohl, M.; Karki, C.; Reed, G.W.; Etzel, C.J.; Greenberg, J.D.; Helliwell, P.S. Utilization of the validated psoriasis epidemiology screening tool to identify signs and symptoms of psoriatic arthritis among those with psoriasis: A cross-sectional analysis from the US-based Corrona Psoriasis Registry. *J. Eur. Acad. Dermatol. Venereol.* **2019**, *33*, 886–892. [CrossRef] [PubMed]
16. Yamamoto, T.; Kawada, A. Clinical characteristics of Japanese patients with psoriatic arthritis: Comparison with East Asian countries. *J. Dermatol.* **2018**, *45*, 273–278. [CrossRef]
17. Yamamoto, T.; Ohtsuki, M.; Sano, S.; Morita, A.; Igarashi, A.; Okuyama, R.; Kawada, A. Late-onset psoriatic arthritis in Japanese patients. *J. Dermatol.* **2019**, *46*, 169–170. [CrossRef]

18.   Yamamoto, T.; Ohtsuki, M.; Sano, S.; Morita, A.; Igarashi, A.; Okuyama, R.; Kawada, A. Switching biologics in the treatment of psoriatic arthritis in Japan. *J. Dermatol.* **2019**, *46*, e113–e114. [CrossRef]

19.   Umezawa, Y.; Yanaba, K.; Asahina, A.; Nakagawa, H.; Fukuda, T.; Fukuda, K. Usefulness of dual-energy computed tomography for the evaluation of psoriatic arthritis accompanied by knee osteoarthritis. *J. Dermatol.* **2019**, *46*, e30–e32. [CrossRef]

20.   Furue, K.; Ito, T.; Tsuji, G.; Kadono, T.; Nakahara, T.; Furue, M. Autoimmunity and autoimmune co-morbidities in psoriasis. *Immunology* **2018**, *154*, 21–27. [CrossRef]

21.   Ho, Y.H.; Hu, H.Y.; Chang, Y.T.; Li, C.P.; Wu, C.Y. Psoriasis is associated with increased risk of bullous pemphigoid: A nationwide population-based cohort study in Taiwan. *J. Dermatol.* **2019**, *46*, 604–609. [CrossRef] [PubMed]

22.   Ichiyama, S.; Hoashi, T.; Kanda, N.; Hashimoto, H.; Matsushita, M.; Nozawa, K.; Ueno, T.; Saeki, H. Psoriasis vulgaris associated with systemic lupus erythematosus successfully treated with apremilast. *J. Dermatol.* **2019**, *46*, e219–e221. [CrossRef] [PubMed]

23.   Chujo, S.; Asahina, A.; Itoh, Y.; Kobayashi, K.; Sueki, H.; Ishiji, T.; Umezawa, Y.; Nakagawa, H. New onset of psoriasis during nivolumab treatment for lung cancer. *J. Dermatol.* **2018**, *45*, e55–e56. [CrossRef] [PubMed]

24.   Kamata, M.; Asano, Y.; Shida, R.; Maeda, N.; Yoshizaki, A.; Miyagaki, T.; Kawashima, T.; Tada, Y.; Sato, S. Secukinumab decreased circulating anti-BP180-NC16a autoantibodies in a patient with coexisting psoriasis vulgaris and bullous pemphigoid. *J. Dermatol.* **2019**, *46*, e216–e217. [CrossRef]

25.   Bayaraa, B.; Imafuku, S. Relationship between environmental factors, age of onset and familial history in Japanese patients with psoriasis. *J. Dermatol.* **2018**, *45*, 715–718. [CrossRef] [PubMed]

26.   Chiu, H.Y.; Chang, W.L.; Shiu, M.N.; Huang, W.F.; Tsai, T.F. Psoriasis is associated with a greater risk for cardiovascular procedure and surgery in patients with hypertension: A nationwide cohort study. *J. Dermatol.* **2018**, *45*, 1381–1388. [CrossRef]

27.   Furue, M.; Kadono, T. "Inflammatory skin march" in atopic dermatitis and psoriasis. *Inflamm. Res.* **2017**, *66*, 833–842. [CrossRef]

28.   Momose, M.; Asahina, A.; Fukuda, T.; Sakuma, T.; Umezawa, Y.; Nakagawa, H. Evaluation of epicardial adipose tissue volume and coronary artery calcification in Japanese patients with psoriasis vulgaris. *J. Dermatol.* **2018**, *45*, 1349–1352. [CrossRef]

29.   Takamura, S.; Takahashi, A.; Inoue, Y.; Teraki, Y. Effects of tumor necrosis factor-α, interleukin-23 and interleukin-17A inhibitors on bodyweight and body mass index in patients with psoriasis. *J. Dermatol.* **2018**, *45*, 1130–1134. [CrossRef]

30.   Wang, C.C.; Tang, C.H.; Huang, K.C.; Huang, S.Y.; Sue, Y.M. Increased risk of incident psoriasis in end-stage renal disease patients on chronic hemodialysis: A nationwide population-based cohort study. *J. Dermatol.* **2018**, *45*, 1063–1070. [CrossRef]

31.   Han, J.H.; Lee, J.H.; Han, K.D.; Kim, H.N.; Bang, C.H.; Park, Y.M.; Lee, J.Y.; Kim, T.Y. Increased risk of psoriasis in subjects with abdominal obesity: A nationwide population-based study. *J. Dermatol.* **2019**, *46*, 695–701. [CrossRef] [PubMed]

32.   Jung, K.J.; Kim, T.G.; Lee, J.W.; Lee, M.; Oh, J.; Lee, S.E.; Chang, H.J.; Jee, S.H.; Lee, M.G. Increased risk of atherosclerotic cardiovascular disease among patients with psoriasis in Korea: A 15-year nationwide population-based cohort study. *J. Dermatol.* **2019**, *46*, 859–866. [CrossRef] [PubMed]

33.   Masaki, S.; Bayaraa, B.; Imafuku, S. Prevalence of inflammatory bowel disease in Japanese psoriatic patients. *J. Dermatol.* **2019**, *46*, 590–594. [CrossRef] [PubMed]

34.   Tokuyama, M.; Shimizu, T.; Yamada, T.; Kondoh, A.; Mabuchi, T. Case of psoriasis vulgaris with atrial fibrillation, heart failure and chronic kidney disease which were found accidentally through blood examination during apremilast treatment. *J. Dermatol.* **2019**, *46*, e239–e240. [CrossRef]

35.   Yamazaki, F.; Takehana, K.; Tamashima, M.; Okamoto, H. Improvement in abnormal coronary arteries estimated by coronary computed tomography angiography after secukinumab treatment in a Japanese psoriatic patient. *J. Dermatol.* **2019**, *46*, e51–e52. [CrossRef]

36.   Wójcik, P.; Biernacki, M.; Wroński, A.; Łuczaj, W.; Waeg, G.; Žarković, N.; Skrzydlewska, E. Altered lipid metabolism in blood mononuclear cells of psoriatic patients indicates differential changes in psoriasis vulgaris and psoriatic arthritis. *Int. J. Mol. Sci.* **2019**, *20*, 4249.

37.   Lee, J.H.; Kim, H.J.; Han, K.D.; Kim, H.N.; Park, Y.M.; Lee, J.Y.; Park, Y.G.; Lee, Y.B. Cancer risk in 892089 patients with psoriasis in Korea: A nationwide population-based cohort study. *J. Dermatol.* **2019**, *46*, 95–102. [CrossRef]

38. Hsu, S.; Papp, K.A.; Lebwohl, M.G.; Bagel, J.; Blauvelt, A.; Duffin, K.C.; Crowley, J.; Eichenfield, L.F.; Feldman, S.R.; Fiorentino, D.F.; et al. Consensus guidelines for the management of plaque psoriasis. *Arch. Dermatol.* **2012**, *148*, 95–102. [CrossRef]

39. Imafuku, S.; Zheng, M.; Tada, Y.; Zhang, X.; Theng, C.; Thevarajah, S.; Zhao, Y.; Song, H.J. Asian consensus on assessment and management of mild to moderate plaque psoriasis with topical therapy. *J. Dermatol.* **2018**, *45*, 805–811. [CrossRef]

40. Meephansan, J.; Subpayasarn, U.; Ponnikorn, S.; Chakkavittumrong, P.; Juntongjin, P.; Komine, M.; Ohtsuki, M.; Poovorawan, Y. Methotrexate, but not narrowband ultraviolet B radiation, suppresses interleukin-33 mRNA levels in psoriatic plaques and protein levels in serum of patients with psoriasis. *J. Dermatol.* **2018**, *45*, 322–325. [CrossRef]

41. Kishimoto, M.; Komine, M.; Hioki, T.; Kamiya, K.; Sugai, J.; Ohtsuki, M. Real-world use of apremilast for patients with psoriasis in Japan. *J. Dermatol.* **2018**, *45*, 1345–1348. [CrossRef] [PubMed]

42. Morita, A. Current developments in phototherapy for psoriasis. *J. Dermatol.* **2018**, *45*, 287–292. [CrossRef] [PubMed]

43. Oh, E.H.; Koh, W.S.; Shin, J.M.; Kim, J.E.; Ko, J.Y.; Ro, Y.S. Clinical experience of cyclosporin treatment in patients with psoriasis and psoriatic arthritis. *J. Dermatol.* **2018**, *45*, 329–330. [CrossRef] [PubMed]

44. Pongparit, K.; Chularojanamontri, L.; Limphoka, P.; Silpa-Archa, N.; Wongpraparat, C. Effectiveness of and factors associated with clinical response to methotrexate under daily life conditions in Asian patients with psoriasis: A retrospective cohort study. *J. Dermatol.* **2018**, *45*, 540–545. [CrossRef] [PubMed]

45. Okazaki, S.; Osawa, R.; Nakajima, H.; Nakajima, K.; Sano, S. Favorable response to apremilast in a patient with refractory psoriasis verrucosa. *J. Dermatol.* **2019**, *46*, 544–547. [CrossRef]

46. Furue, K.; Ito, T.; Furue, M. Differential efficacy of biologic treatments targeting the TNF-α/IL-23/IL-17 axis in psoriasis and psoriatic arthritis. *Cytokine* **2018**, *111*, 182–188. [CrossRef]

47. Furue, K.; Ito, T.; Tsuji, G.; Kadono, T.; Furue, M. Psoriasis and the TNF/IL23/IL17 axis. *G. Ital. Dermatol. Venereol.* **2019**, *154*, 418–424. [CrossRef]

48. Sawyer, L.M.; Malottki, K.; Sabry-Grant, C.; Yasmeen, N.; Wright, E.; Sohrt, A.; Borg, E.; Warren, R.B. Assessing the relative efficacy of interleukin-17 and interleukin-23 targeted treatments for moderate-to-severe plaque psoriasis: A systematic review and network meta-analysis of PASI response. *PLoS ONE* **2019**, *14*, e0220868. [CrossRef]

49. Kamata, M.; Tada, Y. Safety of biologics in psoriasis. *J. Dermatol.* **2018**, *45*, 279–286. [CrossRef]

50. Momose, M.; Asahina, A.; Umezawa, Y.; Nakagawa, H. Long-term clinical efficacy and safety of secukinumab for Japanese patients with psoriasis: A single-center experience. *J. Dermatol.* **2018**, *45*, 318–321.

51. Ogawa, E.; Sato, Y.; Minagawa, A.; Okuyama, R. Pathogenesis of psoriasis and development of treatment. *J. Dermatol.* **2018**, *45*, 264–272. [CrossRef] [PubMed]

52. Ohtsuki, M.; Kubo, H.; Morishima, H.; Goto, R.; Zheng, R.; Nakagawa, H. Guselkumab, an anti-interleukin-23 monoclonal antibody, for the treatment of moderate to severe plaque-type psoriasis in Japanese patients: Efficacy and safety results from a phase 3, randomized, double-blind, placebo-controlled study. *J. Dermatol.* **2018**, *45*, 1053–1062. [CrossRef] [PubMed]

53. Bayaraa, B.; Imafuku, S. Sustainability and switching of biologics for psoriasis and psoriatic arthritis at Fukuoka University Psoriasis Registry. *J. Dermatol.* **2019**, *46*, 389–398. [CrossRef] [PubMed]

54. Kamiya, K.; Karakawa, M.; Komine, M.; Kishimoto, M.; Sugai, J.; Ohtsuki, M. Results of a retrospective study on the efficacy and safety of adalimumab 80 mg administrated every other week in patients with psoriasis at a single Japanese institution. *J. Dermatol.* **2019**, *46*, 199–205. [CrossRef]

55. Komatsu-Fujii, T.; Honda, T.; Otsuka, A.; Kabashima, K. Inverse responses of the skin and nail lesions of psoriatic arthritis to an anti-interleukin-17A antibody and an anti-tumor necrosis factor-α antibody. *J. Dermatol.* **2019**, *46*, e440–e441. [CrossRef]

56. Komatsu-Fujii, T.; Honda, T.; Otsuka, A.; Kabashima, K. Improvement of nail lesions in a patient with psoriatic arthritis by switching the treatment from an anti-interleukin-17A antibody to an anti-tumor necrosis factor-α antibody. *J. Dermatol.* **2019**, *46*, e158–e160. [CrossRef]

57. Lee, M.G.; Huang, Y.H.; Lee, J.H.; Lee, S.C.; Kim, T.G.; Aw, D.C.; Bao, W.; Dee, C.M.A.; Guana, A.; Tsai, T.F. Secukinumab demonstrates superior efficacy and a faster response in clearing skin in Asian subjects with moderate to severe plaque psoriasis compared with ustekinumab: Subgroup analysis from the CLEAR study. *J. Dermatol.* **2019**, *46*, 752–758. [CrossRef]

58. Okubo, Y.; Ohtsuki, M.; Morita, A.; Yamaguchi, M.; Shima, T.; Tani, Y.; Nakagawa, H. Long-term efficacy and safety of secukinumab in Japanese patients with moderate to severe plaque psoriasis: 3-year results of a double-blind extension study. *J. Dermatol.* **2019**, *46*, 186–192. [CrossRef]

59. Shibata, T.; Muto, J.; Takama, H.; Yanagishita, T.; Ito, T.; Watanabe, D. Case of psoriatic erythroderma induced by the discontinuation of the chronic use of topical steroid after dialysis initiation and successfully treated with secukinumab. *J. Dermatol.* **2019**, *46*, e119–e120. [CrossRef]

60. Tada, Y.; Ishii, K.; Kimura, J.; Hanada, K.; Kawaguchi, I. Patient preference for biologic treatments of psoriasis in Japan. *J. Dermatol.* **2019**, *46*, 466–477. [CrossRef]

61. Tsuruta, N.; Narisawa, Y.; Imafuku, S.; Ito, K.; Yamaguchi, K.; Miyagi, T.; Takahashi, K.; Fukamatsu, H.; Morizane, S.; Koketsu, H.; et al. Cross-sectional multicenter observational study of psoriatic arthritis in Japanese patients: Relationship between skin and joint symptoms and results of treatment with tumor necrosis factor-α inhibitors. *J. Dermatol.* **2019**, *46*, 193–198. [CrossRef]

62. Veale, D.J.; Fearon, U. The pathogenesis of psoriatic arthritis. *Lancet* **2018**, *391*, 2273–2284. [CrossRef]

63. Assefa, G.T.; Kaneko, S.; Oguro, H.; Morita, E. Treatment of psoriasis and psoriatic arthritis with secukinumab after unsatisfactory response to ustekinumab in multiple sclerosis patient. *J. Dermatol.* **2019**, *46*, e112–e113. [CrossRef] [PubMed]

64. Mourad, A.; Gniadecki, R. Treatment of dactylitis and enthesitis in psoriatic arthritis with biologic agents: A systematic review and metaanalysis. *J. Rheumatol.* **2019**, *47*, 59–65. [CrossRef] [PubMed]

65. Korman, N.J. Management of psoriasis as a systemic disease: What is the evidence? *Br. J. Dermatol.* **2019**. [CrossRef]

66. Lockshin, B.; Balagula, Y.; Merola, J.F. Interleukin 17, inflammation, and cardiovascular risk in patients with psoriasis. *J. Am. Acad. Dermatol.* **2018**, *79*, 345–352. [CrossRef]

67. Erichsen, C.Y.; Jensen, P.; Kofoed, K. Biologic therapies targeting the interleukin (IL)-23/IL-17 immune axis for the treatment of moderate-to-severe plaque psoriasis: A systematic review and meta-analysis. *J. Eur. Acad. Dermatol. Venereol.* **2020**, *34*, 30–38. [CrossRef]

68. Krueger, J.G.; Brunner, P.M. Interleukin-17 alters the biology of many cell types involved in the genesis of psoriasis, systemic inflammation and associated comorbidities. *Exp. Dermatol.* **2018**, *27*, 115–123. [CrossRef]

69. Krueger, J.G.; Wharton, K.A., Jr.; Schlitt, T.; Suprun, M.; Torene, R.I.; Jiang, X.; Wang, C.Q.; Fuentes-Duculan, J.; Hartmann, N.; Peters, T.; et al. IL-17A inhibition by secukinumab induces early clinical, histopathologic, and molecular resolution of psoriasis. *J. Allergy Clin. Immunol.* **2019**, *144*, 750–763. [CrossRef]

70. Mease, P.J.; Smolen, J.S.; Behrens, F.; Nash, P.; Liu Leage, S.; Li, L.; Tahir, H.; Gooderham, M.; Krishnan, E.; Liu-Seifert, H.; et al. A head-to-head comparison of the efficacy and safety of ixekizumab and adalimumab in biological-naïve patients with active psoriatic arthritis: 24-week results of a randomised, open-label, blinded-assessor trial. *Ann. Rheum. Dis.* **2020**, *79*, 123–131. [CrossRef]

71. Warren, R.B.; Barker, J.; Finlay, A.Y.; Burden, A.D.; Kirby, B.; Armendariz, Y.; Williams, R.; Hatchard, C.; Khare, S.; Griffiths, C.E.M. Secukinumab for patients failing previous TNFα-inhibitor therapy: Results of a randomised open-label study (Signature). *Br. J. Dermatol.* **2019**. [CrossRef] [PubMed]

72. Hawkes, J.E.; Chan, T.C.; Krueger, J.G. Psoriasis pathogenesis and the development of novel targeted immune therapies. *J. Allergy Clin. Immunol.* **2017**, *140*, 645–653. [CrossRef] [PubMed]

73. Hawkes, J.E.; Yan, B.Y.; Chan, T.C.; Krueger, J.G. Discovery of the IL-23/IL-17 signaling pathway and the treatment of psoriasis. *J. Immunol.* **2018**, *201*, 1605–1613. [CrossRef] [PubMed]

74. Langrish, C.L.; Chen, Y.; Blumenschein, W.M.; Mattson, J.; Basham, B.; Sedgwick, J.D.; McClanahan, T.; Kastelein, R.A.; Cua, D.J. IL-23 drives a pathogenic T cell population that induces autoimmune inflammation. *J. Exp. Med.* **2005**, *201*, 233–240. [CrossRef]

75. Shiga, T.; Sato, K.; Kataoka, S.; Sano, S. TNF inhibitors directly target Th17 cells via attenuation of autonomous TNF/TNFR2 signalling in psoriasis. *J. Dermatol. Sci.* **2015**, *77*, 79–81. [CrossRef]

76. Schüler, R.; Brand, A.; Klebow, S.; Wild, J.; Veras, F.P.; Ullmann, E.; Roohani, S.; Kolbinger, F.; Kossmann, S.; Wohn, C.; et al. Antagonization of IL-17A attenuates skin inflammation and vascular dysfunction in mouse models of psoriasis. *J. Investig. Dermatol.* **2019**, *139*, 638–647. [CrossRef]

77. Moos, S.; Mohebiany, A.N.; Waisman, A.; Kurschus, F.C. Imiquimod-induced psoriasis in mice depends on the IL-17 signaling of keratinocytes. *J. Investig. Dermatol.* **2019**, *139*, 1110–1117. [CrossRef]

78. Mabuchi, T.; Takekoshi, T.; Hwang, S.T. Epidermal CCR6+ γδ T cells are major producers of IL-22 and IL-17 in a murine model of psoriasiform dermatitis. *J. Immunol.* **2011**, *187*, 5026–5031. [CrossRef]

79. Mabuchi, T.; Singh, T.P.; Takekoshi, T.; Jia, G.F.; Wu, X.; Kao, M.C.; Weiss, I.; Farber, J.M.; Hwang, S.T. CCR6 is required for epidermal trafficking of γδ-T cells in an IL-23-induced model of psoriasiform dermatitis. *J. Investig. Dermatol.* **2013**, *133*, 164–171. [CrossRef]

80. Nakajima, K.; Sano, S. Mouse models of psoriasis and their relevance. *J. Dermatol.* **2018**, *45*, 252–263. [CrossRef]

81. Brembilla, N.C.; Senra, L.; Boehncke, W.H. The IL-17 family of cytokines in psoriasis: IL-17A and beyond. *Front. Immunol.* **2018**, *9*, 1682. [CrossRef] [PubMed]

82. McGeachy, M.J.; Cua, D.J.; Gaffen, S.L. The IL-17 family of cytokines in health and disease. *Immunity* **2019**, *50*, 892–906. [CrossRef] [PubMed]

83. Buckley, K.M.; Ho, E.C.H.; Hibino, T.; Schrankel, C.S.; Schuh, N.W.; Wang, G.; Rast, J.P. IL17 factors are early regulators in the gut epithelium during inflammatory response to Vibrio in the sea urchin larva. *Elife* **2017**, *6*. [CrossRef] [PubMed]

84. Han, Q.; Das, S.; Hirano, M.; Holland, S.J.; McCurley, N.; Guo, P.; Rosenberg, C.S.; Boehm, T.; Cooper, M.D. Characterization of lamprey IL-17 family members and their receptors. *J. Immunol.* **2015**, *195*, 5440–5451. [CrossRef] [PubMed]

85. Aktar, M.K.; Kido-Nakahara, M.; Furue, M.; Nakahara, T. Mutual upregulation of endothelin-1 and IL-25 in atopic dermatitis. *Allergy* **2015**, *70*, 846–854. [CrossRef]

86. Cua, D.J.; Tato, C.M. Innate IL-17-producing cells: The sentinels of the immune system. *Nat. Rev. Immunol.* **2010**, *10*, 479–489. [CrossRef] [PubMed]

87. Chen, L.; He, Z.; Slinger, E.; Bongers, G.; Lapenda, T.L.S.; Pacer, M.E.; Jiao, J.; Beltrao, M.F.; Soto, A.J.; Harpaz, N.; et al. IL-23 activates innate lymphoid cells to promote neonatal intestinal pathology. *Mucosal Immunol.* **2015**, *8*, 390–402. [CrossRef]

88. Cai, Y.; Shen, X.; Ding, C.; Qi, C.; Li, K.; Li, X.; Jala, V.R.; Zhang, H.G.; Wang, T.; Zheng, J.; et al. Pivotal role of dermal IL-17-producing γδ T cells in skin inflammation. *Immunity* **2011**, *35*, 596–610. [CrossRef]

89. Villanova, F.; Flutter, B.; Tosi, I.; Grys, K.; Sreeneebus, H.; Perera, G.K.; Chapman, A.; Smith, C.H.; Di Meglio, P.; Nestle, F.O. Characterization of innate lymphoid cells in human skin and blood demonstrates increase of NKp44+ ILC3 in psoriasis. *J. Investig. Dermatol.* **2014**, *134*, 984–991. [CrossRef]

90. Matsuzaki, G.; Umemura, M. Interleukin-17 family cytokines in protective immunity against infections: Role of hematopoietic cell-derived and non-hematopoietic cell-derived interleukin-17s. *Microbiol. Immunol.* **2018**, *62*, 1–13. [CrossRef]

91. Chang, S.H.; Reynolds, J.M.; Pappu, B.P.; Chen, G.; Martinez, G.J.; Dong, C. Interleukin-17C promotes Th17 cell responses and autoimmune disease via interleukin-17 receptor E. *Immunity* **2011**, *35*, 611–621. [CrossRef] [PubMed]

92. Hu, Y.; Ota, N.; Peng, I.; Refino, C.J.; Danilenko, D.M.; Caplazi, P.; Ouyang, W. IL-17RC is required for IL-17A- and IL-17F-dependent signaling and the pathogenesis of experimental autoimmune encephalomyelitis. *J. Immunol.* **2010**, *184*, 4307–4316. [CrossRef] [PubMed]

93. Su, Y.; Huang, J.; Zhao, X.; Lu, H.; Wang, W.; Yang, X.O.; Shi, Y.; Wang, X.; Lai, Y.; Dong, C. Interleukin-17 receptor D constitutes an alternative receptor for interleukin-17A important in psoriasis-like skin inflammation. *Sci. Immunol.* **2019**, *4*. [CrossRef]

94. Liu, C.; Swaidani, S.; Qian, W.; Kang, Z.; Sun, P.; Han, Y.; Wang, C.; Gulen, M.F.; Yin, W.; Zhang, C.; et al. A CC′ loop decoy peptide blocks the interaction between Act1 and IL-17RA to attenuate IL-17- and IL-25-induced inflammation. *Sci.Signal* **2011**, *4*, ra72. [CrossRef] [PubMed]

95. Sønder, S.U.; Saret, S.; Tang, W.; Sturdevant, D.E.; Porcella, S.F.; Siebenlist, U. IL-17-induced NF-kappaB activation via CIKS/Act1: Physiologic significance and signaling mechanisms. *J. Biol. Chem.* **2011**, *286*, 12881–12890. [CrossRef] [PubMed]

96. Okada, S.; Puel, A.; Casanova, J.L.; Kobayashi, M. Chronic mucocutaneous candidiasis disease associated with inborn errors of IL-17 immunity. *Clin. Transl. Immunology* **2016**, *5*, e114. [CrossRef] [PubMed]

97. Wang, M.; Zhang, S.; Zheng, G.; Huang, J.; Songyang, Z.; Zhao, X.; Lin, X. Gain-of-function mutation of Card14 leads to spontaneous psoriasis-like skin inflammation through enhanced keratinocyte response to IL-17A. *Immunity* **2018**, *49*, 66–79. [CrossRef] [PubMed]

98. Chen, X.; Cai, G.; Liu, C.; Zhao, J.; Gu, C.; Wu, L.; Hamilton, T.A.; Zhang, C.J.; Ko, J.; Zhu, L.; et al. IL-17R-EGFR axis links wound healing to tumorigenesis in Lrig1(+) stem cells. *J. Exp. Med.* **2019**, *216*, 195–214. [CrossRef]

99.   Tsang, M.; Friesel, R.; Kudoh, T.; Dawid, I.B. Identification of Sef, a novel modulator of FGF signalling. *Nat. Cell Biol.* **2002**, *4*, 165–169. [CrossRef]

100. Calautti, E.; Avalle, L.; Poli, V. Psoriasis: A STAT3-centric view. *Int. J. Mol. Sci.* **2018**, *19*, 171. [CrossRef]

101. Sano, S.; Chan, K.S.; Carbajal, S.; Clifford, J.; Peavey, M.; Kiguchi, K.; Itami, S.; Nickoloff, B.J.; DiGiovanni, J. Stat3 links activated keratinocytes and immunocytes required for development of psoriasis in a novel transgenic mouse model. *Nat. Med.* **2005**, *11*, 43–49. [CrossRef] [PubMed]

102. Miyoshi, K.; Takaishi, M.; Nakajima, K.; Ikeda, M.; Kanda, T.; Tarutani, M.; Iiyama, T.; Asao, N.; DiGiovanni, J.; Sano, S. Stat3 as a therapeutic target for the treatment of psoriasis: A clinical feasibility study with STA-21, a Stat3 inhibitor. *J. Investig. Dermatol.* **2011**, *131*, 108–117. [CrossRef] [PubMed]

103. Bae, H.C.; Jeong, S.H.; Kim, J.H.; Lee, H.; Ryu, W.I.; Kim, M.G.; Son, E.D.; Lee, T.R.; Son, S.W. RIP4 upregulates CCL20 expression through STAT3 signalling in cultured keratinocytes. *Exp. Dermatol.* **2018**, *27*, 1126–1133. [CrossRef] [PubMed]

104. Shi, X.; Jin, L.; Dang, E.; Chang, T.; Feng, Z.; Liu, Y.; Wang, G. IL-17A upregulates keratin 17 expression in keratinocytes through STAT1- and STAT3-dependent mechanisms. *J. Investig. Dermatol.* **2011**, *131*, 2401–2408. [CrossRef]

105. Honma, M.; Minami-Hori, M.; Takahashi, H.; Iizuka, H. Podoplanin expression in wound and hyperproliferative psoriatic epidermis: Regulation by TGF-β and STAT-3 activating cytokines, IFN-γ, IL-6, and IL-22. *J. Dermatol. Sci.* **2012**, *65*, 134–140. [CrossRef]

106. Miyoshi, K.; Takaishi, M.; Digiovanni, J.; Sano, S. Attenuation of psoriasis-like skin lesion in a mouse model by topical treatment with indirubin and its derivastive E804. *J. Dermatol. Sci.* **2012**, *65*, 70–72. [CrossRef]

107. Ekman, A.K.; Bivik Eding, C.; Rundquist, I.; Enerbäck, C. IL-17 and IL-22 promote keratinocyte stemness in the germinative compartment in psoriasis. *J. Investig. Dermatol.* **2019**, *139*, 1564–1573. [CrossRef]

108. Karbach, S.; Croxford, A.L.; Oelze, M.; Schüler, R.; Minwegen, D.; Wegner, J.; Koukes, L.; Yogev, N.; Nikolaev, A.; Reißig, S.; et al. Interleukin 17 drives vascular inflammation, endothelial dysfunction, and arterial hypertension in psoriasis-like skin disease. *Arterioscler. Thromb. Vasc. Biol.* **2014**, *34*, 2658–2668. [CrossRef]

109. Cordoro, K.M.; Hitraya-Low, M.; Taravati, K.; Sandoval, P.M.; Kim, E.; Sugarman, J.; Pauli, M.L.; Liao, W.; Rosenblum, M.D. Skin-infiltrating, interleukin-22-producing T cells differentiate pediatric psoriasis from adult psoriasis. *J. Am. Acad. Dermatol.* **2017**, *77*, 417–424. [CrossRef]

110. Diani, M.; Altomare, G.; Reali, E. T cell responses in psoriasis and psoriatic arthritis. *Autoimmun. Rev.* **2015**, *14*, 286–292. [CrossRef]

111. Puel, A.; Cypowyj, S.; Bustamante, J.; Wright, J.F.; Liu, L.; Lim, H.K.; Migaud, M.; Israel, L.; Chrabieh, M.; Audry, M.; et al. Chronic mucocutaneous candidiasis in humans with inborn errors of interleukin-17 immunity. *Science* **2011**, *332*, 65–68. [CrossRef] [PubMed]

112. Boisson, B.; Wang, C.; Pedergnana, V.; Wu, L.; Cypowyj, S.; Rybojad, M.; Belkadi, A.; Picard, C.; Abel, L.; Fieschi, C.; et al. An ACT1 mutation selectively abolishes interleukin-17 responses in humans with chronic mucocutaneous candidiasis. *Immunity* **2013**, *39*, 676–686. [CrossRef] [PubMed]

113. Ling, Y.; Cypowyj, S.; Aytekin, C.; Galicchio, M.; Camcioglu, Y.; Nepesov, S.; Ikinciogullari, A.; Dogu, F.; Belkadi, A.; Levy, R.; et al. Inherited IL-17RC deficiency in patients with chronic mucocutaneous candidiasis. *J. Exp. Med.* **2015**, *212*, 619–631. [CrossRef] [PubMed]

114. Ferreira, M.C.; Whibley, N.; Mamo, A.J.; Siebenlist, U.; Chan, Y.R.; Gaffen, S.L. Interleukin-17-induced protein lipocalin 2 is dispensable for immunity to oral candidiasis. *Infect. Immun.* **2014**, *82*, 1030–1035. [CrossRef]

115. Conti, H.R.; Shen, F.; Nayyar, N.; Stocum, E.; Sun, J.N.; Lindemann, M.J.; Ho, A.W.; Hai, J.H.; Yu, J.J.; Jung, J.W.; et al. Th17 cells and IL-17 receptor signaling are essential for mucosal host defense against oral candidiasis. *J. Exp. Med.* **2009**, *206*, 299–311. [CrossRef]

116. Conti, H.R.; Gaffen, S.L. IL-17-mediated immunity to the opportunistic fungal pathogen Candida albicans. *J. Immunol.* **2015**, *195*, 780–788. [CrossRef]

117. Li, J.; Vinh, D.C.; Casanova, J.L.; Puel, A. Inborn errors of immunity underlying fungal diseases in otherwise healthy individuals. *Curr. Opin. Microbiol.* **2017**, *40*, 46–57. [CrossRef]

118. Sparber, F.; De Gregorio, C.; Steckholzer, S.; Ferreira, F.M.; Dolowschiak, T.; Ruchti, F.; Kirchner, F.R.; Mertens, S.; Prinz, I.; Joller, N.; et al. The skin commensal yeast Malassezia triggers a type 17 response that

coordinates anti-fungal immunity and exacerbates skin inflammation. *Cell Host Microbe* **2019**, *25*, 389–403. [CrossRef]

119. Wohn, C.; Brand, A.; van Ettinger, K.; Brouwers-Haspels, I.; Waisman, A.; Laman, J.D.; Clausen, B.E. Gradual development of psoriatic skin lesions by constitutive low-level expression of IL-17A. *Cell. Immunol.* **2016**, *308*, 57–65. [CrossRef]

120. Aggarwal, S.; Ghilardi, N.; Xie, M.H.; de Sauvage, F.J.; Gurney, A.L. Interleukin-23 promotes a distinct CD4 T cell activation state characterized by the production of interleukin-17. *J. Biol. Chem.* **2003**, *278*, 1910–1914. [CrossRef]

121. Ivanov, I.I.; McKenzie, B.S.; Zhou, L.; Tadokoro, C.E.; Lepelley, A.; Lafaille, J.J.; Cua, D.J.; Littman, D.R. The orphan nuclear receptor RORgammat directs the differentiation program of proinflammatory IL-17+ T helper cells. *Cell* **2006**, *126*, 1121–1133. [CrossRef] [PubMed]

122. Gaffen, S.L. Structure and signalling in the IL-17 receptor family. *Nat. Rev. Immunol.* **2009**, *9*, 556–567. [CrossRef] [PubMed]

123. Villegas, J.A.; Bayer, A.C.; Ider, K.; Bismuth, J.; Truffault, F.; Roussin, R.; Santelmo, N.; Le Panse, R.; Berrih-Aknin, S.; Dragin, N. Il-23/Th17 cell pathway: A promising target to alleviate thymic inflammation maintenance in myasthenia gravis. *J. Autoimmun.* **2019**, *98*, 59–73. [CrossRef] [PubMed]

124. Chan, J.R.; Blumenschein, W.; Murphy, E.; Diveu, C.; Wiekowski, M.; Abbondanzo, S.; Lucian, L.; Geissler, R.; Brodie, S.; Kimball, A.B.; et al. IL-23 stimulates epidermal hyperplasia via TNF and IL-20R2-dependent mechanisms with implications for psoriasis pathogenesis. *J. Exp. Med.* **2006**, *203*, 2577–2587. [CrossRef]

125. Furue, M.; Kadono, T. The contribution of IL-17 to the development of autoimmunity in psoriasis. *Innate Immun.* **2019**, *25*, 337–343. [CrossRef]

126. Arakawa, A.; Siewert, K.; Stöhr, J.; Besgen, P.; Kim, S.M.; Rühl, G.; Nickel, J.; Vollmer, S.; Thomas, P.; Krebs, S.; et al. Melanocyte antigen triggers autoimmunity in human psoriasis. *J. Exp. Med.* **2015**, *212*, 2203–2212. [CrossRef]

127. Lee, E.; Trepicchio, W.L.; Oestreicher, J.L.; Pittman, D.; Wang, F.; Chamian, F.; Dhodapkar, M.; Krueger, J.G. Increased expression of interleukin 23 p19 and p40 in lesional skin of patients with psoriasis vulgaris. *J. Exp. Med.* **2004**, *199*, 125–130. [CrossRef]

128. Zaba, L.C.; Cardinale, I.; Gilleaudeau, P.; Sullivan-Whalen, M.; Suárez-Fariñas, M.; Fuentes-Duculan, J.; Novitskaya, I.; Khatcherian, A.; Bluth, M.J.; Lowes, M.A.; et al. Amelioration of epidermal hyperplasia by TNF inhibition is associated with reduced Th17 responses. *J. Exp. Med.* **2007**, *204*, 3183–3194. [CrossRef]

129. Piskin, G.; Sylva-Steenland, R.M.; Bos, J.D.; Teunissen, M.B. In vitro and in situ expression of IL-23 by keratinocytes in healthy skin and psoriasis lesions: Enhanced expression in psoriatic skin. *J. Immunol.* **2006**, *176*, 1908–1915. [CrossRef]

130. Li, H.; Yao, Q.; Mariscal, A.G.; Wu, X.; Hülse, J.; Pedersen, E.; Helin, K.; Waisman, A.; Vinkel, C.; Thomsen, S.F.; et al. Epigenetic control of IL-23 expression in keratinocytes is important for chronic skin inflammation. *Nat. Commun.* **2018**, *9*, 1420. [CrossRef]

131. Tu, Z.; Zhang, S.; Zhou, G.; Zhou, L.; Xiang, Q.; Chen, Q.; Zhao, P.; Zhan, H.; Zhou, H.; Sun, L. LMO4 is a disease-provocative transcription coregulator activated by IL-23 in psoriatic keratinocytes. *J. Investig. Dermatol.* **2018**, *138*, 1078–1087. [CrossRef] [PubMed]

132. McInnes, I.B.; Kavanaugh, A.; Gottlieb, A.B.; Puig, L.; Rahman, P.; Ritchlin, C.; Brodmerkel, C.; Li, S.; Wang, Y.; Mendelsohn, A.M.; et al. Efficacy and safety of ustekinumab in patients with active psoriatic arthritis: 1 year results of the phase 3, multicentre, double-blind, placebo-controlled PSUMMIT 1 trial. *Lancet* **2013**, *382*, 780–789. [CrossRef]

133. Papp, K.A.; Blauvelt, A.; Bukhalo, M.; Gooderham, M.; Krueger, J.G.; Lacour, J.P.; Menter, A.; Philipp, S.; Sofen, H.; Tyring, S.; et al. Risankizumab versus ustekinumab for moderate-to-severe plaque psoriasis. *N. Engl. J. Med.* **2017**, *376*, 1551–1560. [CrossRef] [PubMed]

134. Blauvelt, A.; Papp, K.A.; Griffiths, C.E.; Randazzo, B.; Wasfi, Y.; Shen, Y.K.; Li, S.; Kimball, A.B. Efficacy and safety of guselkumab, an anti-interleukin-23 monoclonal antibody, compared with adalimumab for the continuous treatment of patients with moderate to severe psoriasis: Results from the phase III, double-blinded, placebo- and active comparator-controlled VOYAGE 1 trial. *J. Am. Acad. Dermatol.* **2017**, *76*, 405–417.

135. Reich, K.; Papp, K.A.; Blauvelt, A.; Tyring, S.K.; Sinclair, R.; Thaçi, D.; Nograles, K.; Mehta, A.; Cichanowitz, N.; Li, Q.; et al. Tildrakizumab versus placebo or etanercept for chronic plaque psoriasis (reSURFACE 1 and reSURFACE 2): Results from two randomised controlled, phase 3 trials. *Lancet* **2017**, *390*, 276–288. [CrossRef]

136. Johansen, C.; Usher, P.A.; Kellerup, R.B.; Lundsgaard, D.; Iversen, L.; Kragballe, K. Characterization of the interleukin-17 isoforms and receptors in lesional psoriatic skin. *Br. J. Dermatol.* **2009**, *160*, 319–324. [CrossRef]

137. Johnston, A.; Fritz, Y.; Dawes, S.M.; Diaconu, D.; Al-Attar, P.M.; Guzman, A.M.; Chen, C.S.; Fu, W.; Gudjonsson, J.E.; McCormick, T.S.; et al. Keratinocyte overexpression of IL-17C promotes psoriasiform skin inflammation. *J. Immunol.* **2013**, *190*, 2252–2262. [CrossRef]

138. Martin, D.A.; Towne, J.E.; Kricorian, G.; Klekotka, P.; Gudjonsson, J.E.; Krueger, J.G.; Russell, C.B. The emerging role of IL-17 in the pathogenesis of psoriasis: Preclinical and clinical findings. *J. Investig. Dermatol.* **2013**, *133*, 17–26. [CrossRef]

139. Ramirez-Carrozzi, V.; Sambandam, A.; Luis, E.; Lin, Z.; Jeet, S.; Lesch, J.; Hackney, J.; Kim, J.; Zhou, M.; Lai, J.; et al. IL-17C regulates the innate immune function of epithelial cells in an autocrine manner. *Nat. Immunol.* **2011**, *12*, 1159–1166. [CrossRef]

140. Vandeghinste, N.; Klattig, J.; Jagerschmidt, C.; Lavazais, S.; Marsais, F.; Haas, J.D.; Auberval, M.; Lauffer, F.; Moran, T.; Ongenaert, M.; et al. Neutralization of IL-17C reduces skin inflammation in mouse models of psoriasis and atopic dermatitis. *J. Investig. Dermatol.* **2018**, *138*, 1555–1563. [CrossRef]

141. Guttman-Yassky, E.; Krueger, J.G. IL-17C: A unique epithelial cytokine with potential for targeting across the spectrum of atopic dermatitis and psoriasis. *J. Investig. Dermatol.* **2018**, *138*, 1467–1469. [CrossRef] [PubMed]

142. Tsoi, L.C.; Rodriguez, E.; Degenhardt, F.; Baurecht, H.; Wehkamp, U.; Volks, N.; Szymczak, S.; Swindell, W.R.; Sarkar, M.K.; Raja, K.; et al. Atopic dermatitis is an IL-13-dominant disease with greater molecular heterogeneity compared to psoriasis. *J. Investig. Dermatol.* **2019**, *139*, 1480–1489. [CrossRef] [PubMed]

143. Pène, J.; Chevalier, S.; Preisser, L.; Vénéreau, E.; Guilleux, M.H.; Ghannam, S.; Molès, J.P.; Danger, Y.; Ravon, E.; Lesaux, S.; et al. Chronically inflamed human tissues are infiltrated by highly differentiated Th17 lymphocytes. *J. Immunol.* **2008**, *180*, 7423–7430. [CrossRef]

144. Lande, R.; Botti, E.; Jandus, C.; Dojcinovic, D.; Fanelli, G.; Conrad, C.; Chamilos, G.; Feldmeyer, L.; Marinari, B.; Chon, S.; et al. The antimicrobial peptide LL37 is a T-cell autoantigen in psoriasis. *Nat. Commun.* **2014**, *5*, 5621. [CrossRef] [PubMed]

145. Fuentes-Duculan, J.; Bonifacio, K.M.; Hawkes, J.E.; Kunjravia, N.; Cueto, I.; Li, X.; Gonzalez, J.; Garcet, S.; Krueger, J.G. Autoantigens ADAMTSL5 and LL37 are significantly upregulated in active Psoriasis and localized with keratinocytes, dendritic cells and other leukocytes. *Exp. Dermatol.* **2017**, *26*, 1075–1082. [CrossRef] [PubMed]

146. Yunusbaeva, M.; Valiev, R.; Bilalov, F.; Sultanova, Z.; Sharipova, L.; Yunusbayev, B. Psoriasis patients demonstrate HLA-Cw*06:02 allele dosage-dependent T cell proliferation when treated with hair follicle-derived keratin 17 protein. *Sci. Rep.* **2018**, *8*, 6098. [CrossRef] [PubMed]

147. Cheung, K.L.; Jarrett, R.; Subramaniam, S.; Salimi, M.; Gutowska-Owsiak, D.; Chen, Y.L.; Hardman, C.; Xue, L.; Cerundolo, V.; Ogg, G. Psoriatic T cells recognize neolipid antigens generated by mast cell phospholipase delivered by exosomes and presented by CD1a. *J. Exp. Med.* **2016**, *213*, 2399–2412. [CrossRef] [PubMed]

148. Chiricozzi, A.; Suárez-Fariñas, M.; Fuentes-Duculan, J.; Cueto, I.; Li, K.; Tian, S.; Brodmerkel, C.; Krueger, J.G. Increased expression of interleukin-17 pathway genes in nonlesional skin of moderate-to-severe psoriasis vulgaris. *Br. J. Dermatol.* **2016**, *174*, 136–145. [CrossRef] [PubMed]

149. Weisman, S.; Pollack, C.R.; Gottschalk, R.W. Psoriasis disease severity measures: Comparing efficacy of treatments for severe psoriasis. *J. Dermatolog. Treat.* **2003**, *14*, 158–165. [CrossRef] [PubMed]

150. Langley, R.G.; Elewski, B.E.; Lebwohl, M.; Reich, K.; Griffiths, C.E.; Papp, K.; Puig, L.; Nakagawa, H.; Spelman, L.; Sigurgeirsson, B.; et al. Secukinumab in plaque psoriasis—results of two phase 3 trials. *N. Engl. J. Med.* **2014**, *371*, 326–338. [CrossRef] [PubMed]

151. Gordon, K.B.; Blauvelt, A.; Papp, K.A.; Langley, R.G.; Luger, T.; Ohtsuki, M.; Reich, K.; Amato, D.; Ball, S.G.; Braun, D.K.; et al. Phase 3 trials of ixekizumab in moderate-to-severe plaque psoriasis. *N. Engl. J. Med.* **2016**, *375*, 345–356. [CrossRef] [PubMed]

152. Lebwohl, M.; Strober, B.; Menter, A.; Gordon, K.; Weglowska, J.; Puig, L.; Papp, K.; Spelman, L.; Toth, D.; Kerdel, F.; et al. Phase 3 studies comparing brodalumab with ustekinumab in psoriasis. *N. Engl. J. Med.* **2015**, *373*, 1318–1328. [CrossRef] [PubMed]

153. Paramio, J.M.; Casanova, M.L.; Segrelles, C.; Mittnacht, S.; Lane, E.B.; Jorcano, J.L. Modulation of cell proliferation by cytokeratins K10 and K16. *Mol. Cell Biol.* **1999**, *19*, 3086–3094. [CrossRef] [PubMed]

154. Krueger, J.G.; Ferris, L.K.; Menter, A.; Wagner, F.; White, A.; Visvanathan, S.; Lalovic, B.; Aslanyan, S.; Wang, E.E.; Hall, D.; et al. Anti-IL-23A mAb BI 655066 for treatment of moderate-to-severe psoriasis: Safety, efficacy, pharmacokinetics, and biomarker results of a single-rising-dose, randomized, double-blind, placebo-controlled trial. *J. Allergy Clin. Immunol.* **2015**, *136*, 116–124. [CrossRef] [PubMed]

155. Kulke, R.; Tödt-Pingel, I.; Rademacher, D.; Röwert, J.; Schröder, J.M.; Christophers, E. Co-localized overexpression of GRO-alpha and IL-8 mRNA is restricted to the suprapapillary layers of psoriatic lesions. *J. Investig. Dermatol.* **1996**, *106*, 526–530. [CrossRef] [PubMed]

156. Furue, K.; Yamamura, K.; Tsuji, G.; Mitoma, C.; Uchi, H.; Nakahara, T.; Kido-Nakahara, M.; Kadono, T.; Furue, M. Highlighting interleukin-36 signalling in plaque psoriasis and pustular psoriasis. *Acta Derm. Venereol.* **2018**, *98*, 5–13. [CrossRef] [PubMed]

157. Johnston, A.; Xing, X.; Guzman, A.M.; Riblett, M.; Loyd, C.M.; Ward, N.L.; Wohn, C.; Prens, E.P.; Wang, F.; Maier, L.E.; et al. IL-1F5, -F6, -F8, and -F9: A novel IL-1 family signaling system that is active in psoriasis and promotes keratinocyte antimicrobial peptide expression. *J. Immunol.* **2011**, *186*, 2613–2622. [CrossRef]

158. Homey, B.; Dieu-Nosjean, M.C.; Wiesenborn, A.; Massacrier, C.; Pin, J.J.; Oldham, E.; Catron, D.; Buchanan, M.E.; Müller, A.; de Waal Malefyt, R.; et al. Up-regulation of macrophage inflammatory protein-3 alpha/CCL20 and CC chemokine receptor 6 in psoriasis. *J. Immunol.* **2000**, *164*, 6621–6632. [CrossRef]

159. Kim, T.G.; Jee, H.; Fuentes-Duculan, J.; Wu, W.H.; Byamba, D.; Kim, D.S.; Kim, D.Y.; Lew, D.H.; Yang, W.I.; Krueger, J.G.; et al. Dermal clusters of mature dendritic cells and T cells are associated with the CCL20/CCR6 chemokine system in chronic psoriasis. *J. Investig. Dermatol.* **2014**, *134*, 1462–1465. [CrossRef]

160. Furue, K.; Ito, T.; Tsuji, G.; Nakahara, T.; Furue, M. The CCL20 and CCR6 axis in psoriasis. *Scand. J. Immunol.* **2019**. [CrossRef]

161. Bando, J.K.; Gilfillan, S.; Song, C.; McDonald, K.G.; Huang, S.C.; Newberry, R.D.; Kobayashi, Y.; Allan, D.S.J.; Carlyle, J.R.; Cella, M.; et al. The tumor necrosis factor superfamily member RANKL suppresses effector cytokine production in group 3 innate lymphoid cells. *Immunity* **2018**, *48*, 1208–1219. [CrossRef]

162. Talayero, P.; Mancebo, E.; Calvo-Pulido, J.; Rodríguez-Muñoz, S.; Bernardo, I.; Laguna-Goya, R.; Cano-Romero, F.L.; García-Sesma, A.; Loinaz, C.; Jiménez, C.; et al. Innate lymphoid cells groups 1 and 3 in the epithelial compartment of functional human intestinal allografts. *Am. J. Transplant.* **2016**, *16*, 72–82. [CrossRef]

163. Diani, M.; Casciano, F.; Marongiu, L.; Longhi, M.; Altomare, A.; Pigatto, P.D.; Secchiero, P.; Gambari, R.; Banfi, G.; Manfredi, A.A.; et al. Increased frequency of activated CD8(+) T cell effectors in patients with psoriatic arthritis. *Sci. Rep.* **2019**, *9*, 10870. [CrossRef]

164. Steel, K.J.A.; Srenathan, U.; Ridley, M.; Durham, L.E.; Wu, S.Y.; Ryan, S.E.; Hughes, C.D.; Chan, E.; Kirkham, B.W.; Taams, L.S. Synovial IL-17A+ CD8+ T cells display a polyfunctional, pro-inflammatory and tissue-resident memory phenotype and function in psoriatic arthritis. *Arthritis Rheumatol.* **2019**. [CrossRef]

165. Campbell, J.J.; Ebsworth, K.; Ertl, L.S.; McMahon, J.P.; Newland, D.; Wang, Y.; Liu, S.; Miao, Z.; Dang, T.; Zhang, P.; et al. IL-17-secreting γδ T Cells are completely dependent upon CCR6 for homing to inflamed skin. *J. Immunol.* **2017**, *199*, 3129–3136. [CrossRef]

166. Ishida-Yamamoto, A.; Iizuka, H. Differences in involucrin immunolabeling within cornified cell envelopes in normal and psoriatic epidermis. *J. Investig. Dermatol.* **1995**, *104*, 391–395. [CrossRef]

167. Caldwell, C.J.; Hobbs, C.; McKee, P.H. The relationship of Ki67 and involucrin expression in proliferative, pre-neoplastic and neoplastic skin. *Clin. Exp. Dermatol.* **1997**, *22*, 11–16. [CrossRef]

168. Krueger, J.G.; Fretzin, S.; Suárez-Fariñas, M.; Haslett, P.A.; Phipps, K.M.; Cameron, G.S.; McColm, J.; Katcherian, A.; Cueto, I.; White, T.; et al. IL-17A is essential for cell activation and inflammatory gene circuits in subjects with psoriasis. *J. Allergy Clin. Immunol.* **2012**, *130*, 145–154.e9. [CrossRef] [PubMed]

169. Chiricozzi, A.; Nograles, K.E.; Johnson-Huang, L.M.; Fuentes-Duculan, J.; Cardinale, I.; Bonifacio, K.M.; Gulati, N.; Mitsui, H.; Guttman-Yassky, E.; Suárez-Fariñas, M.; et al. IL-17 induces an expanded range of downstream genes in reconstituted human epidermis model. *PLoS ONE* **2014**, *9*, e90284. [CrossRef] [PubMed]

170. Ha, H.L.; Wang, H.; Pisitkun, P.; Kim, J.C.; Tassi, I.; Tang, W.; Morasso, M.I.; Udey, M.C.; Siebenlist, U. IL-17 drives psoriatic inflammation via distinct, target cell-specific mechanisms. *Proc. Natl. Acad. Sci. USA* **2014**, *111*, E3422–E3431. [CrossRef] [PubMed]

171. Ma, W.Y.; Jia, K.; Zhang, Y. IL-17 promotes keratinocyte proliferation via the downregulation of C/EBPα. *Exp. Ther. Med.* **2016**, *11*, 631–636. [CrossRef] [PubMed]

172. Zenobia, C.; Hajishengallis, G. Basic biology and role of interleukin-17 in immunity and inflammation. *Periodontol. 2000.* **2015**, *69*, 142–159. [CrossRef] [PubMed]

173. Chiricozzi, A.; Guttman-Yassky, E.; Suárez-Fariñas, M.; Nograles, K.E.; Tian, S.; Cardinale, I.; Chimenti, S.; Krueger, J.G. Integrative responses to IL-17 and TNF-α in human keratinocytes account for key inflammatory pathogenic circuits in psoriasis. *J. Investig. Dermatol.* **2011**, *131*, 677–687. [CrossRef] [PubMed]

174. Lawrence, T. The nuclear factor NF-kappaB pathway in inflammation. *Cold Spring Harb. Perspect. Biol.* **2009**, *1*, a001651. [CrossRef] [PubMed]

175. House, J.S.; Zhu, S.; Ranjan, R.; Linder, K.; Smart, R.C. C/EBPalpha and C/EBPbeta are required for Sebocyte differentiation and stratified squamous differentiation in adult mouse skin. *PLoS ONE* **2010**, *5*, e9837. [CrossRef] [PubMed]

176. Crish, J.F.; Gopalakrishnan, R.; Bone, F.; Gilliam, A.C.; Eckert, R.L. The distal and proximal regulatory regions of the involucrin gene promoter have distinct functions and are required for in vivo involucrin expression. *J. Investig. Dermatol.* **2006**, *126*, 305–314. [CrossRef] [PubMed]

177. Witte, E.; Kokolakis, G.; Witte, K.; Philipp, S.; Doecke, W.D.; Babel, N.; Wittig, B.M.; Warszawska, K.; Kurek, A.; Erdmann-Keding, M.; et al. IL-19 is a component of the pathogenetic IL-23/IL-17 cascade in psoriasis. *J. Investig. Dermatol.* **2014**, *134*, 2757–2767. [CrossRef]

178. Sun, D.P.; Yeh, C.H.; So, E.; Wang, L.Y.; Wei, T.S.; Chang, M.S.; Hsing, C.H. Interleukin (IL)-19 promoted skin wound healing by increasing fibroblast keratinocyte growth factor expression. *Cytokine* **2013**, *62*, 360–368. [CrossRef]

179. Yang, L.; Fan, X.; Cui, T.; Dang, E.; Wang, G. Nrf2 promotes keratinocyte proliferation in psoriasis through up-regulation of keratin 6, keratin 16, and keratin 17. *J. Investig. Dermatol.* **2017**, *137*, 2168–2176. [CrossRef]

180. Paladini, R.D.; Coulombe, P.A. Directed expression of keratin 16 to the progenitor basal cells of transgenic mouse skin delays skin maturation. *J. Cell Biol.* **1998**, *142*, 1035–1051. [CrossRef]

181. Acciani, T.H.; Suzuki, T.; Trapnell, B.C.; Le Cras, T.D. Epidermal growth factor receptor signalling regulates granulocyte-macrophage colony-stimulating factor production by airway epithelial cells and established allergic airway disease. *Clin. Exp. Allergy* **2016**, *46*, 317–328. [CrossRef] [PubMed]

182. Furue, K.; Ito, T.; Tanaka, Y.; Hashimoto-Hachiya, A.; Takemura, M.; Murata, M.; Kido-Nakahara, M.; Tsuji, G.; Nakahara, T.; Furue, M. The EGFR-ERK/JNK-CCL20 pathway in scratched keratinocytes may underpin koebnerization in psoriasis atients. *Int. J. Mol. Sci.* **2020**, *21*, 434. [CrossRef] [PubMed]

183. Johnston, A.; Gudjonsson, J.E.; Aphale, A.; Guzman, A.M.; Stoll, S.W.; Elder, J.T. EGFR and IL-1 signaling synergistically promote keratinocyte antimicrobial defenses in a differentiation-dependent manner. *J. Investig. Dermatol.* **2011**, *131*, 329–337. [CrossRef] [PubMed]

184. Goepel, L.; Jacobi, A.; Augustin, M.; Radtke, M.A. Rapid improvement of psoriasis in a patient with lung cancer after treatment with erlotinib. *J. Eur. Acad. Dermatol. Venereol.* **2018**, *32*, e311–e313. [CrossRef] [PubMed]

185. Overbeck, T.R.; Griesinger, F. Two cases of psoriasis responding to erlotinib: Time to revisiting inhibition of epidermal growth factor receptor in psoriasis therapy? *Dermatology* **2012**, *225*, 179–182. [CrossRef]

186. Trivin, F.; Boucher, E.; Raoul, J.L. Complete sustained regression of extensive psoriasis with cetuximab combination chemotherapy. *Acta Oncol.* **2004**, *43*, 592–593. [CrossRef]

187. Neyns, B.; Meert, V.; Vandenbroucke, F. Cetuximab treatment in a patient with metastatic colorectal cancer and psoriasis. *Curr. Oncol.* **2008**, *15*, 196–197. [CrossRef]

188. Carrier, Y.; Ma, H.L.; Ramon, H.E.; Napierata, L.; Small, C.; O'Toole, M.; Young, D.A.; Fouser, L.A.; Nickerson-Nutter, C.; Collins, M.; et al. Inter-regulation of Th17 cytokines and the IL-36 cytokines in vitro and in vivo: Implications in psoriasis pathogenesis. *J. Investig. Dermatol.* **2011**, *131*, 2428–2437. [CrossRef]

189. Gläser, R.; Meyer-Hoffert, U.; Harder, J.; Cordes, J.; Wittersheim, M.; Kobliakova, J.; Fölster-Holst, R.; Proksch, E.; Schröder, J.M.; Schwarz, T. The antimicrobial protein psoriasin (S100A7) is upregulated in atopic dermatitis and after experimental skin barrier disruption. *J. Investig. Dermatol.* **2009**, *129*, 641–649. [CrossRef]

190. Nograles, K.E.; Zaba, L.C.; Guttman-Yassky, E.; Fuentes-Duculan, J.; Suárez-Fariñas, M.; Cardinale, I.; Khatcherian, A.; Gonzalez, J.; Pierson, K.C.; White, T.R.; et al. Th17 cytokines interleukin (IL)-17 and IL-22 modulate distinct inflammatory and keratinocyte-response pathways. *Br. J. Dermatol.* **2008**, *159*, 1092–1102. [CrossRef]

191. Baggiolini, M. Chemokines in pathology and medicine. *J. Intern. Med.* **2001**, *250*, 91–104. [CrossRef] [PubMed]

192. Johnston, A.; Xing, X.; Wolterink, L.; Barnes, D.H.; Yin, Z.; Reingold, L.; Kahlenberg, J.M.; Harms, P.W.; Gudjonsson, J.E. IL-1 and IL-36 are dominant cytokines in generalized pustular psoriasis. *J. Allergy Clin. Immunol.* **2017**, *140*, 109–120. [CrossRef] [PubMed]

193. Nedoszytko, B.; Sokołowska-Wojdyło, M.; Ruckemann-Dziurdzińska, K.; Roszkiewicz, J.; Nowicki, R.J. Chemokines and cytokines network in the pathogenesis of the inflammatory skin diseases: Atopic dermatitis, psoriasis and skin mastocytosis. *Postepy. Dermatol. Alergol.* **2014**, *31*, 84–91. [CrossRef] [PubMed]

194. Li, N.; Yamasaki, K.; Saito, R.; Fukushi-Takahashi, S.; Shimada-Omori, R.; Asano, M.; Aiba, S. Alarmin function of cathelicidin antimicrobial peptide LL37 through IL-36γ induction in human epidermal keratinocytes. *J. Immunol.* **2014**, *193*, 5140–5148. [CrossRef] [PubMed]

195. Henry, C.M.; Sullivan, G.P.; Clancy, D.M.; Afonina, I.S.; Kulms, D.; Martin, S.J. Neutrophil-derived proteases escalate inflammation through activation of IL-36 family cytokines. *Cell Rep.* **2016**, *14*, 708–722. [CrossRef]

196. Pfaff, C.M.; Marquardt, Y.; Fietkau, K.; Baron, J.M.; Lüscher, B. The psoriasis-associated IL-17A induces and cooperates with IL-36 cytokines to control keratinocyte differentiation and function. *Sci. Rep.* **2017**, *7*, 15631. [CrossRef]

197. Muhr, P.; Zeitvogel, J.; Heitland, I.; Werfel, T.; Wittmann, M. Expression of interleukin (IL)-1 family members upon stimulation with IL-17 differs in keratinocytes derived from patients with psoriasis and healthy donors. *Br. J. Dermatol.* **2011**, *165*, 189–193. [CrossRef]

198. Gabay, C.; Towne, J.E. Regulation and function of interleukin-36 cytokines in homeostasis and pathological conditions. *J. Leukoc. Biol.* **2015**, *97*, 645–652. [CrossRef]

199. Madonna, S.; Girolomoni, G.; Dinarello, C.A.; Albanesi, C. The significance of IL-36 hyperactivation and IL-36R targeting in psoriasis. *Int. J. Mol. Sci.* **2019**, *20*, 3318. [CrossRef]

200. Bachelez, H.; Choon, S.E.; Marrakchi, S.; Burden, A.D.; Tsai, T.F.; Morita, A.; Turki, H.; Hall, D.B.; Shear, M.; Baum, P.; et al. Inhibition of the interleukin-36 pathway for the treatment of generalized pustular psoriasis. *N. Engl. J. Med.* **2019**, *380*, 981–983. [CrossRef]

201. Furue, K.; Ito, T.; Tanaka, Y.; Yumine, A.; Hashimoto-Hachiya, A.; Takemura, M.; Murata, M.; Yamamura, K.; Tsuji, G.; Furue, M. Cyto/chemokine profile of in vitro scratched keratinocyte model: Implications of significant upregulation of CCL20, CXCL8 and IL36G in Koebner phenomenon. *J. Dermatol. Sci.* **2019**, *94*, 244–251. [CrossRef] [PubMed]

202. Maecker, H.T.; McCoy, J.P.; Nussenblatt, R. Standardizing immunophenotyping for the Human Immunology Project. *Nat. Rev. Immunol.* **2012**, *12*, 191–200. [CrossRef]

203. Singh, S.P.; Zhang, H.H.; Foley, J.F.; Hedrick, M.N.; Farber, J.M. Human T cells that are able to produce IL-17 express the chemokine receptor CCR6. *J. Immunol.* **2008**, *180*, 214–221. [CrossRef] [PubMed]

204. Harper, E.G.; Guo, C.; Rizzo, H.; Lillis, J.V.; Kurtz, S.E.; Skorcheva, I.; Purdy, D.; Fitch, E.; Iordanov, M.; Blauvelt, A. Th17 cytokines stimulate CCL20 expression in keratinocytes in vitro and in vivo: Implications for psoriasis pathogenesis. *J. Investig. Dermatol.* **2009**, *129*, 2175–2183. [CrossRef] [PubMed]

205. Bouma, G.; Zamuner, S.; Hicks, K.; Want, A.; Oliveira, J.; Choudhury, A.; Brett, S.; Robertson, D.; Felton, L.; Norris, V.; et al. CCL20 neutralization by a monoclonal antibody in healthy subjects selectively inhibits recruitment of CCR6(+) cells in an experimental suction blister. *Br. J. Clin. Pharmacol.* **2017**, *83*, 1976–1990. [CrossRef] [PubMed]

206. Robert, R.; Ang, C.; Sun, G.; Juglair, L.; Lim, E.X.; Mason, L.J.; Payne, N.L.; Bernard, C.C.; Mackay, C.R. Essential role for CCR6 in certain inflammatory diseases demonstrated using specific antagonist and knockin mice. *JCI. Insight* **2017**, *2*. [CrossRef]

207. Tawaraishi, T.; Sakauchi, N.; Hidaka, K.; Yoshikawa, K.; Okui, T.; Kuno, H.; Chisaki, I.; Aso, K. Identification of a novel series of potent and selective CCR6 inhibitors as biological probes. *Bioorg. Med. Chem. Lett.* **2018**, *28*, 3067–3072. [CrossRef]

208. Campbell, J.J.; Ebsworth, K.; Ertl, L.S.; McMahon, J.P.; Wang, Y.; Yau, S.; Mali, V.R.; Chhina, V.; Kumamoto, A.; Liu, S.; et al. Efficacy of chemokine receptor inhibition in treating IL-36α-induced psoriasiform inflammation. *J. Immunol.* **2019**, *202*, 1687–1692. [CrossRef]

209. Mose, M.; Kang, Z.; Raaby, L.; Iversen, L.; Johansen, C. TNFα- and IL-17A-mediated S100A8 expression is regulated by p38 MAPK. *Exp. Dermatol.* **2013**, *22*, 476–481. [CrossRef]

210. Liang, S.C.; Tan, X.Y.; Luxenberg, D.P.; Karim, R.; Dunussi-Joannopoulos, K.; Collins, M.; Fouser, L.A. Interleukin (IL)-22 and IL-17 are coexpressed by Th17 cells and cooperatively enhance expression of antimicrobial peptides. *J. Exp. Med.* **2006**, *203*, 2271–2279. [CrossRef]

211. D'Amico, F.; Skarmoutsou, E.; Granata, M.; Trovato, C.; Rossi, G.A.; Mazzarino, M.C. S100A7: A rAMPing up AMP molecule in psoriasis. *Cytokine Growth Factor Rev.* **2016**, *32*, 97–104. [CrossRef] [PubMed]

212. Sa, S.M.; Valdez, P.A.; Wu, J.; Jung, K.; Zhong, F.; Hall, L.; Kasman, I.; Winer, J.; Modrusan, Z.; Danilenko, D.M.; et al. The effects of IL-20 subfamily cytokines on reconstituted human epidermis suggest potential roles in cutaneous innate defense and pathogenic adaptive immunity in psoriasis. *J. Immunol.* **2007**, *178*, 2229–2240. [CrossRef] [PubMed]

213. Hegyi, Z.; Zwicker, S.; Bureik, D.; Peric, M.; Koglin, S.; Batycka-Baran, A.; Prinz, J.C.; Ruzicka, T.; Schauber, J.; Wolf, R. Vitamin D analog calcipotriol suppresses the Th17 cytokine-induced proinflammatory S100 "alarmins" psoriasin (S100A7) and koebnerisin (S100A15) in psoriasis. *J. Investig. Dermatol.* **2012**, *132*, 1416–1424. [CrossRef] [PubMed]

214. Hsu, K.; Champaiboon, C.; Guenther, B.D.; Sorenson, B.S.; Khammanivong, A.; Ross, K.F.; Geczy, C.L.; Herzberg, M.C. Anti-infective protective properties of S100 calgranulins. *Antiinflamm. Antiallergy Agents Med. Chem.* **2009**, *8*, 290–305. [CrossRef]

215. Kolbinger, F.; Loesche, C.; Valentin, M.A.; Jiang, X.; Cheng, Y.; Jarvis, P.; Peters, T.; Calonder, C.; Bruin, G.; Polus, F.; et al. β-Defensin 2 is a responsive biomarker of IL-17A-driven skin pathology in patients with psoriasis. *J. Allergy Clin. Immunol.* **2017**, *139*, 923–932. [CrossRef]

216. Yan, W.X.; Armishaw, C.; Goyette, J.; Yang, Z.; Cai, H.; Alewood, P.; Geczy, C.L. Mast cell and monocyte recruitment by S100A12 and its hinge domain. *J. Biol. Chem.* **2008**, *283*, 13035–13043. [CrossRef]

217. Nukui, T.; Ehama, R.; Sakaguchi, M.; Sonegawa, H.; Katagiri, C.; Hibino, T.; Huh, N.H. S100A8/A9, a key mediator for positive feedback growth stimulation of normal human keratinocytes. *J. Cell Biochem.* **2008**, *104*, 453–464. [CrossRef]

218. Muta, T. IkappaB-zeta: An inducible regulator of nuclear factor-kappaB. *Vitam. Horm.* **2006**, *74*, 301–316.

219. Bertelsen, T.; Iversen, L.; Johansen, C. The human IL-17A/F heterodimer regulates psoriasis-associated genes through IκBζ. *Exp. Dermatol.* **2018**, *27*, 1048–1052. [CrossRef]

220. Muromoto, R.; Hirao, T.; Tawa, K.; Hirashima, K.; Kon, S.; Kitai, Y.; Matsuda, T. IL-17A plays a central role in the expression of psoriasis signature genes through the induction of IκB-ζ in keratinocytes. *Int. Immunol.* **2016**, *28*, 443–452. [CrossRef]

221. Dorschner, R.A.; Pestonjamasp, V.K.; Tamakuwala, S.; Ohtake, T.; Rudisill, J.; Nizet, V.; Agerberth, B.; Gudmundsson, G.H.; Gallo, R.L. Cutaneous injury induces the release of cathelicidin anti-microbial peptides active against group A Streptococcus. *J. Investig. Dermatol.* **2001**, *117*, 91–97. [CrossRef] [PubMed]

222. Reinholz, M.; Ruzicka, T.; Schauber, J. Cathelicidin LL-37: An antimicrobial peptide with a role in inflammatory skin disease. *Ann. Dermatol.* **2012**, *24*, 126–135. [CrossRef] [PubMed]

223. Tomasinsig, L.; Pizzirani, C.; Skerlavaj, B.; Pellegatti, P.; Gulinelli, S.; Tossi, A.; Di Virgilio, F.; Zanetti, M. The human cathelicidin LL-37 modulates the activities of the P2X7 receptor in a structure-dependent manner. *J. Biol. Chem.* **2008**, *283*, 30471–30481. [CrossRef] [PubMed]

224. Di Nardo, A.; Braff, M.H.; Taylor, K.R.; Na, C.; Granstein, R.D.; McInturff, J.E.; Krutzik, S.; Modlin, R.L.; Gallo, R.L. Cathelicidin antimicrobial peptides block dendritic cell TLR4 activation and allergic contact sensitization. *J. Immunol.* **2007**, *178*, 1829–1834. [CrossRef]

225. Tokumaru, S.; Sayama, K.; Shirakata, Y.; Komatsuzawa, H.; Ouhara, K.; Hanakawa, Y.; Yahata, Y.; Dai, X.; Tohyama, M.; Nagai, H.; et al. Induction of keratinocyte migration via transactivation of the epidermal growth factor receptor by the antimicrobial peptide LL-37. *J. Immunol.* **2005**, *175*, 4662–4668. [CrossRef]

226. Hu, S.C.; Yu, H.S.; Yen, F.L.; Lin, C.L.; Chen, G.S.; Lan, C.C. Neutrophil extracellular trap formation is increased in psoriasis and induces human β-defensin-2 production in epidermal keratinocytes. *Sci. Rep.* **2016**, *6*, 31119. [CrossRef]

227. Lande, R.; Gregorio, J.; Facchinetti, V.; Chatterjee, B.; Wang, Y.H.; Homey, B.; Cao, W.; Wang, Y.H.; Su, B.; Nestle, F.O.; et al. Plasmacytoid dendritic cells sense self-DNA coupled with antimicrobial peptide. *Nature* **2007**, *449*, 564–569. [CrossRef]

228. Mabuchi, T.; Hirayama, N. Binding affinity and interaction of LL-37 with HLA-C*06:02 in psoriasis. *J. Investig. Dermatol.* **2016** *136*, 1901–1903. [CrossRef]

229. Takahashi, T.; Kulkarni, N.N.; Lee, E.Y.; Zhang, L.J.; Wong, G.C.L.; Gallo, R.L. Cathelicidin promotes inflammation by enabling binding of self-RNA to cell surface scavenger receptors. *Sci. Rep.* **2018**, *8*, 4032. [CrossRef]
230. Ong, P.Y.; Ohtake, T.; Brandt, C.; Strickland, I.; Boguniewicz, M.; Ganz, T.; Gallo, R.L.; Leung, D.Y. Endogenous antimicrobial peptides and skin infections in atopic dermatitis. *N. Engl. J. Med.* **2002**, *347*, 1151–1160. [CrossRef]
231. de Jongh, G.J.; Zeeuwen, P.L.; Kucharekova, M.; Pfundt, R.; van der Valk, P.G.; Blokx, W.; Dogan, A.; Hiemstra, P.S.; van de Kerkhof, P.C.; Schalkwijk, J. High expression levels of keratinocyte antimicrobial proteins in psoriasis compared with atopic dermatitis. *J. Investig. Dermatol.* **2005**, *125*, 1163–1173. [CrossRef] [PubMed]
232. Nomura, I.; Goleva, E.; Howell, M.D.; Hamid, Q.A.; Ong, P.Y.; Hall, C.F.; Darst, M.A.; Gao, B.; Boguniewicz, M.; Travers, J.B.; et al. Cytokine milieu of atopic dermatitis, as compared to psoriasis, skin prevents induction of innate immune response genes. *J. Immunol.* **2003**, *171*, 3262–3269. [CrossRef] [PubMed]
233. Yang, D.; Chertov, O.; Bykovskaia, S.N.; Chen, Q.; Buffo, M.J.; Shogan, J.; Anderson, M.; Schröder, J.M.; Wang, J.M.; Howard, O.M.; et al. Beta-defensins: Linking innate and adaptive immunity through dendritic and T cell CCR6. *Science* **1999**, *286*, 525–528. [CrossRef] [PubMed]
234. Ghannam, S.; Dejou, C.; Pedretti, N.; Giot, J.P.; Dorgham, K.; Boukhaddaoui, H.; Deleuze, V.; Bernard, F.X.; Jorgensen, C.; Yssel, H.; et al. CCL20 and β-defensin-2 induce arrest of human Th17 cells on inflamed endothelium in vitro under flow conditions. *J. Immunol.* **2011**, *186*, 1411–1420. [CrossRef] [PubMed]

7

Systemic Dermatitis Model Mice Exhibit Atrophy of Visceral Adipose Tissue and Increase Stromal Cells via Skin-Derived Inflammatory Cytokines

Kento Mizutani [1,†], **Eri Shirakami** [1,2,†], **Masako Ichishi** [3], **Yoshiaki Matsushima** [1], **Ai Umaoka** [1], **Karin Okada** [1], **Yukie Yamaguchi** [4], **Masatoshi Watanabe** [3], **Eishin Morita** [2] and **Keiichi Yamanaka** [1,*]

[1] Department of Dermatology, Graduate School of Medicine, Mie University, Mie, Tsu 514-8507, Japan; k-mizutani@clin.medic.mie-u.ac (K.M.); white818@med.shimane-u.ac.jp (E.S.); matsushima-y@clin.medi.mie-u.ac (Y.M.); ai618lovemyfamily@yahoo.co.jp (A.U.); okadakarin@clin.medic.mie-u.ac.jp (K.O.)

[2] Department of Dermatology, Faculty of Medicine, Shimane University, Shimane, Izumo 693-8501, Japan; emorita@med.shimane-u.ac.jp

[3] Department of Oncologic Pathology, Graduate School of Medicine, Mie University, Mie, Tsu 514-8507, Japan; masako-i@doc.medic.mie-u.ac.jp (M.I.); mawata@doc.medic.mie-u.ac.jp (M.W.)

[4] Department of Environmental Immuno-Dermatology, School of Medicine, Yokohama City University Graduate, Yokohama 236-0027, Japan; yui1783@yokohama-cu.ac.jp

* Correspondence: yamake@clin.medic.mie-u.ac.jp

† These authors contributed equally to this work.

Abstract: Adipose tissue (AT) is the largest endocrine organ, producing bioactive products called adipocytokines, which regulate several metabolic pathways, especially in inflammatory conditions. On the other hand, there is evidence that chronic inflammatory skin disease is closely associated with vascular sclerotic changes, cardiomegaly, and severe systemic amyloidosis in multiple organs. In psoriasis, a common chronic intractable inflammatory skin disease, several studies have shown that adipokine levels are associated with disease severity. Chronic skin disease is also associated with metabolic syndrome, including abnormal tissue remodeling; however, the mechanism is still unclear. We addressed this problem using keratin 14-specific caspase-1 overexpressing transgenic (KCASP1Tg) mice with severe erosive dermatitis from 8 weeks of age, followed by re-epithelization. The whole body and gonadal white AT (GWAT) weights were decreased. Each adipocyte was large in number, small in size and irregularly shaped; abundant inflammatory cells, including activated CD4+ or CD8+ T cells and toll-like receptor 4/CD11b-positive activated monocytes, infiltrated into the GWAT. We assumed that inflammatory cytokine production in skin lesions was the key factor for this lymphocyte/monocyte activation and AT dysregulation. We tested our hypothesis that the AT in a mouse dermatitis model shows an impaired thermogenesis ability due to systemic inflammation. After exposure to 4 °C, the mRNA expression of the thermogenic gene uncoupling protein 1 in adipocytes was elevated; however, the body temperature of the KCASP1Tg mice decreased rapidly, revealing an impaired thermogenesis ability of the AT due to atrophy. Tumor necrosis factor (TNF)-α, IL-1β and interferon (INF)-γ levels were significantly increased in KCASP1Tg mouse ear skin lesions. To investigate the direct effects of these cytokines, BL/6 wild mice were administered intraperitoneal TNF-α, IL-1β and INF-γ injections, which resulted in small adipocytes with abundant stromal cell infiltration, suggesting those cytokines have a synergistic effect on adipocytes. The systemic dermatitis model mice showed atrophy of AT and increased stromal cells. These findings were reproducible by the intraperitoneal administration of inflammatory cytokines whose production was increased in inflamed skin lesions.

Keywords: skin inflammation; cytokine; adipose tissue; adiponectin; leptin; thermogenesis

---

1. Introduction

Adipose tissue (AT) is the largest endocrine organ, producing bioactive products called adipocytokines, which regulate several metabolic pathways [1]. AT inflammation induces the dysregulation of adipocytokine production, which plays a critical role in the pathophysiology of atherosclerosis [2]. It is well known that obesity induces AT inflammation and contributes to vascular and AT changes, which may lead to the development of metabolic syndrome. Metabolic syndrome induces insulin resistance that causes hyperglycemia and diabetes, and causes dyslipidemia such as hypertriglyceridemia and low HDL cholesterol, which are risk factors for cardiovascular disorders [3]. In addition, obese AT causes increased angiogenesis, immune cell infiltration, the overproduction of extracellular matrix, and the increased production of pro-inflammatory adipocytokines [4]. As a result, the risks of ischemic heart disease and cerebral strokes increase.

Chronic inflammatory skin disease is also associated with metabolic syndrome [5–7]. However, the mechanism is under discussion, and the contribution of AT is still unclear. We addressed this problem by using keratin 14-specific human caspase-1 overexpressing transgenic (KCASP1Tg) mice, which are accepted as a spontaneous dermatitis model [8]. Caspase-1 is a cytoplasmic cysteine protease characterized by its ability to process the inactive pro-interleukin-1β (IL-1β) into the biologically active IL-1β [9]. IL-1β is an inflammatory cytokine that plays a key role in inflammation and keratinocyte activation. KCASP1Tg mice show severe erosive dermatitis from 8 weeks old, followed by re-epithelization and the development of parakeratotic scale-crust [8]. It was previously reported that a sustained circulating low level of IL-1α/β derived from severe dermatitis causes vascular sclerotic changes, cardiomegaly, and severe systemic amyloidosis in multiple organs [10].

In this study, we aimed to investigate the influence of chronic dermatitis in the pathological and functional changes in AT using a KCASP1Tg mouse model.

2. Results

2.1. GWAT Weight Is Decreased, and Inflammation Affects AT Atrophy

We measured whole-body and GWAT weights with a precision electronic balance to evaluate the effect of dermatitis on the AT. The whole-body and GWAT weights were significantly lower in KCASP1Tg than in wild littermate mice at 10 weeks of age (Figure 1A,B). Next, we evaluated the phenotype of adipocytes in GWAT using hematoxylin and eosin staining (HE). In KCASP1Tg mice, adipocytes were small in size and irregularly shaped compared to in wild type mice (Figure 1C). Abundant mononuclear cell infiltration compared to in control mice suggests the so-called burnout or worn out condition of the adipocytes. We performed immunohistochemical (IHC) staining to identify the stromal cells of AT such as T cells, monocytes and neutrophils. The infiltration of inflammatory cells such as lymphocytes, monocytes and neutrophils was slightly higher in KCASP1Tg mice compared to that in wild type littermates (Figure 1D).

Figure 1. *Cont.*

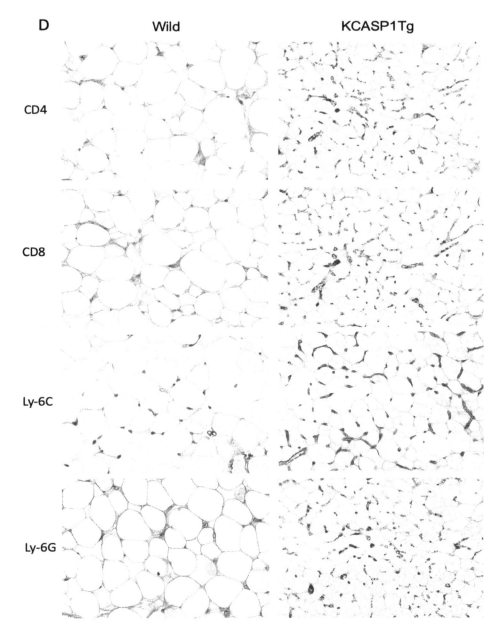

Figure 1. KCASP1Tg mice showed low gonadal white adipose tissue (GWAT) weights and degenerated adipose tissue (AT). (**A**) The whole body and (**B**) GWAT weights were decreased in KCASP1Tg compared to wild littermate mice at 10 weeks of age. (**C**) Representative photomicrographs of the hematoxylin and eosin (HE) (×400) staining of the GWAT of wild littermate and KCASP1Tg mice at 10 weeks of age. Histological sections were 3.5 μm thick. Adipocyte number and adipocyte area were measured by using ImageJ and Adiposoft (three parts of each slide, $n = 3$ in each group). Adipocytes were significantly smaller and larger in number in KCASP1Tg. (**D**) Immunohistochemical staining (×400) was performed to characterize stromal cells. Lymphocytes, monocytes and neutrophils were slightly higher in KCASP1Tg but not significantly so. ** $p < 0.01$, **** $p < 0.0001$ versus control.

2.2. Activated T Cells and Monocytes Infiltrated the AT

We assessed the number or proportion and characteristic composition of the stromal cells infiltrating the GWAT by flow cytometry. The number of infiltrated stromal cells, including lymphocytes and monocytes, was significantly increased in KCASP1Tg mice (Figure 2A). Next, we verified the characteristics of the lymphocytes and monocytes. We measured the proportion of the CD25+ T cells (Figure 2B). Activated T cells, both CD4+ and CD8+, were increased in KCASP1Tg mice (Figure 2C).

Additionally, we measured the proportion of regulatory T cells by using CD127, CD4, CD25 and Foxp3 antibodies (Figure 2D). The regulatory T cells were increased in KCASP1Tg, but there was no significant difference (Figure 2E). Finally, we measured the number of TLR4+ CD11b+ monocytes and proportion of Ly-6C+ CD11b+ monocytes TLR4+ CD11b+ monocytes were significantly increased in KCASP1Tg, and Ly-6C+ CD11b+ monocytes were also increased (Figure 2F,G).

Figure 2. AT cell infiltration in KCASP1Tg mice. (**A**) Flow cytometric analysis of infiltrated stromal cells in GWAT. The black and red circles correspond to the lymphocyte and monocyte populations, respectively, in the left figure. Stromal cell infiltration, including lymphocytes and monocytes, was significantly increased in KCASP1Tg mice. (**B,C**) The population of CD25+ activated lymphocytes was measured in CD4+ or CD8+ lymphocytes. Activated T cells were significantly increased in KCASP1Tg. (**D,E**) The proportion of regulatory T cells in AT was measured. There was no significant difference between KCASP1Tg and wild mice. (**F,G**) The proportion of Ly-6C+ CD11b+ and number of TLR4+ CD11b+ activated monocytes were evaluated and increased in the AT of KCASP1Tg mice. $n = 5$–6 in each group. * $p < 0.05$, ** $p < 0.01$ versus control.

2.3. Expression of Inflammation-Related Cytokine Levels in AT

An adipocytokine is a physiologically active substance secreted from adipocytes, and the amount secreted also changes depending on the environment of the adipocytes. Representative adipocytokines such as adiponectin, TNF-α, leptin and MCP-1 were analyzed in the adipocytes of GWAT using a specific ELISA kit (Figure 3). The TNF-α level was significantly elevated in KCASP1Tg mice compared to in controls. Conversely, KCASP1Tg mice showed a lower leptin level.

Figure 3. Adipokine expression in AT. We quantified adipocytokines such as adiponectin, TNF-α, leptin and MCP-1 from the adipocytes of GWAT by using a specific ELISA kit. The TNF-α level was elevated in KCASP1Tg mice compared to in controls; conversely, the leptin level was decreased in KCASP1Tg ($n = 5$ in each group). * $p < 0.05$ and ** $p < 0.01$ versus control.

2.4. Changes in UCP1 Expression after Cold Exposure

HSP90, IL-33 and UCP-1 are deeply involved in thermogenesis in adipocytes, and their expression is increased by cold exposure or adrenergic stimulation. We investigated the heat production upon cold exposure challenge and the expression of these thermogenic genes. After 4 °C cold exposure, the mRNA expression of HSP90, IL-33 and UCP1 in adipocytes was quantified using real time-PCR. The mRNA expression of HSP90 and IL-33 was significantly decreased in KCASP1Tg mice (Figure 4A). Although the mRNA expression of UCP1 was significantly increased in KCASP1Tg mice (Figure 4A), the body temperature decreased more rapidly upon exposure to the cold environment, and the KCASP1Tg mice could not survive for a long time (Figure 4B).

Figure 4. mRNA expression of heat-related proteins in GWAT after cold exposure. (**A**) The mRNA expression of HSP90 and IL-33 was decreased, while that of UCP1 was increased in the adipocytes of KCASP1Tg mice after exposure to 4 °C ($n = 5$, each group). (**B**) The body temperature of mice exposed to 4 °C was measured every 1 hour using thermal imaging camera. The body temperature of the KCASP1Tg mice decreased more rapidly in a cold environment ($n = 5$, each group). * $p < 0.05$, ** $p < 0.01$ versus control.

2.5. Pro-Inflammatory Cytokines Produced in Response to Dermatitis Caused AT Atrophy and Increased Activated Monocyte Infiltration In Vivo

We hypothesized that cytokines produced in inflamed skin affect AT and measured the mRNA expression levels of inflammatory cytokines in the skin of KCASP1Tg and control mice. The mRNA expression levels of TNF-α, IL-1β and IFN-γ in ear skin were measured by real-time PCR. All cytokine levels were significantly increased in KCASP1Tg mice (Figure 5A). To clarify the direct effect of skin-derived cytokines on GWAT, we treated wild-type mice by the intraperitoneal administration of inflammatory cytokines including TNF-α, IL-1β and IFN-γ. The GWATs of the TNF-α-treated wild-type mice were similar to those of KCASP1Tg mice; the adipocytes were large in number, small and irregularly shaped; IL-1β- and IFN-γ-injected mice also showed a similar trend (Figure 5B). The number of infiltrating stromal cells tended to increase in mice that were administered cytokines (Figure 5C); additionally, TLR4+ CD11b+ monocytes were significantly increased in IFN-γ treated mice (Figure 5D).

Figure 5. Production of inflammatory cytokines in the skin and the direct effect on AT. (**A**) The TNFα, IL-1β and INF-γ levels were significantly increased in KCASP1Tg mouse ear skin lesions. (**B**) Eight-week-old BL/6 wild mice were treated by intraperitoneal injections of TNF-α, IL-1β, IFN-γ (250 μg/kg body weight/each time) or PBS three times per week for two weeks. The AT of TNF-α-treated mice showed a similar appearance to that of KCASP1Tg mice; IL-1β- and IFN-γ-administrated mice also showed a similar trend; adipocytes were large in number, small and irregularly shaped (HE, ×400). (**C,D**) The number of infiltrating cells in GWAT was counted, and the infiltrating cells were analyzed by flowcytometry. The number of infiltrating cells in GWAT was increased in cytokine-administrated mice, while TLR4+ CD11b+ activated monocytes were significantly increased in IFN-γ-treated mice. $n = 5$ per group. * $p < 0.05$, ** $p < 0.01$ versus control.

3. Discussion

In the current study, we demonstrated that severe dermatitis induces AT atrophy accompanied by abundant lymphocyte and activated monocyte infiltration, the dysregulation of adipocytokine production and maladaptation to cold environments. We observed not only histopathological AT remodeling but also a GWAT functional change when skin is inflamed. Inflammatory skin disorders are not only skin-related but also involve systemic organ impairment. A previous study showed chronic skin inflammation induces the aberrant remodeling of vascular tissues, potentially resulting in atherosclerosis [11]. Systemic amyloidosis with functional deterioration has also been seen in inflammatory skin conditions [12]. The erupted skin of KCASP1Tg mice produces significantly higher amounts of IL-1α and β compared to normal skin, while the supernatant from skin lesions leads to a severe reduction in lipid particles in an adipocyte culture system [10]. Computed tomography imaging of KCASP1Tg mice at 6 months of age revealed a dramatic decrease in visceral fat compared to in normal controls [10]. Based on these findings, it was hypothesized that persistent dermatitis had a negative effect on visceral AT, and we investigated the state of GWAT using dermatitis model mice.

In KCASP1Tg mice, the whole body and GWAT weights were decreased compared to in wild littermate mice. Each adipocyte was small and irregularly shaped, and showed abundant inflammatory cell infiltration in GWAT. Since increased inflammatory cell infiltration and atrophy of adipocytes were observed, it was considered that AT was strongly inflamed under chronic dermatitis. The stromal cells that infiltrate into GWAT are mainly lymphocytes and monocytes, but it was difficult to quantify them by examination using immunohistochemical staining. We performed stromal cell classification using flow cytometry. It was found that lymphocytes and monocytes, which infiltrated into GWAT, were increased in KCASP1Tg mice. In the lymphocyte fraction, both CD4+ and CD8+ T cells were activated compared to in the control. Moreover, although there was no significant difference, regulatory T cells also tended to increase in the inflamed AT. The CD11b antigen is expressed when premature monocytes are activated to become differentiated monocytes and represents the best molecular marker of the macrophage lineage [13]. In monocytes, the expression of TLR4 is important in mediating inflammatory cytokine production in AT inflammation. In humans, TNF-α suppresses the expression of TLR4 on monocytes; however, IL-6 or IFN-γ mediates the upregulation of TLR4 expression [14]. The number of lymphocytes and TLR4+ CD11b+ activated monocytes was significantly higher in the AT of the KCASP1Tg mice.

AT plays an essential role in metabolic homeostasis by storing and releasing lipids and secreting bioactive proteins and peptides called adipokines, including adiponectin, leptin, MCP-1 and TNF-α in response to environmental changes. Both leptin and adiponectin are mainly produced by adipocytes. The main function of leptin seems to be to provide an afferent signal of nutritional and fat mass status to the hypothalamus, thus controlling energy fat stores and regulating appetite and body weight [15]. Leptin reduces the appetite; increased adipocyte storage leads to higher leptin production, which results in a further loss of appetite. On the other hand, adiponectin helps to repair damaged blood vessel walls, prevent arteriosclerosis, increase insulin's action and lower blood pressure. However, clinically, blood adiponectin concentration is inversely correlated to visceral fat mass; the mechanism behind this relationship has not been elucidated so far. In psoriasis, one of the most common chronic intractable inflammatory skin diseases, several studies showed that adipokine levels are associated with disease severity [16]. AT plays an important role in the development of psoriasis. Leptin induces IL-6, CXCL-1, IL-8 and MCP-1 production, which is involved in the hyperproliferation of the epidermis in psoriasis [17]. To the contrary, adiponectin is an anti-inflammatory adipocytokine, and when dermatitis is caused in adiponectin knock out mice, the expression of IL-17A, IL-17F and IL-22 increases [18]. Moreover, an increased circulating level of IL-1 has been shown to be accompanied by the local overexpression of TNF-α and IL-12/23 p40 [19], as was also seen in our model mice. However, although our model mice exhibited AT atrophy, psoriasis patients are often obese. BMI is also known to be a risk factor for developing psoriasis [20]. The lower leptin level in KCASP1Tg mice may be responsible for the upregulation of body weight. Additionally, adiponectin production from GWAT was significantly increased because adipocytes oversecrete adiponectin in chronic dermatitis. The effects of systemic dermatitis on AT in our study differ from those in psoriasis and may resemble those in erythroderma, which often results in weight loss. However, a recent report shows that psoriasis patients treated with anti-TNF-α antibodies experience weight gain [21]. If it occurs more often in patients with severe psoriasis and high improvement rates for psoriasis, it is likely that dermatitis has a considerable impact on weight loss.

We speculated that the AT in a dermatitis model shows an impaired thermogenesis ability due to systemic inflammation. After exposure to 4 °C, the mRNA expression of heat-related proteins such as HSP90, IL-33 and UCP1 in GWAT was measured. Heat shock proteins (HSPs) are primary mitigators of cell stress HSPs expression is also induced by cold exposure in brown adipose tissue [22]. It is well known that brown adipocytes play an important role in heat production in mice [23]. When white adipocytes face various stimuli such as cold exposure and adrenergic stimulation, they form beige adipocytes and induce UCP1, producing brown adipocytes [24]. This process can be induced by IL-33, which is released from various cells in response to stress and injury in adult mice and activates type 2 innate lymphocytes (ILC2) [25]. In our study, although IL-33 levels were lower in the KCASP1Tg mice, UCP1 expression was significantly increased after exposure to the 4 °C environment. Therefore, heat production occurred correctly; however, the body temperature of the KCASP1Tg mice decreased more rapidly in the cold environment, and these mice died earlier than the wild-type mice, meaning survival in a cold environment may be harder due to AT atrophy.

We assumed that increased inflammatory cytokine production in the skin lesions was the key factor for this lymphocyte/monocyte activation and AT dysregulation. In fact, TNFα, IL-1β and INF-γ levels were significantly increased in KCASP1Tg mouse ear skin lesions (Figure 5A). To investigate the direct effects of these cytokines, BL/6 wild mice were administrated intraperitoneal injections of TNF-α, IL-1β and IFN-γ, revealing small adipocytes and abundant stromal cell infiltration, suggesting those cytokines exert a synergistic effect on adipocytes (Figure 5B–D). According to our results, inflammatory cytokines whose production is increased by the eczema lesions cause AT atrophy and increased inflammatory cell infiltration in AT. We have reported, in previous studies, that the inhibition of IL-1 can prevent cerebrovascular disease [26]. In this study, we did not prove the prevention of AT damage by treating dermatitis. However, controlling dermatitis with topical corticosteroids, immunosuppressants or anti-cytokine antibodies probably reduce damage to AT. Of course, the long-term use of topical steroids can cause side effects such as skin atrophy, rosacea-like dermatitis and dermatomycosis [27,28], and immunosuppressants or anti-cytokine antibodies may cause severe infections and malignant tumors. We should realize that dermatitis causes damage to various organs and the importance of the active treatment of dermatitis.

There are only a few studies evaluating AT pathology and function in inflammatory skin disease. We found that skin-derived inflammatory cytokines led to the secretion of pro-inflammatory proteins from adipocytes. As a result, activated monocytes and lymphocytes infiltrated into the AT, which lead to AT atrophy and increased the difficulty in the metabolic adaptation to cold temperatures. Our study suggested that inflammatory skin diseases lead to organ damage and require careful attention.

4. Materials and Methods

4.1. Mouse Study

We used 8–10-week-old spontaneous dermatitis transgenic female KCASP1Tg mice, while female littermate C57BL/6 mice were used as controls. The experimental protocol was approved by the Mie University Board Committee for Animal Care and Use (Protocol #22-39-2, approved date, 1 October 2014). Eight-week-old female wild mice were also administered intraperitoneal injections of recombinant tumor necrosis factor-alpha (TNF-α), recombinant IL-1β, recombinant interferon-gamma (IFN-γ) or phosphate-buffered saline (PBS). The cytokines were diluted in PBS and 250 μg/kg of body weight each time were injected three times per week for two weeks. All the recombinant compounds were purchased from Biolegend (San Diego, CA). All the mice were sacrificed the day after the sixth injection. For the cold stimulation study, 10-week-old KCASP1Tg and littermate mice were housed, one per cage, at a temperature of 22 °C. All the mice were transferred to a 4 °C room, and body temperature was measured every hour using thermal imaging camera FLIR i5 (Extech Instruments, Waltham, MA, USA). After eight hours, all the mice were sacrificed and AT was sampled.

4.2. Tissue Sampling

Isolated adipocytes were prepared as previously reported with minor modifications [29,30]. In brief, extracted gonadal white AT (GWAT) was minced and incubated in PBS with 0.5% bovine serum albumin (BSA, Sigma-Aldrich, St. Louis, MO, USA), 10 mM $CaCl_2$, and 2 mg/mL of collagenase type II (Worthington Biochemical Corporation, Lakewood, NJ, USA) at 37 °C for 20 min at 200 rpm. The suspension was filtered through a 100-μm nylon filter and centrifuged at room temperature at 400 rpm for one minute; the floating cells (adipocytes) were then collected. The remaining suspension was further centrifuged at 1500 rpm for 10 min. The supernatant was decanted and the remaining cell pellets were resuspended with 0.5% BSA/PBS. We counted the number of viable cells based on trypan blue exclusion and diluted the cell suspensions to final concentrations of $5–10 \times 10^6$ cells/mL as adipose-infiltrated stromal cells.

4.3. Histological and Immunohistochemistry Analysis

Tissue was fixed in 10% formalin neutral buffer solution (Wako, Osaka, Japan), embedded in paraffin, cut into 3.5-μm sections and stained with hematoxylin and eosin (HE). Immunohistochemistry (IHC) was performed with primary antibodies—rabbit anti-mouse CD4 antibody (Cell Signaling Technology, Danvers, MA, USA), rabbit anti-mouse CD8a antibody (Cell Signaling Technology), rabbit anti-Ly6G antibody (Abcam, Cambridge, UK) and rat anti-Ly6C antibody (abcam)—and secondary antibodies—goat anti-rabbit immunoglobulins/biotinylated (Dako, Santa Clara, CA, USA) and simple stain MAX-PO (rat) (Nichirei Biosciences, Tokyo, Japan). The adipocytes were observed with 400× HE and counted, and the area was measured using ImageJ and Adiposoft (NIH, Bethesda, MD, USA).

4.4. Flow Cytometry Analysis

AT-infiltrating stromal cells were stained with FITC anti-mouse CD3ε antibody, PE anti-mouse CD4 antibody, PE/Cy7 anti-mouse CD25 antibody, APC anti-mouse CD8a antibody, FITC anti-mouse CD127 antibody, PerCP/Cy5.5 anti-mouse CD4 antibody, APC anti-mouse CD25 antibody (these antibodies were purchased from Biolegend, San Diego, CA, USA), PE anti-mouse/Foxp3 antibody (Invitrogen, Carlsbad, CA, USA), PE anti-mouse CD11b antibody (Biolegend), PE/Cy7 anti-mouse Ly-6C antibody (Biolegend, San Diego, CA, USA) and APC anti-toll-like receptor 4 (TLR4) antibody (Invitrogen, Waltham, MA, USA), and analyzed using an Accuri C6 (Becton, Dickinson and Company, Franklin Lakes, NJ, USA).

4.5. Real-Time Polymerase Chain Reaction (PCR)

Total RNA was extracted from ear skin and AT using TRI Reagent (Molecular Research Center, Cincinnati, OH) according to the manufacturer's protocol. The RNA concentration was measured using a NanoDrop Lite spectrophotometer (Thermo Fisher Scientific, Worsham, MA, USA) and 1 μg of total RNA was converted to cDNA using the High-Capacity RNA-to-cDNA Kit (Applied Biosystems, Foster City, CA, USA). The TaqMan Universal PCR Master Mix II with UNG (Applied Biosystems, Foster City, CA, USA) was used to measure the mRNA expression of TNF-α (Mm00443258_m1), IL-1β (Mm01336189_m1), IFN-γ (Mm01168134_m), heat shock protein 90 (HSP90, Mm00658568_gH), IL-33 (Mm00505403_m1) and uncoupling protein 1 (UCP-1, Mm01244861_m1). All probes were purchased from Applied Biosystems and glyceraldehyde-3-phosphate dehydrogenase (Mm99999915_g1) was used as the internal control. Amplification was performed in a LightCycler 96 System (Roche Diagnostics, Basel, Switzerland). The cycling parameters were as follows: 95 °C for 30 s, followed by 40 cycles of amplification at 95 °C for 5 s and 60 °C for 30 s.

4.6. Enzyme-Linked Immunosorbent Assay (ELISA)

The total protein content from adipocytes was extracted using a radioimmunoprecipitation assay buffer (Nacalai tesque, Kyoto, Japan). Adiponectin, TNF-α, leptin and monocyte chemotactic protein-1 (MCP-1) levels were measured using specific ELISA kits (R&D systems Minneapolis, MN) according to the manufacturer's protocol, and the data were normalized to GWAT weight. The absorbance was measured using MULTISKAN JX (Thermo Fisher Scientific, Worsham, MA, USA). The values were analyzed using Ascent Software for Multiskan Ascent (Thermo Fisher Scientific, Worsham, MA, USA).

4.7. Statistical Analysis

Statistical analysis was performed using the PRISM software version 8 (GraphPad, San Diego, CA, USA). The Mann–Whitney U test was used to compare variables between groups. Differences were considered significant at $p < 0.05$.

5. Conclusions

The systemic dermatitis model mice showed atrophy of AT and an increased infiltration of activated T cells and monocytes into the AT. These were reproducible by the intraperitoneal administration of inflammatory cytokines such as TNF-α, IL-1β and IFN-g, whose production was increased in inflamed skin lesions. The persistence of skin inflammation can potentially cause negative reactions in AT.

Author Contributions: K.M. and E.S. performed the experiments and wrote the paper. M.I. performed part of the histopathological analysis, and Y.M., A.U., K.O., and A.U. performed the experiments. Y.Y., M.W., E.M., and K.Y. designed and supervised the experiments. All authors have read and agreed to the published version of the manuscript.

Abbreviations

AT	adipose tissue
BSA	bovine serum albumin
ELISA	enzyme-linked immunosorbent assay
KCASP1Tg	keratin 14-specific caspase-1 overexpressing transgenic mouse
GWAT	gonadal white adipose tissue
HSP90	heat shock protein 90
IL	interleukin
INF	interferon
MCP-1	monocyte chemotactic protein-1
PBS	phosphate-buffered saline
PCR	polymerase chain reaction
TLR	toll-like receptor
TNF	tumor necrosis factor
UCP	uncoupling protein 1

References

1.　Scherer, P.E. Adipose tissue: From lipid storage compartment to endocrine organ. *Diabetes* **2006**, *55*, 1537–1545. [CrossRef] [PubMed]

2.　Gerdes, S.; Rostami-Yazdi, M.; Mrowietz, U. Adipokines and psoriasis. *Exp. Dermatol.* **2011**, *20*, 81–87. [CrossRef] [PubMed]

3.　Blaton, V. How is the metabolic syndrome related to the dyslipidemia? *EJIFCC* **2007**, *18*, 15–22. [CrossRef]

4.　Suganami, T.; Ogawa, Y. Adipose tissue macrophages: Their role in adipose tissue remodeling. *J. Leukoc. Biol.* **2010**, *88*, 33–39. [CrossRef] [PubMed]

5.   Caton, P.W.; Evans, E.A.; Philpott, M.P.; Hannen, R.F. Can the skin make you fat? A role for the skin in regulating adipose tissue function and whole-body glucose and lipid homeostasis. *Curr. Opin. Pharmacol.* **2017**, *37*, 59–64. [CrossRef] [PubMed]

6.   Coimbra, S.; Catarino, C.; Santos-Silva, A. The triad psoriasis-obesity-adipokine profile. *J. Eur. Acad. Dermatol. Venereol.* **2016**, *30*, 1876–1885. [CrossRef] [PubMed]

7.   Nakamizo, S.; Honda, T.; Adachi, A.; Nagatake, T.; Kunisawa, J.; Kitoh, A.; Otsuka, A.; Dainichi, T.; Nomura, T.; Ginhoux, F.; et al. High fat diet exacerbates murine psoriatic dermatitis by increasing the number of IL-17-producing gammadelta T cells. *Sci. Rep.* **2017**, *7*, 14076. [CrossRef] [PubMed]

8.   Yamanaka, K.; Tanaka, M.; Tsutsui, H.; Kupper, T.S.; Asahi, K.; Okamura, H.; Nakanishi, K.; Suzuki, M.; Kayagaki, N.; Black, R.A.; et al. Skin-specific caspase-1-transgenic mice show cutaneous apoptosis and pre-endotoxin shock condition with a high serum level of IL-18. *J. Immunol.* **2000**, *165*, 997–1003. [CrossRef]

9.   Black, R.A.; Kronheim, S.R.; Cantrell, M.; Deeley, M.C.; March, C.J.; Prickett, K.S.; Wignall, J.; Conlon, P.J.; Cosman, D.; Hopp, T.P.; et al. Generation of biologically active interleukin-1 beta by proteolytic cleavage of the inactive precursor. *J. Biol. Chem.* **1988**, *263*, 9437–9442.

10. Yamanaka, K.; Nakanishi, T.; Saito, H.; Maruyama, J.; Isoda, K.; Yokochi, A.; Imanaka-Yoshida, K.; Tsuda, K.; Kakeda, M.; Okamoto, R.; et al. Persistent release of IL-1s from skin is associated with systemic cardio-vascular disease, emaciation and systemic amyloidosis: The potential of anti-IL-1 therapy for systemic inflammatory diseases. *PLoS ONE* **2014**, *9*, e104479. [CrossRef]

11. Herrero, L.; Shapiro, H.; Nayer, A.; Lee, J.; Shoelson, S.E. Inflammation and adipose tissue macrophages in lipodystrophic mice. *Proc. Natl. Acad. Sci. USA* **2010**, *107*, 240–245. [CrossRef] [PubMed]

12. Yamanaka, K.; Okada, K.; Nakanishi, T.; Mizutani, K.; Matsushima, Y.; Kondo, M.; Habe, K.; Mizutani, H.; Seo, N. Skin inflammation leads immunoglobulin G aggregation and deposition in multiple organs. *J. Dermatol. Sci.* **2017**, *88*, 146–148. [CrossRef] [PubMed]

13. Leenen, P.J.; de Bruijn, M.F.; Voerman, J.S.; Campbell, P.A.; van Ewijk, W. Markers of mouse macrophage development detected by monoclonal antibodies. *J. Immunol. Methods* **1994**, *174*, 5–19. [CrossRef]

14. Guzzo, C.; Ayer, A.; Basta, S.; Banfield, B.W.; Gee, K. IL-27 enhances LPS-induced proinflammatory cytokine production via upregulation of TLR4 expression and signaling in human monocytes. *J. Immunol.* **2012**, *188*, 864–873. [CrossRef]

15. Schwartz, M.W.; Woods, S.C.; Porte, D.; Seeley, R.J.; Baskin, D.G. Central nervous system control of food intake. *Nature* **2000**, *404*, 661–671. [CrossRef]

16. Nakajima, H.; Nakajima, K.; Tarutani, M.; Morishige, R.; Sano, S. Kinetics of circulating Th17 cytokines and adipokines in psoriasis patients. *Arch. Dermatol. Res.* **2011**, *303*, 451–455. [CrossRef]

17. Ommen, P.; Stjernholm, T.; Kragstrup, T.; Raaby, L.; Johansen, C.; Stenderup, K.; Iversen, L.; Rosada, C. The role of leptin in psoriasis comprises a proinflammatory response by the dermal fibroblast. *Br. J. Dermatol.* **2016**, *174*, 187–190. [CrossRef]

18. Shibata, S.; Tada, Y.; Hau, C.S.; Mitsui, A.; Kamata, M.; Asano, Y.; Sugaya, M.; Kadono, T.; Masamoto, Y.; Kurokawa, M.; et al. Adiponectin regulates psoriasiform skin inflammation by suppressing IL-17 production from gammadelta-T cells. *Nat. Commun.* **2015**, *6*, 7687. [CrossRef]

19. Yu, A.P.; Tang, J.; Xie, J.; Wu, E.Q.; Gupta, S.R.; Bao, Y.; Mulani, P.M. Economic burden of psoriasis compared to the general population and stratified by disease severity. *Curr. Med. Res. Opin.* **2009**, *25*, 2429–2438. [CrossRef]

20. Budu-Aggrey, A.; Brumpton, B.; Tyrrell, J.; Watkins, S.; Modalsli, E.H.; Celis-Morales, C.; Ferguson, L.D.; Vie, G.Å.; Palmer, T.; Fritsche, L.G.; et al. Evidence of a causal relationship between body mass index and psoriasis: A mendelian randomization study. *PLoS Med.* **2019**, *16*, e1002739. [CrossRef]

21. Wu, M.-Y.; Yu, C.-L.; Yang, S.-J.; Chi, C.-C. Change in body weight and body mass index in psoriasis patients receiving biologics: A systematic review and network meta-analysis. *J. Am. Acad. Dermatol.* **2020**, *82*, 101–109. [CrossRef] [PubMed]

22. Matz, J.M.; Blake, M.J.; Tatelman, H.M.; Lavoi, K.P.; Holbrook, N.J. Characterization and regulation of cold-induced heat shock protein expression in mouse brown adipose tissue. *Am. J. Physiol. Regul. Integr. Comp. Physiol.* **1995**, *269*, R38–R47. [CrossRef] [PubMed]

23. Nedergaard, J.; Cannon, B. Brown adipose tissue as a heat-producing thermoeffector. *Handb. Clin. Neurol.* **2018**, *156*, 137–152. [CrossRef] [PubMed]

24. Wong, W. A signal to warm up to. *Sci. Signal.* **2016**, *9*, ec190. [CrossRef]

25. Mathis, D. IL-33, imprimatur of adipocyte thermogenesis. *Cell* **2016**, *166*, 794–795. [CrossRef] [PubMed]

26. Kato, S.; Matsushima, Y.; Mizutani, K.; Kawakita, F.; Fujimoto, M.; Okada, K.; Kondo, M.; Habe, K.; Suzuki, H.; Mizutani, H.; et al. The stenosis of cerebral arteries and impaired brain glucose uptake by long-lasting inflammatory cytokine release from dermatitis is rescued by Anti-IL-1 therapy. *J. Investig. Dermatol.* **2018**, *138*, 2280–2283. [CrossRef]

27. Tatu, A.L.; Ionescu, M.A.; Clatici, V.G.; Cristea, V.C. Bacillus cereus strain isolated from Demodex folliculorum in patients with topical steroid-induced rosaceiform facial dermatitis. *Bras. Dermatol.* **2016**, *91*, 676–678. [CrossRef]

28. Meena, S.; Gupta, L.K.; Khare, A.K.; Balai, M.; Mittal, A.; Mehta, S.; Bhatri, G. Topical corticosteroids abuse: A clinical study of cutaneous adverse effects. *Indian J. Dermatol.* **2017**, *62*, 675. [CrossRef]

29. Orr, J.S.; Kennedy, A.J.; Hasty, A.H. Isolation of adipose tissue immune cells. *J. Vis. Exp.* **2013**. [CrossRef]

30. Lumeng, C.N.; Deyoung, S.M.; Bodzin, J.L.; Saltiel, A.R. Increased inflammatory properties of adipose tissue macrophages recruited during diet-induced obesity. *Diabetes* **2007**, *56*, 16–23. [CrossRef]

8

Differences in Osteoimmunological Biomarkers Predictive of Psoriatic Arthritis among a Large Italian Cohort of Psoriatic Patients

Marco Diani [1,†], Silvia Perego [2,†], Veronica Sansoni [2,†], Lucrezia Bertino [3], Marta Gomarasca [2], Martina Faraldi [2], Paolo Daniele Maria Pigatto [1,4], Giovanni Damiani [1,4,5,6,*], Giuseppe Banfi [2,7], Gianfranco Altomare [1] and Giovanni Lombardi [2,8]

[1] Department of Dermatology and Venereology, IRCCS Istituto Ortopedico Galeazzi, 20161 Milan, Italy; marco.diani@unimi.it (M.D.); paolo.pigatto@unimi.it (P.D.M.P.); gianfranco.altomare@unimi.it (G.A.)
[2] Laboratory of Experimental Biochemistry and Molecular Biology, IRCCS Istituto Ortopedico Galeazzi, 20161 Milan, Italy; silvia.perego@grupposandonato.it (S.P.); veronica.sansoni@grupposandonato.it (V.S.); marta.gomarasca@grupposandonato.it (M.G.); martina.faraldi@grupposandonato.it (M.F.); banfi.giuseppe@fondazionesanraffaele.it (G.B.); giovanni.lombardi@grupposandonato.it (G.L.)
[3] Department of Clinical and Experimental Medicine, section of Dermatology, University of Messina, 98122 Messina, Italy; bertino.lucrezia@gmail.com
[4] Department of Biomedical, Surgical and Dental Sciences, University of Milan, 20122 Milano, Italy
[5] Department of Dermatology, Case Western Reserve University, Cleveland, OH 44106, USA
[6] Young Dermatologists Italian Network, Centro Studi GISED, 24121 Bergamo, Italy
[7] Vita-Salute San Raffaele University, 20132 Milan, Italy
[8] Department of Physiology and Pharmacology, Gdańsk University of Physical Education and Sport, 80336 Gdańsk, Poland
* Correspondence: dr.giovanni.damiani@gmail.com
† These authors contributed equally to this work.

Abstract: (1) Background: In literature it is reported that 20–30% of psoriatic patients evolve to psoriatic arthritis over time. Currently, no specific biochemical markers can either predict progression to psoriatic arthritis or response to therapies. This study aimed to identify osteoimmunological markers applicable to clinical practice, giving a quantitative tool for evaluating pathological status and, eventually, to provide prognostic support in diagnosis. (2) Methods: Soluble (serum) bone and cartilage markers were quantified in 50 patients with only psoriasis, 50 psoriatic patients with psoriatic arthritis, and 20 healthy controls by means of multiplex and enzyme-linked immunoassays. (3) Results: Differences in the concentrations of matrix metalloproteases (MMPs), tissue inhibitors of metalloproteinases (TIMPs), receptor activator of nuclear factor kappa-B- ligand (RANK-L), procollagen type I N propeptide (PINP), C-terminal telopeptide of type I collagen (CTx-I), dickkopf-related protein 1 (DKK1), and sclerostin (SOST) distinguished healthy controls from psoriasis and psoriatic arthritis patients. We found that MMP2, MMP12, MMP13, TIMP2, and TIMP4 distinguished psoriasis from psoriatic arthritis patients undergoing a systemic treatment, with a good diagnostic accuracy (Area under the ROC Curve (AUC) > 0.7). Then, chitinase-3-like protein 1 (CHI3L1) and MMP10 distinguished psoriasis from psoriatic arthritis not undergoing systemic therapy and, in the presence of onychopathy, MMP8 levels were higher in psoriasis than in psoriatic arthritis. However, in these latter cases, the diagnostic accuracy of the identified biomarkers was low (0.5 < AUC < 0.7). (4) Conclusions. By highlighting never exploited differences, the wide osteoimmunological biomarkers panel provides a novel clue to the development of diagnostic paths in psoriasis and psoriasis-associated arthropathic disease.

Keywords: psoriasis; psoriatic arthritis; osteoimmunological markers; bone resorption

1. Introduction

Adult psoriatic disease depicts a continuum encompassing disease progression from psoriasis (Ps) to psoriatic arthritis (PsA) [1]. In contrast to children, in adults, PsA manifests mainly after Ps and its musculoskeletal damages may be prevented with an early diagnosis and treatment [1,2]. Remarkably, 20–30% of Ps patients develop PsA but the non-clinically oriented instrumental screening of psoriatic patients is neither routinely adopted nor recommended due to the connected costs [1]. Thus, both clinical signs, such as psoriatic onychopathy and non-specific inflammatory parameters, are considered to identify Ps patients with a putative higher risk of developing PsA [3]. This is also accompanied by other proposed tools, such as the psoriasis epidemiology screening tool (PEST) questionnaire, evaluating the risk of developing PsA [4]. However, epidemiological studies based on clinical health records comparing Ps and PsA cohorts displayed contrasting results about the possible risk factors implicated in the evolution from Ps to PsA [5].

A biochemical marker that clearly predicts PsA in a cohort of Ps patients is still elusive. A biomarker is defined as a measurable characteristic indicating a biological or pathophysiological process and can be used to identify the risk to develop a certain disease [6]. Several studies investigated the association of different biomarkers with PsA. This condition has been associated with higher levels of cartilage oligomeric matrix protein (COMP), osteoprotegerin (OPG), matrix metalloproteinase 3 (MMP3), and the ratio between C-propeptide of type II collagen (CIIP) and collagen fragment neoepitope Col2–3/4 (C2C) [7]. Other studies found higher levels of CXCL10 in PsA patients compared to Ps patients [8], interleukin (IL)-6 [9], Dikkopf-1 (DKK-1), and macrophage-colony stimulating factor (M-CSF) [10]. However, the clinical significance of these studies is somehow limited due to the restricted panel of biomarkers considered and, more importantly, the lack of consideration of the therapeutic regimens and comorbidities/clinical signs (e.g., nail involvement).

Based on this background, this study aimed to investigate the possible association between a wide panel of osteoimmunological biomarkers with Ps and PsA, and in the relative sub-cohorts in order to identify a possible laboratory tool that could support PsA diagnosis and early prediction.

2. Results

2.1. Clinical Features of the Study Cohorts

Table 1 summarizes the study population demographics and clinical features.

Table 1. Clinical features of patients at the time of recruitment.

Variables	Total Cases (n = 100)	Ps Group (n = 50)	PsA Group (n = 50)	CTRL Group (n = 20)
Age median (IQR), years	49 (19–82)	48 (19–82)	48 (28–79)	48 (29–67)
Female, n (%)	28 (28)	17 (34)	11 (22)	10 (50)
Male, n (%)	72 (72)	33 (66)	39 (78)	10 (50)
BMI median (IQR), kg/m^2	25 (23–28)	25 (23–29)	26 (23–28)	24 (22–25)
Ps duration median (IQR), months	195 (83–319)	200 (67–347)	195 (110–317)	-
Eruptive/stable Ps, (n)	-	39/11		-
PsA duration median (IQR), months	-	-	25 (4–110)	-
PASI median (IQR)	5 (2–8)	6 (5–12)	4 (1–7)	-
Onychopathy (n)	43	19	24	-
Non systemic therapy (n)	64	31	33	-
Systemic therapy (n)	36	19	17	-
Acitretin (n) (dose)	1 (20 mg/die)	1 (20 mg/die)	0	-
CsA (n) (dose)	6 (237.5 (221.3–257.5) mg/die)	5 (250 (220–260) mg/die)	1 (225 mg/die)	-
MTX (n) (dose)	28 (15 (15–17.5) mg/week)	13 (15 (15–17.5) mg/die)	15 (15 (15–16.25) mg/die)	-
Systemic prednisone (n) (dose)	1 (10 mg/die)	-	1 (10 mg/die)	-

BMI: Body mass index, CsA: Cyclosporin, CTRL: Controls, IQR: Interquartile range, MTX: Methotrexate, n: number, Ps: Psoriasis, PsA: Psoriatic arthritis.

In both Ps and PsA groups, a prevalence of male subjects, 66% and 78%, respectively, was observed despite no gender prevalence being reported. Median ages were 48 (19–82) years in Ps, 51(28–79) years in PsA, and 48 (29–67) years in controls. The body mass index (BMI), in the three groups, was 25 (23–29), 26 (23–28), and 24 (22–25) kg/m^2, respectively.

The Psoriasis Area Severity Score (PASI) was higher in Ps (6 (5–12)) than in PsA (4 (1–7)).

Onychopathic signs were present in 38% of Ps subjects and 48% of PsA subjects, according to the literature [11,12], PsA occurred after the diagnosis of Ps in 88% of patients. At recruitment, patients undergoing systemic therapy (ST) were 38% Ps and 34% PsA patients, respectively. Among these, 28 patients were treated with methotrexate (MTX, 13 Ps and 15 PsA), 6 with cyclosporine (CsA, 5 Ps and 1 PsA), 1 with acitretin (Ps), and 1 with cortisone (PsA).

2.2. Biochemical Characterization of the Study Cohorts

When considered in their entirety, without any subgrouping for treatment status, no significant differences were observed for any of the tested markers between Ps and PsA. Conversely, compared to the control group (CTRL), both Ps and PsA groups differed for most of the analyzed molecules, except for MMP3, MMP7, MMP12, tissue inhibitors of metalloproteinase (TIMP)-1, TIMP-2, OPG, C-telopeptide of type II collagen (CTx-II), and chitinase-3-like protein 1 (CHI3L1) (Table 2).

Table 2. Concentration of serum osteoimmunological markers measured in the study cohorts.

Markers	CTRL Group (n = 20)	Ps Group (n = 50)	PsA Group (n = 50)	CTRL vs. Ps p-Value	CTRL vs. PsA p-Value
MMP1 (pg/mL)	35.00 (35.00–35.00)	471.20 (159.10–1033.00)	608.00 (35.00–1266.00)	$p < 0.001$ ⇑	$p = 0.001$ ⇑
MMP2 (ng/mL)	91.70 (74.58–102.26)	21.18 (7.8–76.60)	16.52 (4.75–78.11)	$p < 0.001$ ⇓	$p < 0.001$ ⇓
MMP3 (ng/mL)	6.27 (3.10–11.67)	2.39 (1.14–4.93)	2.29 (0.74–4.44)	n.s	n.s
MMP7 (ng/mL)	0.86 (0.47–1.16)	0.42 (0.22–1.08)	0.38 (0.19–1.31)	n.s	n.s
MMP8 (ng/mL)	0.61 (0.51–0.71)	1.35 (0.83–3.01)	1.32 (0.71–3.15)	$p = 0.001$ ⇑	$p = 0.009$ ⇑
MMP9 (ng/mL)	0.83 (0.61–1.25)	8.22 (3.31–11.72)	6.59 (3.35–11.63)	$p < 0.001$ ⇑	$p < 0.001$ ⇑
MMP10 (pg/mL)	1.60 (1.60–1.60)	317 (1.60–824.30)	257.47 (1.60–541.60)	$p < 0.001$ ⇑	$p < 0.001$ ⇑
MMP12 (pg/mL)	1.00 (1.00–444.20)	86.63 (11.76–165.40)	76.99 (7.65–144.10)	n.s	n.s
MMP13 (pg/mL)	4.90 (4.90–4.90)	24.8 5(4.90–63.21)	4.90 (4.90–49.19)	$p = 0.004$ ⇑	n.s
TIMP1 (ng/mL)	78.74 (66.65–109.45)	101.19 (17.17–114.69)	85.53 (17.71–113.35)	n.s	n.s
TIMP2 (ng/mL)	90.71 (72.38–105.16)	70.77 (10.09–83.73)	59.83 (8.91–76.81)	$p = 0.011$ ⇓	$p < 0.001$ ⇓
TIMP3 (ng/mL)	0.09 (0.09–1.66)	8.79 (0.76–10.73)	6.98 (0.61–9.17)	$p < 0.001$ ⇑	$p < 0.001$ ⇑
TIMP4 (pg/mL)	1072.75 (701.90–1934.00)	27.11 (1.70–320.90)	1.70 (1.70–175.20)	$p < 0.001$ ⇓	$p < 0.001$ ⇓
OPG (pmol/L)	6.46 (3.83–8.51)	5.58 (4.23–6.99)	5.67 (4.51–6.95)	n.s	n.s
RANKL (pmol/L)	393.95 (295.50–943.00)	148.20 (81.75–293.20)	165.40 (86.79–235.20)	$p < 0.001$ ⇓	$p < 0.001$ ⇓
PINP (ng/mL)	46.17 (33.55–62.88)	5.94 (5.01–7.40)	7.08 (4.87–8.22)	$p < 0.001$ ⇓	$p < 0.001$ ⇓
CTx-I (ng/mL)	1.70 (1.38–2.14)	0.55 (0.44–0.61)	0.51 (0.40–0.62)	$p < 0.001$ ⇓	$p < 0.001$ ⇓
CTx-II (ng/mL)	0.25 (0.19–0.29)	0.26 (0.20–0.31)	0.26 (0.20–0.30)	n.s	n.s
DKK1 (ng/mL)	0.27 (0.23–0.37)	2.79 (2.30–3.74)	2.80 (2.02–3.53)	$p < 0.001$ ⇑	$p < 0.001$ ⇑
SOST (pg/mL)	55.17 (35.37–97.10)	147.95 (111.20–186.70)	154.20 (126.90–196.60)	$p < 0.001$ ⇑	$p < 0.001$ ⇑
CHI3L1 (pg/mL)	70.19 (31.87–118.80)	65.98 (47.81–107.00)	83.11 (47.33–114.90)	n.s	n.s

Measures are expressed as median (IQR). CHI3L1: chitinase-3-like protein 1, CTRL: controls, CTx-I: C-terminal cross-linked telopetide of type I collagen, CTx-II: C-terminal cross-linked telopeptides of type II collagen, DKK1: Dickkopf-related protein 1, IQR: Interquartile range, MMP: Matrix metalloproteinases, n.s.: Not significant, PINP: procollagen type I N-terminal propeptide, Ps: Psoriasis, PsA: Psoriatic arthritis, RANKL: receptor activator of NF-κB ligand, TIMP: tissue inhibitor of metalloproteinases, SOST: sclerostin.

Furthermore, statistically significant correlations were found between markers' concentration and duration of both Ps and PsA: MMP2, MMP12, MMP13, TIMP1, TIMP2, TIMP3, sclerostin (SOST), and CHI3L1 in Ps (positive correlation) and with MMP10 and TIMP2 in PsA (negative correlation). Moreover, in Ps group, MMP8, MMP10, and CTx-I positively correlated with PASI score, while TIMP4 was negatively correlated (Table 3).

Table 3. Correlation analysis between osteoimmunological biomarker concentrations and duration of disease or PASI score. Correlations reaching statistical significance are given in bold.

Markers	Ps Duration		PsA Duration		Ps PASI		PsA PASI	
	p	r	p	r	p	r	p	r
MMP1	0.486	−0.10	0.790	−0.04	0.216	0.18	0.647	0.07
MMP2	**0.001**	**0.46**	0.929	0.01	0.322	−0.14	0.205	−0.18
MMP3	0.549	0.09	0.458	0.11	0.459	−0.11	0.829	−0.03
MMP7	0.651	0.07	0.120	−0.23	0.316	0.14	0.746	−0.05
MMP8	0.177	0.19	0.098	−0.24	0.040	0.29	0.054	0.27
MMP9	0.630	0.07	0.306	−0.15	0.257	0.16	0.226	0.17
MMP10	0.876	0.02	**0.025**	**−0.32**	**0.004**	**0.40**	0.057	0.27
MMP12	**0.001**	**0.45**	0.418	−0.12	0.372	−0.13	0.313	−0.15
MMP13	**0.010**	**0.36**	0.392	−0.13	0.667	−0.06	0.781	−0.04
TIMP1	**0.016**	**0.34**	**0.049**	**−0.29**	0.935	0.01	0.361	−0.13
TIMP2	**0.037**	**0.30**	0.203	−0.19	0.871	0.02	0.372	−0.13
TIMP3	**0.042**	**0.29**	0.087	−0.25	0.946	0.01	0.709	−0.05
TIMP4	0.065	0.26	0.052	0.28	**0.041**	**−0.29**	0.497	−0.10
OPG	0.341	0.14	0.176	0.20	0.067	−0.26	0.448	−0.11
RANKL	0.335	−0.14	0.616	−0.07	0.450	−0.11	0.680	0.06
PINP	0.571	−0.08	0.638	−0.07	0.999	0.00	0.480	0.10
CTX-I	0.215	−0.18	0.341	0.14	**0.048**	**0.28**	0.440	0.11
CTX-II	0.398	0.12	0.956	−0.01	0.124	−0.22	0.161	−0.20
DKK1	0.233	0.17	0.684	−0.06	0.474	−0.10	0.985	0.00
SOST	**0.015**	**0.34**	0.343	−0.14	0.286	−0.15	0.421	−0.12
CHI3L1	**0.010**	**0.36**	0.384	0.13	0.284	−0.15	0.596	0.08

CHI3L1: Chitinase-3-like protein 1, CTx-I: C-terminal cross-linked telopetide of type I collagen, CTx-II: C-terminal cross-linked telopeptides of type II collagen, DKK1: Dickkopf-related protein 1, MMP: Matrix metalloproteinases, PASI: Psoriasis area severity index, p: p value, PINP: Procollagen type I N-terminal propeptide, Ps: Psoriasis, PsA: Psoriatic arthritis, RANKL: Receptor activator of NF-κB ligand, r: Pearson coefficient, TIMP: Tissue inhibitor of metalloproteinases, SOST: Sclerostin.

2.3. Effect of Systemic Treatments

The Ps and PsA cohorts were further divided based on the therapy regimen (subjects undergone to systemic treatments (ST) and not systemically treated (NST)).

When Ps and PsA subjects ST ($n = 19$ and $n = 17$, respectively) were compared, MMP2 (57.47 vs. 11.50 ng/mL, $p = 0.006$), MMP12 (124.10 vs. 76.43 pg/mL, $p = 0.013$), MMP13 (62.48 vs. 4.90 pg/mL, $p = 0.029$), TIMP2 (80.00 vs. 50.34 ng/mL, $p = 0.001$), and TIMP4 (177.7 vs. 1.7 pg/mL, $p = 0.012$) were higher in Ps to PsA (Figure 1A). As expected, PASI score was higher in Ps than in PsA patients (5.5 vs. 1.8, $p = 0.004$).

The Relative Operating Characteristic (ROC) analysis shows that the area under the ROC curve (AUC) for both the single markers (MMP2: 0.768, MMP12: 0.743, TIMP2: 0.811, TIMP4: 0.724) and their combination (0.755 to 0.845) display a moderately accurate diagnostic potential in discriminating Ps from PsA ST patients. Noteworthy, the combination of all these markers gave the highest diagnostic accuracy (AUC = 0.845) (Figure S1).

By focusing on the NST group, Ps NST ($n = 31$) and PsA NST ($n = 33$) significantly differed for MMP10 (340.9 vs. 224.9 pg/mL, $p = 0.031$), and CHI3L1 (65.21 vs. 91.54 pg/mL, $p = 0.042$) (Figure 1B), with the PASI score being always higher in Ps than in PsA (7 vs. 4, $p = 0.002$).

Figure 1. (a) Changes in PASI and serum profile of osteoimmunological markers in Ps ST group (hashed box) and PsA ST group (gray box). (b) Changes in PASI and serum profile of osteoimmunological markers in Ps NST group (hashed box) and PsA NST group (gray box). The box and whiskers plot identify, respectively, the value of the median (intermediate line), the 25th and 75th percentile (box), and the minimum and maximum value (whiskers). Asterisks indicate significant intergroup differences (* $p < 0.05$, ** $p < 0.01$). CHI3L1: Chitinase-3-like protein 1, MMP: Matrix metalloproteinases, NST: not systemically treated, PASI: Psoriasis area severity index, Ps: Psoriasis, PsA: Psoriatic arthritis, ST: systemically treated, TIMP: Tissue inhibitor of metalloproteinases.

In Ps NST, MMP10 positively correlated with CHI3L1 (r = 0.446, $p = 0.011$), and negatively with PsA duration (r = −0.32, $p = 0.024$).

From the ROC analysis emerges the AUC for these markers and their combinations are below 0.700 (Figure S2). Compared to Ps NST ($n = 31$), Ps ST ($n = 19$) had significantly increased serum levels of MMP2 (57.47 vs. 10.37 ng/mL, $p = 0.007$), MMP3 (3.52 vs. 1.65 ng/mL, $p = 0.026$), MMP12 (124.1 vs. 31.84 pg/mL, $p = 0.002$), MMP13 (62.48 vs. 12.21 pg/mL, $p = 0.013$), TIMP2 (80.00 vs. 14.34 ng/mL, $p = 0.003$), TIMP3 (9.83 vs. 1.33 ng/mL, $p = 0.022$), and CTx-I (265.2 vs. 246.8 pg/mL, $p = 0.01$) (Figure 2).

Interestingly, no osteoimmunological biomarkers were statistically different in the comparison PsA ST ($n = 17$) vs. PsA NST ($n = 33$).

Figure 2. Changes in the serum profile of osteoimmunological markers in Ps ST group (hashed box) and Ps NST group (grey box). The box and whiskers plot identifies, respectively, the value of the median (intermediate line), the 25th and 75th percentile (box), and the minimum and maximum value (whiskers). Asterisks indicate significant intergroup differences (* $p < 0.05$, ** $p < 0.01$). CTx-I: C-terminal cross-linked telopetide of type I collagen, MMP: Matrix metalloproteinases, NST: not systemically treated, Ps: Psoriasis, PsA: Psoriatic arthritis, ST: systemically treated, TIMP: Tissue inhibitor of metalloproteinases.

2.4. Onychopathy Biochemical Signature

Ps patients with onychopathy (Ps O) had higher PASI (6.5 vs. 3.7 $p = 0.009$) and higher circulating MMP8 (1.96 vs. 1.26 ng/mL, $p = 0.028$) compared to onychopathic PsA patients (PsA O) (Figure 3). ROC analysis gave an AUC below 0.700, for MMP8 (Figure S3).

Non-onychopathic Ps compared to PsA counterparts achieved significance only for PASI (6.6 vs. 1.7 $p = 0.002$).

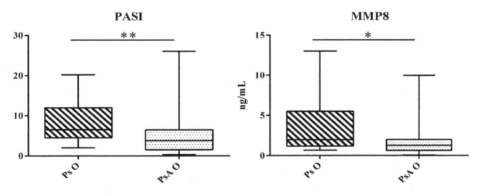

Figure 3. Changes in PASI and serum profile of MMP8 in Ps O group (hashed box) and PsA O group (dotted box). The box and whiskers plot identifies, respectively, the value of the median (intermediate line), the 25th and 75th percentile (box), and the minimum and maximum value (whiskers). Asterisks indicate significant intergroup differences (* $p < 0.05$, ** $p < 0.01$). MMP: Matrix metalloproteinasis, PASI: Psoriasis area severity index, Ps O: Psoriatic onychopathy, PsA O: Psoriatic arthritis with onychopathy.

3. Discussion

The present study investigated two different possible sets of osteoimmunological biomarkers to screen for PsA among Ps. This is of particular interest because Ps patients, especially those with a mild cutaneous involvement, having a subclinical PsA are hardly identifiable using standard measures. The consequent delayed diagnosis of PsA results in a more severe impact on the joint status. Imaging techniques have a high diagnostic potential, but they are intrinsically limited in terms of predictability.

Contrarily, since biochemical markers expression anticipates the micro/macro-structural changes, they have a predictive potential. However, markers discriminating between Ps and PsA have not been identified, although advances have been gained in the biochemical differential characterization between RA and seronegative arthropathies [13].

Previous findings gave controversy results, eventually due to the high within-cohort heterogeneity. Indeed, in our study, when the entire cohorts are considered, the main differences were between Ps and PsA and healthy controls. Similarly, previous studies failed in determining any difference between Ps and PsA in sRANKL, COMP, and OPG concentrations. A possible explanation of differences found comparing Ps and PsA patients with their healthy counterparts is that, actually, some Ps patients that are asymptomatic for PsA are, instead, suffering from subclinical cartilage and bone changing [14]. In particular, the pathological changes in cartilage and bone can be associated with enthesitis, dactylitis, nail dystrophy, and new bone apposition. Importantly, aberrant bone formation characterizes and clearly differentiates PsA from rheumatoid arthritis (RA) and other inflammatory arthritis where resorptive phenomena prevail [15,16]. On the other hand, the inclusion of patients under different treatment regimens and/or with different clinical features within the same cohorts makes the comparison less fine.

A first set of biomarkers, composed matrix metalloproteinases, and their tissue inhibitors comprises of MMP2, MMP12, MMP13, TIMP2, and TIMP4 whose circulating levels are higher in Ps undergoing systemic therapy compared to the parallel PsA cohort. Moreover, the ROC analysis of both single and differently combined markers (even more, the combination of all five) gave a good diagnostic accuracy. Consequently, this panel is particularly promising because of the wide use of MTX in both Ps and PsA. The effects of systemic treatments on the osteoimmune function is clearly depicted, in our study, by the decrease in the circulating levels of most of the markers here considered.

A second set of biomarkers seems to be useful in differentiating between Ps and PsA that have never undergone systemic treatments (NST). Given their naïve condition, the comparison of Ps NST and PsA NST patients could be considered as the most useful. This set comprises of MMP10 and CHI3L1 whose levels are, moreover, reciprocally correlated. CHI3L1 is an inactive chitinase due to the lack of the catalytic domain whose physiological functions have not been fully clarified, although it may play a role in inflammation [17–19]. Biological activities of CHI3L1 include regulation of cell proliferation, adhesion, migration, and activation. Furthermore, CHI3L1 is produced by a variety of inflammatory cells, including neutrophils, monocytes/macrophages, and osteoclasts [20], and its induction has been reported in patients suffering from many diseases, including several autoimmune disorders [21]. In addition, elevated plasma levels of CHI3L1 have also been found in RA [22]. According to previous findings, Ps patients experience higher CHI3L1 circulating levels than healthy subjects [23]. Our result seems to indicate that this protein could be a new inflammatory biomarker associated with PsA.

Nail psoriasis is, among others, a risk factor for the development of PsA, especially within the distal interphalangeal joints, as suggested by McGonagle and colleagues [24,25]. Remarkably, the enthesistis of the extensor tendon of the finger in the distal interphalangeal joint of the hand may clinically manifest with psoriatic onychopathy [26]. Although it is reported in literature that psoriatic onychopathy appears in 50% of Ps and in 93% of PsA patients [27], PsA is diagnosed after Ps development in 88% of adult patients. Several epidemiological studies associated psoriatic onychopathy with Ps duration, Ps early onset, high PASI, and concurrent PsA [28]. Systemic therapies, both biologics and non-biological, are regarded as effective and as a possible secondary treatment step in case of lack/loss of response to topical therapies in patients with high PASI or high DLQI (the dermatology life quality index) or PsA [29]. MTX and CsA can improve the nail lesions, with MTX being more effective in treating nail matrix changes, while CsA is more effective in improving nail bed scores [30].

In those subjects presenting onychopathy signs, MMP8 concentrations were higher in Ps than in PsA. Being a collagenase, MMP8 preferentially cleaves the interstitial type I collagen and is the first collagenase that appears during dermal wound-healing [31,32]. MMP8 is expressed by keratinocytes, fibroblasts, and granulocytes, at the level of the cutaneous lesions, and by synovial cells. In this latter case it was hypothesized that MMP8 solves a function in osteo-articular remodeling [33]. It is known that MMP-expressing cells are found in high amounts in the flogotic joint [34]. Therefore, it could be hypothesized that the circulating levels of MMP8 in PsA patients with onychopathy, compared to their Ps counterparts, were low because of its release into the close joint structures rather than into the blood stream. In fact, in PsA patients, as in those with RA, the levels of MMPs are elevated within the joint, which is a closed environment [35]. On the contrary, in Ps subjects without any joint involvement, MMP8 is released directly into the bloodstream, since expressed at the skin level which is, instead, an open system. Although possible, this speculation needs to be demonstrated.

The cross-sectional nature of this study and the somehow limited sample size (pilot study) represent the main limitations, although this is compensated by the great homogeneity of the selected cohorts that limits the number of variables potentially affecting the circulating levels of the analyzed biomarkers. Remarkably, due to the exiguity of the sample, it was not possible to evaluate the influences of drugs and severity on the biomarker's levels. Future studies are mandatory to assess the osteoimmunological biomarker specificity for PsA and further compare the present findings with other autoimmune diseases involving joints, such as RA or gout.

4. Methods

4.1. Ethical Committee

The clinical trial was approved by the ethical committee (BioArp, Ospedale San Raffaele, Milano, Italia), and registered at clinicaltrials.gov (NCT03455166). The study was carried out following the rules of the Declaration of Helsinki of 1975, revised in 2008 (https://www.wma.net/what-we-do/medical-ethics/declaration-of-helsinki/).

A written consent to the use of clinical data was obtained from all patients after being informed about the study procedures, their benefits, and eventual risks.

4.2. Patients Selection and Study Design

Patients with a diagnosis of plaque psoriasis (Ps, $n = 50$) and patients with Ps and PsA (PsA, $n = 50$) were enrolled at the department of dermatology and venereology of the IRCCS Istituto Ortopedico Galeazzi (Milan, Italy), starting from June 2015 until April 2017, during routine clinical activities. Inclusion criteria for Ps patients were plaque psoriasis (no erythrodermic, inverse, or guttate forms) for more than six months, neither current nor previous treatment with biological drugs, and no joint involvement.

Inclusion criteria for PsA patients fulfilling classification for psoriatic arthritis (CASPAR) criteria [36] were active peripheral (disease activity index for psoriatic arthritis (DAPSA) [37] ≥5 points) and axial arthropathy (Bath ankylosing spondylitis disease activity index (BASDAI) [38] ≥4 points), as well as enthesitis (Leeds enthesitis index (LEI) [39] >0 points), and dactylitis (dactylitis severity score (DSS) [40] >2 points) with cutaneous involvement (PASI >3), neither current treatment with biological drugs nor biological treatment. For PsA, we included a new diagnosis of PsA in order, but also of patients without an experience with biologics or patients unresponsive to biological treatments willing to start a new systemic treatment, or, if they experienced biologics, they stopped them in favor of a systemic conventional treatment for a minimum of 4 months before entering in this study. Remarkably, patients should have suspended topical therapy for at least 4 weeks.

Psoriatic onychopathy was included only if nail psoriasis severity index (NAPSI) [41] ≥ 3 points.

Exclusion criteria, common to the two groups, included pregnancy, current or previous malignancies, other acute or chronic inflammatory diseases, infectious diseases (human immunodeficiency virus (HIV), hepatitis B and C [42], tuberculosis), other rheumatologic diseases, primary bone metabolic diseases, recent bone fractures (within 6 months), anxiety, psychosis, or depressive disorders, supplementations, or particular diets (included fasting) [43–45].

4.3. Dermatology and Rheumatology Assessment of Patients

During the outpatient visit, Ps history, disease onset and evolution were evaluated. The most prevalent type of Ps was determined, along with the body sites involved and the presence of the onychopathic trait. A psoriasis area and severity index (PASI) score was assigned by two independent board-certified dermatologists.

PsA diagnosis was formulated by two independent board certified rheumatologists prior to the dermatological examination, based on anamnestic and clinical evaluations of the patient's inflammatory and imaging indexes. In particular, based on CASPAR criteria [36] and ultrasound (US) or nuclear magnetic resonance imaging (NMRI), the specialist evaluated the presence of Ps, signs and symptoms of joint inflammation (i.e., dactylitis, enthesitis), and reduced joint mobility.

Finally, laboratory analyses completed the diagnostic path by investigating markers useful in the differential diagnosis with other forms of inflammatory arthritis (e.g., rheumatoid factor, anti-CCP, inflammatory indices).

4.4. Blood Sampling and Biochemical Determinations

Blood samples were collected by standard venipuncture of the antecubital vein in SST II Advance Vacutainer® (Becton, Dickinson and Co., Franklin Lakes, NJ, USA). Blood was immediately centrifuged at $1300 \times g$ (10 min, 15 °C) and serum was aliquoted and stored at −80 °C until assayed. Serum samples from 20 healthy Caucasian age- and sex-matched subjects (10 males and 10 females, Cliniscience, Nanterre, FR, EU) were used as a control (CTRL).

Serum matrix metalloproteinases (MMP1, MMP2, MMP3, MMP7, MMP8, MMP9, MMP10, MMP12, MMP13) and their tissue inhibitors (TIMP1, TIMP2, TIMP3, TIMP4) were quantified using a multiplex assay on a Bio-Plex® Multiplex System (Bio-Rad Laboratories Inc., Hercules, CA, USA).

Osteoimmune markers, OPG, and RANKL, concentrations were measured in serum using monoclonal antibody-based immunoassays (ELISA) (BioVendor-Laboratorni Medicina A.S., Brno, CZ, EU). A marker of bone resorption, CTx-I, and a marker of bone formation, PINP, were measured in serum by monoclonal antibody-based immunoassays (Cloud-Clone Corp©, Houston, TX, USA). Serum markers of cartilage degradation and inflammation, CTx-II and CHI3L1, also known as YKL-40, were measured by a competitive enzyme immunoassay (Cloud-Clone Corp©) and a sandwich enzyme immunoassay (BioVendor-Laboratorni Medicina A.S.), respectively. Inhibitors of the Wnt signaling pathway, DKK1, and SOST, were assayed in serum by a solid-phase ELISA (Quantikine® R&D Systems Inc., Minneapolis, MN, USA).

The lower limits of detection (LOD) were 0.03 pmol/L for OPG, 0.4 pmol/L for RANKL, 44.3 pg/mL for CTx-I, 12.4 pg/mL for PINP, 52.3 pg/mL for CTx-II, 5.0 pg/mL for CHI3L1, 4.20 pg/mL for DKK1, and 1.78 pg/mL for SOST. Intra-assay (CV_w) and inter-assay (CV_b) variations were: 2.5–4.9% and 1.7–9.0% for OPG, 7.25–11.51% and 11.21–12.77% for RANKL, <10% and <12% for CTx-I, PINP, CTx-II, CHI3L1, 4.2% and 7.6% for DKK1, 2.1% and 10.8% for SOST.

Strict warnings were applied during the pre-analytical phase (i.e., collection, handling, and storage) in order to limit variability in the final analytical output [12,13].

4.5. Statistical Analysis

Shapiro–Wilk's normality test was performed on data from the entire cohort. Since the non-parametrical distribution of the values, quantitative parameters are expressed as the median and the interquartile range in the descriptive analysis. The within-group comparisons were performed using Mann–Whitney U-test. Kruskall–Wallis test was used for multiple comparison. Spearman's rank correlation test was applied to evaluate correlations that were considered significant when $r \geq 0.25$.

Diagnostic accuracy of those markers displaying a statistically significant difference in the subgroup's comparison was determined by the ROC (receiver operating characteristic) curves analysis. The AUC (area under curve)-based accuracy was classified according to Swets JA [14].

The significance was set at $p < 0.05$. Analyses were performed using SPSS software (IBM, Armonk, NY, USA).

5. Conclusions

This study, comparing a large panel of osteoimmunological biomarkers, highlighted profound differences between Ps, PsA, and healthy controls. These phenotypic differences, which are attenuated in the comparison between Ps and PsA, reinforces the thesis according to which these two diseases belong to the same pathological spectrum. However, we also identified important differences in the expression of specific tissue-remodeling associated enzymatic activities in selected sub-cohorts of Ps and PsA subjects that seem to be dependent upon the treatment (systemic vs. topic) and the presence nail involvement (onychopathy).

Author Contributions: Conceptualization, G.A. and G.L.; methodology, M.D., S.P., V.S., L.B., M.G., M.F.; validation, G.B., G.A., G.L., and G.D.; formal analysis, S.P., V.S., and G.D.; investigation, M.D., S.P., V.S., and L.B.; data curation, S.P., V.S., G.A., and G.L.; writing—original draft preparation, M.D., S.P., V.S., and G.D.; writing—review and editing, P.D.M.P., G.B., G.A., and G.L.; supervision, P.D.M.P., G.B., and G.L.; project administration, G.A. and G.L.; funding acquisition, P.D.M.P., G.B., G.A., and G.L.

References

1. Ritchlin, C.T.; Colbert, R.A.; Gladman, D.D. Psoriatic Arthritis. *N. Eng. J. Med.* **2017**, *376*, 957–970. [CrossRef] [PubMed]

2. Kane, D.; Stafford, L.; Bresnihan, B.; FitzGerald, O. A prospective, clinical and radiological study of early psoriatic arthritis: An early synovitis clinic experience. *Rheumatology* **2003**, *42*, 1460–1468. [CrossRef] [PubMed]

3. Haneke, E. Nail psoriasis: Clinical features, pathogenesis, differential diagnoses, and management. *Psoriasis* **2017**, *7*, 51–63. [CrossRef]

4. Ibrahim, G.H.; Buch, M.H.; Lawson, C.; Waxman, R.; Helliwell, P.S. Evaluation of an existing screening tool for psoriatic arthritis in people with psoriasis and the development of a new instrument: The Psoriasis Epidemiology Screening Tool (PEST) questionnaire. *Clin. Exp. Rheumatol.* **2009**, *27*, 469–474. [PubMed]

5. Ogdie, A. The preclinical phase of PsA: A challenge for the epidemiologist. *Ann. Rheum. Dis.* **2017**, *76*, 1481–1483. [CrossRef] [PubMed]

6. Biomarkers Definitions Working Group. Biomarkers and surrogate endpoints: Preferred definitions and conceptual framework. *Clin. Pharmacol. Ther.* **2001**, *69*, 89–95. [CrossRef]

7. Chandran, V.; Cook, R.J.; Edwin, J.; Shen, H.; Pellett, F.J.; Shanmugarajah, S.; Rosen, C.F.; Gladman, D.D. Soluble biomarkers differentiate patients with psoriatic arthritis from those with psoriasis without arthritis. *Rheumatology* **2010**, *49*, 1399–1405. [CrossRef]

8. Abji, F.; Pollock, R.A.; Liang, K.; Chandran, V.; Gladman, D.D. CXCL10 Is a Possible Biomarker for the Development of Psoriatic Arthritis among Patients with Psoriasis. *Arthritis Rheumatol.* **2016**, *68*, 2911–2916. [CrossRef]

9. Alenius, G.M.; Eriksson, C.; Rantapaa Dahlqvist, S. Interleukin-6 and soluble interleukin-2 receptor alpha-markers of inflammation in patients with psoriatic arthritis? *Clin. Exp. Rheumatol.* **2009**, *27*, 120–123.

10. Dalbeth, N.; Pool, B.; Smith, T.; Callon, K.E.; Lobo, M.; Taylor, W.J.; Cornish, J.; McQueen, F.M. Circulating mediators of bone remodeling in psoriatic arthritis: Implications for disordered osteoclastogenesis and bone erosion. *Arthritis Res. Ther.* **2010**, *12*, R164. [CrossRef]

11. Armesto, S.; Esteve, A.; Coto-Segura, P.; Drake, M.; Galache, C.; Martinez-Borra, J.; Santos-Juanes, J. [Nail psoriasis in individuals with psoriasis vulgaris: A study of 661 patients]. *Actas Dermo-Sifiliogr.* **2011**, *102*, 365–372. [CrossRef] [PubMed]

12. Augustin, M.; Reich, K.; Blome, C.; Schafer, I.; Laass, A.; Radtke, M.A. Nail psoriasis in Germany: Epidemiology and burden of disease. *Br. J. Dermatol.* **2010**, *163*, 580–585. [CrossRef] [PubMed]

13. Sakellariou, G.; Lombardi, G.; Vitolo, B.; Gomarasca, M.; Faraldi, M.; Caporali, R.; Banfi, G.; Montecucco, C. Serum calprotectin as a marker of ultrasound-detected synovitis in early psoriatic and rheumatoid arthritis: Results from a cross-sectional retrospective study. *Clin. Exp. Rheumatol.* **2019**, *37*, 429–436. [PubMed]

14. Bartosinska, J.; Michalak-Stoma, A.; Juszkiewicz-Borowiec, M.; Kowal, M.; Chodorowska, G. The Assessment of Selected Bone and Cartilage Biomarkers in Psoriatic Patients from Poland. *Mediat. Inflamm.* **2015**, *2015*, 194535. [CrossRef]

15. Merola, J.F.; Espinoza, L.R.; Fleischmann, R. Distinguishing rheumatoid arthritis from psoriatic arthritis. *RMD Open* **2018**, *4*, e000656. [CrossRef]

16. Mc Ardle, A.; Flatley, B.; Pennington, S.R.; FitzGerald, O. Early biomarkers of joint damage in rheumatoid and psoriatic arthritis. *Arthritis Res. Ther.* **2015**, *17*, 141. [CrossRef]

17. Lee, C.G.; Hartl, D.; Lee, G.R.; Koller, B.; Matsuura, H.; Da Silva, C.A.; Sohn, M.H.; Cohn, L.; Homer, R.J.; Kozhich, A.A.; et al. Role of breast regression protein 39 (BRP-39)/chitinase 3-like-1 in Th2 and IL-13-induced tissue responses and apoptosis. *J. Exp. Med.* **2009**, *206*, 1149–1166. [CrossRef]

18. Di Rosa, M.; Distefano, G.; Zorena, K.; Malaguarnera, L. Chitinases and immunity: Ancestral molecules with new functions. *Immunobiology* **2016**, *221*, 399–411. [CrossRef]

19. Rathcke, C.N.; Johansen, J.S.; Vestergaard, H. YKL-40, a biomarker of inflammation, is elevated in patients with type 2 diabetes and is related to insulin resistance. *Inflamm. Res.* **2006**, *55*, 53–59. [CrossRef]

20. Di Rosa, M.; Tibullo, D.; Vecchio, M.; Nunnari, G.; Saccone, S.; Di Raimondo, F.; Malaguarnera, L. Determination of chitinases family during osteoclastogenesis. *Bone* **2014**, *61*, 55–63. [CrossRef]

21. Coffman, F.D. Chitinase 3-Like-1 (CHI3L1): A putative disease marker at the interface of proteomics and glycomics. *Crit. Rev. Clin. Lab. Sci.* **2008**, *45*, 531–562. [CrossRef] [PubMed]

22. Andersen, O.A.; Dixon, M.J.; Eggleston, I.M.; van Aalten, D.M. Natural product family 18 chitinase inhibitors. *Nat. Prod. Rep.* **2005**, *22*, 563–579. [CrossRef] [PubMed]

23. Imai, Y.; Tsuda, T.; Aochi, S.; Futatsugi-Yumikura, S.; Sakaguchi, Y.; Nakagawa, N.; Iwatsuki, K.; Yamanishi, K. YKL-40 (chitinase 3-like-1) as a biomarker for psoriasis vulgaris and pustular psoriasis. *J. Dermatol. Sci.* **2011**, *64*, 75–77. [CrossRef] [PubMed]

24. Tan, A.L.; Benjamin, M.; Toumi, H.; Grainger, A.J.; Tanner, S.F.; Emery, P.; McGonagle, D. The relationship between the extensor tendon enthesis and the nail in distal interphalangeal joint disease in psoriatic arthritis–a high-resolution MRI and histological study. *Rheumatology* **2007**, *46*, 253–256. [CrossRef] [PubMed]

25. Aydin, S.Z.; Castillo-Gallego, C.; Ash, Z.R.; Marzo-Ortega, H.; Emery, P.; Wakefield, R.J.; Wittmann, M.; McGonagle, D. Ultrasonographic assessment of nail in psoriatic disease shows a link between onychopathy and distal interphalangeal joint extensor tendon enthesopathy. *Dermatology* **2012**, *225*, 231–235. [CrossRef] [PubMed]

26. Sandre, M.K.; Rohekar, S. Psoriatic arthritis and nail changes: Exploring the relationship. *Semin. Arthritis Rheum.* **2014**, *44*, 162–169. [CrossRef] [PubMed]

27. Skroza, N.; Proietti, I.; Pampena, R.; La Viola, G.; Bernardini, N.; Nicolucci, F.; Tolino, E.; Zuber, S.; Soccodato, V.; Potenza, C. Correlations between psoriasis and inflammatory bowel diseases. *BioMed Res. Int.* **2013**, *2013*, 983902. [CrossRef]

28. Schons, K.R.; Beber, A.A.; Beck Mde, O.; Monticielo, O.A. Nail involvement in adult patients with plaque-type psoriasis: Prevalence and clinical features. *An. Bras. Dermatol.* **2015**, *90*, 314–319. [CrossRef]

29. Lombardi, G.; Perego, S.; Sansoni, V.; Diani, M.; Banfi, G.; Altomare, G. Anti-adalimumab antibodies in psoriasis: Lack of clinical utility and laboratory evidence. *BMJ Open* **2016**, *6*, e011941. [CrossRef]

30. Sobolewski, P.; Walecka, I.; Dopytalska, K. Nail involvement in psoriatic arthritis. *Reumatologia* **2017**, *55*, 131–135. [CrossRef]

31. Nwomeh, B.C.; Liang, H.X.; Diegelmann, R.F.; Cohen, I.K.; Yager, D.R. Dynamics of the matrix metalloproteinases MMP-1 and MMP-8 in acute open human dermal wounds. *Wound Repair Regen.* **1998**, *6*, 127–134. [CrossRef] [PubMed]

32. Mezentsev, A.; Nikolaev, A.; Bruskin, S. Matrix metalloproteinases and their role in psoriasis. *Gene* **2014**, *540*, 1–10. [CrossRef] [PubMed]

33. Hitchon, C.A.; Danning, C.L.; Illei, G.G.; El-Gabalawy, H.S.; Boumpas, D.T. Gelatinase expression and activity in the synovium and skin of patients with erosive psoriatic arthritis. *J. Rheumatol.* **2002** *29*, 107–117.

34. Ritchlin, C. Psoriatic disease-from skin to bone. *Nat. Clin. Pract. Rheumatol.* **2007**, *3*, 698–706. [CrossRef] [PubMed]

35. Alenius, G.M.; Jonsson, S.; Wallberg Jonsson, S.; Ny, A.; Rantapaa Dahlqvist, S. Matrix metalloproteinase 9 (MMP-9) in patients with psoriatic arthritis and rheumatoid arthritis. *Clin. Exp. Rheumatol.* **2001**, *19*, 760. [PubMed]

36. Palazzi, C.; Lubrano, E.; D'Angelo, S.; Olivieri, I. Beyond early diagnosis: Occult psoriatic arthritis. *J. Rheumatol.* **2010**, *37*, 1556–1558. [CrossRef] [PubMed]

37. Schoels, M.M.; Aletaha, D.; Alasti, F.; Smolen, J.S. Disease activity in psoriatic arthritis (PsA): Defining remission and treatment success using the DAPSA score. *Ann. Rheum. Dis.* **2016**, *75*, 811–818. [CrossRef]

38. Garrett, S.; Jenkinson, T.; Kennedy, L.G.; Whitelock, H.; Gaisford, P.; Calin, A. A new approach to defining disease status in ankylosing spondylitis: The Bath Ankylosing Spondylitis Disease Activity Index. *J. Rheumatol.* **1994**, *21*, 2286–2291.

39. Healy, P.J.; Helliwell, P.S. Measuring clinical enthesitis in psoriatic arthritis: Assessment of existing measures and development of an instrument specific to psoriatic arthritis. *Arthritis Rheum.* **2008**, *59*, 686–691. [CrossRef]

40. Helliwell, P.S.; Firth, J.; Ibrahim, G.H.; Melsom, R.D.; Shah, I.; Turner, D.E. Development of an assessment tool for dactylitis in patients with psoriatic arthritis. *J. Rheumatol.* **2005**, *32*, 1745–1750.

41. Rich, P.; Scher, R.K. Nail Psoriasis Severity Index: A useful tool for evaluation of nail psoriasis. *J. Am. Acad. Dermatol.* **2003**, *49*, 206–212. [CrossRef]

42. Damiani, G.; Franchi, C.; Pigatto, P.; Altomare, A.; Pacifico, A.; Petrou, S.; Leone, S.; Pace, M.C.; Fiore, M. Outcomes assessment of hepatitis C virus-positive psoriatic patients treated using pegylated interferon in combination with ribavirin compared to new Direct-Acting Antiviral agents. *World J. Hepatol.* **2018**, *10*, 329–336. [CrossRef] [PubMed]

43. Adawi, M.; Damiani, G.; Bragazzi, N.L.; Bridgewood, C.; Pacifico, A.; Conic, R.R.Z.; Morrone, A.; Malagoli, P.; Pigatto, P.D.M.; Amital, H.; et al. The Impact of Intermittent Fasting (Ramadan Fasting) on Psoriatic Arthritis Disease Activity, Enthesitis, and Dactylitis: A Multicentre Study. *Nutrients* **2019**, *11*, 601. [CrossRef] [PubMed]

44. Damiani, G.; Watad, A.; Bridgewood, C.; Pigatto, P.D.M.; Pacifico, A.; Malagoli, P.; Bragazzi, N.L.; Adawi, M. The Impact of Ramadan Fasting on the Reduction of PASI Score, in Moderate-To-Severe Psoriatic Patients: A Real-Life Multicenter Study. *Nutrients* **2019**, *11*, 277. [CrossRef] [PubMed]

45. Kocic, H.; Damiani, G.; Stamenkovic, B.; Tirant, M.; Jovic, A.; Tiodorovic, D.; Peris, K. Dietary compounds as potential modulators of microRNA expression in psoriasis. *Ther. Adv. Chronic Dis.* **2019**, *10*. [CrossRef]

9

Multifaceted Analyses of Epidermal Serine Protease Activity in Patients with Atopic Dermatitis

Hayato Nomura [1], Mutsumi Suganuma [2], Takuya Takeichi [2], Michihiro Kono [3], Yuki Isokane [1], Ko Sunagawa [1], Mina Kobashi [1], Satoru Sugihara [1], Ai Kajita [1], Tomoko Miyake [1], Yoji Hirai [1], Osamu Yamasaki [1], Masashi Akiyama [2] and Shin Morizane [1,*]

[1]   Department of Dermatology, Okayama University Graduate School of Medicine, Dentistry, and Pharmaceutical Science, 2-5-1 Shikata-cho, Kitaku, Okayama 700-8558, Japan; rsa32585@gmail.com (H.N.); pz7h9ipi@s.okayama-u.ac.jp (Y.I.); p5eh8nav@s.okayama-u.ac.jp (K.S.); x58437@gmail.com (M.K.); suginami0816@gmail.com (S.S.); gmd421029@s.okayama-u.ac.jp (A.K.); toco_my@cc.okayama-u.ac.jp (T.M.); gmd20033@s.okayama-u.ac.jp (Y.H.); yamasa-o@cc.okayama-u.ac.jp (O.Y.)

[2]   Department of Dermatology, Nagoya University Graduate School of Medicine, 65 Tsurumai-cho, Showa-ku, Nagoya 466-8550, Japan; msuga@med.nagoya-u.ac.jp (M.S.); takeichi@med.nagoya-u.ac.jp (T.T.); makiyama@med.nagoya-u.ac.jp (M.A.)

[3]   Department of Dermatology and Plastic Surgery, Akita University Graduate School of Medicine, Hondo 1-1-1, Akita-shi, Akita 010-8543, Japan; miro@med.akita-u.ac.jp

*   Correspondence: zanemori@cc.okayama-u.ac.jp

Abstract: The serine proteases kallikrein-related peptidase (KLK) 5 and KLK7 cleave cell adhesion molecules in the epidermis. Aberrant epidermal serine protease activity is thought to play an important role in the pathogenesis of atopic dermatitis (AD). We collected the stratum corneum (SC) from healthy individuals ($n = 46$) and AD patients ($n = 63$) by tape stripping and then measuring the trypsin- and chymotrypsin-like serine protease activity. We also analyzed the p.D386N and p.E420K of *SPINK5* variants and loss-of-function mutations of *FLG* in the AD patients. The serine protease activity in the SC was increased not only in AD lesions but also in non-lesions of AD patients. We found, generally, that there was a positive correlation between the serine protease activity in the SC and the total serum immunoglobulin E (IgE) levels, serum thymus and activation-regulated chemokine (TARC) levels, and peripheral blood eosinophil counts. Moreover, the p.D386N or p.E420K in *SPINK5* and *FLG* mutations were not significantly associated with the SC's serine protease activity. Epidermal serine protease activity was increased even in non-lesions of AD patients. Such activity was found to correlate with a number of biomarkers of AD. Further investigations of serine proteases might provide new treatments and prophylaxis for AD.

Keywords: atopic dermatitis; serine proteases; kallikrein-related peptidases; epidermal barrier dysfunction; lympho-epithelial Kazal-type-related inhibitor (LEKTI); *SPINK5*; filaggrin

---

1. Introduction

Atopic dermatitis (AD) is a chronic, pruritic inflammatory skin disease that affects up to 25% of children and 2–3% of adults [1]. AD has a complex pathogenesis involving genetic, immunologic, and environmental factors which lead to a dysfunctional skin barrier and dysregulation of the immune system [1]. Aberrant epidermal serine protease activity is related to the pathogenesis of inflammatory skin diseases such as Netherton syndrome, AD, psoriasis, and rosacea [2–8]. Kallikrein-related peptidases (KLKs) are a family of 15 trypsin- or chymotrypsin-like serine proteases encoded by a cluster of protease-encoded genes (*KLK1-15*) in the human genome [9]. KLK5, a trypsin-like serine protease, and KLK7, a chymotrypsin-like serine protease, are major epidermal KLKs. These proteases have roles in the desquamation of epidermis by decomposing cell adhesion molecules such as corneodesmosin, desmoglein 1, and desmocollin 1 [10]. It has been reported that the expression and activity of several KLKs is increased in AD lesions [5,8,11]. Research suggests that KLK5 and KLK7 are particularly involved in the pathogenesis of AD. For instance, KLK5, but not KLK7, directly activates proteinase-activated receptor 2 and induces nuclear factor κB-mediated overexpression of thymic stromal lymphopoietin (TSLP) [12]. Moreover, transgenic-KLK5 mice display cutaneous and systemic hallmarks of severe inflammation and allergy with pruritus [13]. Transgenic mice expressing human KLK7 in epidermal keratinocytes have been found to develop pathologic skin changes with increased epidermal thickness, hyperkeratosis, dermal inflammation, and severe pruritus [14]. Our group demonstrated that Th2 cytokines increase the KLK7 expression and function in epidermal keratinocytes, suggesting an association between allergic inflammation and epidermal barrier function [15].

Serine protease activity in the skin is tightly regulated by not only KLKs but also serine protease inhibitors such as lympho-epithelial Kazal-type-related inhibitor (LEKTI), secretory leukocyte protease inhibitor (SLPI), and elafin [16]. LEKTI, encoded by the *serine protease inhibitor Kazal-type 5* (*SPINK5*) gene, is composed of 15 Kazal-type domains, all of which are capable of inhibiting serine protease activity including KLK5 and KLK7 [17,18]. Individuals with mutations of *SPINK5* develop Netherton syndrome, characterized by ichthyosis, hair abnormality, and atopic manifestations [19]. Nonsynonymous variants of *SPINK5* such as the p.D386N (c.G1156A, in exon 13) and p.E420K (c.G1258A, in exon 14) have been reported to be associated with the pathogenesis of AD [20–25]. The p.D386N variants disrupt the role of domain (D) 6 of LEKTI which suppresses the induction of TSLP by KLK5 [25]. The p.E420K variant increases the furin cleavage rate at the LEKTI linker region D6–D7 and prevents the formation of the LEKTI fragment D6D9, known to display the strongest inhibitory activity against KLK5-mediated desmoglein 1 degradation [20].

Profilaggrin is dephosphorylated and degraded to produce monomeric filaggrin in the SC and then further proteolyzed to release its component amino acids [26]. Profilaggrin, filaggrin and the amino acids each make different contributions to the epidermal structure and barrier function [26]. In 2006, loss-of-function mutations in the filaggrin gene (*FLG*) were identified as the cause of ichthyosis vulgaris [27]. The same year, it was first reported that loss-of-function genetic variants in *FLG* are predisposing factors in the context of AD [28]. In 2009, it was reported that 27% of Japanese AD patients carried *FLG* mutations [29]. To date, ten *FLG* mutations have been identified in the Japanese population [30]. Although *FLG* mutations are well known to affect epidermal barrier functions, the association between the mutations and the epidermal serine protease activity has not been investigated.

Here, we performed multifaceted analyses of epidermal serine protease activity in patients with AD. We focused particularly on the relationship between the epidermal serine protease activity and biomarkers of AD or AD-related gene variants.

2. Results

2.1. Serine Protease Activity in the SC of AD Is Increased in Both Non-Lesions and Lesions

We examined trypsin- and chymotrypsin-like serine protease activity in SC samples from normal healthy volunteers and AD patients. The activity of trypsin- and chymotrypsin-like serine proteases in the SC samples from both non-lesions and lesions of the AD patients were significantly higher than those from the healthy individuals (Figure 1A,B). The trypsin-like serine protease activity of the AD lesions was higher than that of the non-lesions (Figure 1A). A significant positive correlation between trypsin- and chymotrypsin-like serine protease activity was observed in both the non-lesions and lesions of the AD patients (Figure 1C,D).

Figure 1. Serine protease activity in the stratum corneum (SC) of atopic dermatitis (AD) patients was increased in both non-lesions and lesions. (**A,B**) Trypsin- and chymotrypsin-like serine protease activity in the SC of normal healthy volunteers ($n = 46$) and both non-lesions (AD-NL) and lesions (AD-L) of AD patients ($n = 63$) were measured. ** $p < 0.01$, *** $p < 0.001$. (**C,D**) The correlations between trypsin- and chymotrypsin-like serine protease activity in the non-lesions and lesions of AD patients were analyzed by Spearman's rank correlation coefficient.

2.2. The Association between Serine Protease Activity in the SC of AD and Medical Treatments

We next analysed the association between serine protease activity in the SC in lesions of AD patients ($n = 63$) and various medical treatments. The treatments were as follows: topical corticosteroid ($n = 44$), topical tacrolimus ($n = 15$), oral antihistamine ($n = 36$), oral corticosteroid ($n = 6$) and oral cyclosporine ($n = 4$). The trypsin-like serine protease activity in the SC of patients with topical corticosteroid therapy was significantly higher than those without topical corticosteroid therapy (Figure 2A). On the other hand, the chymotrypsin-like serine protease activity in the SC was not significantly different with or without topical corticosteroid therapy (Figure 2B). Neither trypsin- and chymotrypsin-like serine protease activity in the SC was significantly different with or without topical tacrolimus, oral antihistamine, oral corticosteroid or oral cyclosporine therapies (Figure 2C–J).

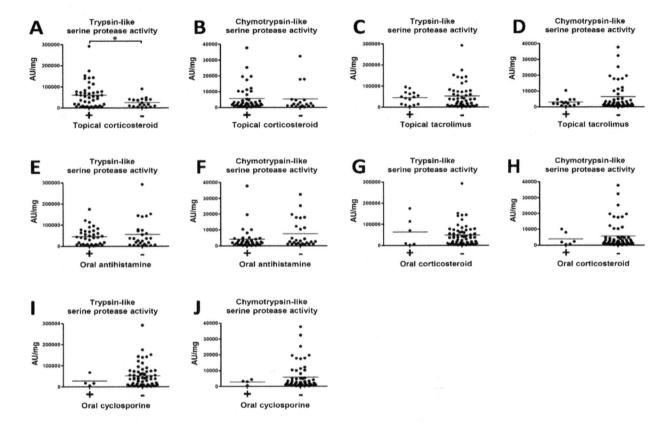

Figure 2. The association between serine protease activity in the SC in lesions of AD patients and medical treatments. Trypsin- or chymotrypsin-like serine protease activity in lesions were compared with and without topical corticosteroid (**A,B**), topical tacrolimus (**C,D**), oral antihistamine (**E,F**), oral corticosteroid (**G,H**) and oral cyclosporine therapies (**I,J**). * $p < 0.05$.

2.3. Serine Protease Activity in the SC of AD Correlate with Biomarkers of AD

We further examined the correlation between serine protease activity in the SC and the biomarkers of AD. We observed that the serum total immunoglobulin E (IgE) levels were highly correlated with the trypsin-like serine protease activity in non-lesions of the AD patients, but not with the chymotrypsin-like serine protease activity in non-lesions or the trypsin- or chymotrypsin-like serine protease activity in AD lesions (Figure 3A–D). The serum levels of thymus and activation-regulated chemokine (TARC) were highly correlated with the trypsin- or chymotrypsin-like serine protease activity in the non-lesions of the AD patients and the trypsin-like serine protease activity in AD lesions, but not with the chymotrypsin-like serine protease activity in AD lesions (Figure 3E–H). Our study found, further, that peripheral blood eosinophil counts were highly correlated with the trypsin-like serine protease activity in the non-lesions and lesions of the AD patients, but not with the chymotrypsin-like serine protease activity in the AD non-lesions or lesions (Figure 3I–L).

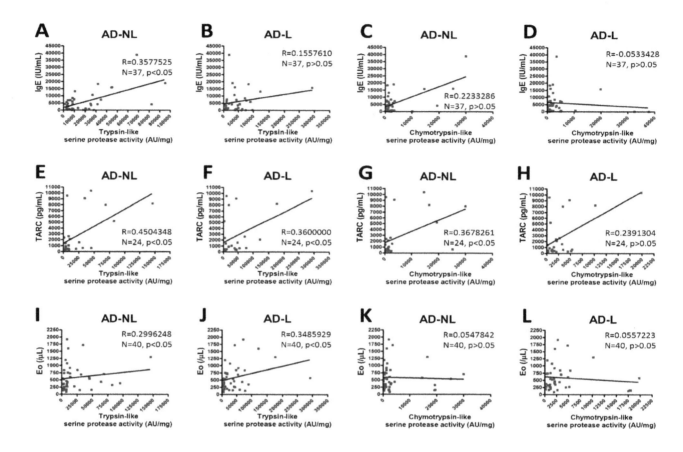

Figure 3. The correlations between serine protease activity in the SC and biomarkers of AD. The correlations between trypsin- or chymotrypsin-like serine protease activity in non-lesions (AD-NL) or lesions (AD-L) and the serum total IgE levels (**A–D**), serum TARC levels (**E–H**) and the peripheral blood eosinophil counts (Eo) (**I–L**) of the AD patients were analyzed by Spearman's rank correlation coefficient.

2.4. p.D386N and p.E420K of SPINK5 and Loss-Of-Function Mutations in FLG Do Not Affect the Serine Protease Activity in the SC

To clarify the association between serine protease activity in the SC and the AD-related gene variants, we analyzed *FLG* mutations in the AD patients. Eighteen of the 115 patients (15.7%) had one of the ten *FLG* mutations. We were able to perform protease assays with the SC samples from 61 of the AD patients. Ten of the 61 patients (16.4%) had the *FLG* mutations: p.Q1701X ($n = 1$), p.S2554X ($n = 1$), p.S2889X ($n = 4$), p.S3296X ($n = 2$) and p.K4022X ($n = 2$). We also analyzed p.D386N (c.G1156A) and p.E420K (c.G1258A) of *SPINK5* in the AD patients. In respect of p.D386N, the numbers of the genotypes were as follows: GG ($n = 21$), GA ($n = 28$), and AA ($n = 12$). For p.E420K, the numbers of the genotypes were as follows: GG ($n = 14$), GA ($n = 31$), and AA ($n = 16$). The trypsin- and chymotrypsin-like serine protease activity in the SC was not significantly different among the subgroups of p.D386N (Figure 4A,B) or p.E420K (Figure 4C,D). In addition, *FLG* mutations did not significantly affect the trypsin- or chymotrypsin-like serine protease activity of the SC in the AD patients (Figure 4E,F).

Figure 4. Serine protease activity in the SC of the subgroups of patients with the variants of the *SPINK5* gene and *FLG* gene in AD patients. Trypsin- and chymotrypsin-like serine protease activity in non-lesions and lesions was compared among the subgroups of the p.D386N (**A–B**) or p.E420K (**C–D**) of *SPINK5* and among the subgroups with or without loss-of-function mutations of *FLG* (**E–F**).

3. Discussion

It has been reported that the expression and activity of several KLKs are increased in AD lesions and trigger or enhance epidermal barrier dysfunction [5,8,11]. In this context, we examined the serine protease activity in the SC of both non-lesions and lesions of AD patients. Our findings demonstrated for the first time that serine protease activity is increased not only in lesions but also in non-lesions of AD patients.

Our results are consistent with previous reports that the quantity and activity of serine proteases are increased in AD lesions [5,8]. Our new finding that serine protease activity is also increased in non-lesions suggests two possibilities: (1) Serine protease activity may be influenced by some genetic factors; and (2) Non-lesions of AD patients have subclinical inflammation that may induce the enhancement of serine protease activity.

Considering the fact that Th2 cytokines such as interleukin (IL)-4 and IL-13 increase the expression and function of KLK7 in epidermal keratinocytes [15], the upregulation of chymotrypsin-like serine protease activity may be induced by systemic Th2 inflammation. However, the trypsin-like serine protease activity is not affected by Th2 cytokines [15]. Our present analyses showed that trypsin-like serine protease activity is also increased in both non-lesions and lesions of AD. Further analyses are needed to clarify the mechanism underlying the increase in trypsin-like serine protease activity.

We next investigated the association between serine protease activity in the SC and the content of therapy for AD. The trypsin-like serine protease activity in the SC of patients with topical corticosteroid therapy was significantly higher than those without topical corticosteroid therapy. These results suggest the possibility that patients with clinically severe AD needed to be treated with topical corticosteroid and clinically mild patients were able to be treated with topical tacrolimus or moisturizer only. Thus far, it is unknown why there is a difference between trypsin-like and chymotrypsin-like serine protease activity even though they are positively correlated (see Figure 1). Furthermore, it was unclear whether all the patients strictly took ointments or oral medicines. In addition, we did not prepare a wash-out period before collecting samples. These questions will guide future investigations.

We also investigated the correlation between serine protease activity in the SC and several biomarkers of AD. Not all serine protease activity was significantly correlated with the serum total IgE levels, serum TARC levels, or peripheral blood eosinophil counts, but there were tendencies for these to correlate positively. The absence of statistical significance in several of the comparisons might be due to the insufficiency of the sample number considered for the analysis or the technical instability of our protease assays. Serum total IgE reflects the degree of allergen sensitization [31,32]. Serum TARC is the most sensitive clinical biomarker of AD [33]. Peripheral blood eosinophil numbers also correlate roughly with disease severity [34]. Our results suggest that serine protease activity in the SC correlates with the clinical severity of AD and allergen sensitization due to epidermal barrier dysfunction.

We investigated whether nonsynonymous variants of *SPINK5* and loss-of-function mutations in *FLG* are involved in serine protease activity in the SC. p.D386N and p.E420K polymorphisms of *SPINK5* were each reported to be associated with the pathogenesis of AD [20–25]. We found, specifically, that the p.D386N variant disrupts the role of D6 of LEKTI which suppresses the induction of TSLP by KLK5 [25]. Moreover, the p.E420K substitution increases the furin cleavage rate at the LEKTI linker region D6–D7 and prevents the formation of the LEKTI fragment D6D9, known to display the strongest inhibitory activity against KLK5-mediated desmoglein 1 degradation [20]. However, our analyses revealed that p.D386N and p.E420K do not change the trypsin- or chymotrypsin-like serine protease activity of the SC in AD patients. Japanese AD patients might exhibit another genetic particularity related to serine protease activity that neutralizes the effects of p.D386N and p.E420K.

The *FLG* mutations are well known to be strongly associated with the pathogenesis of AD [28,29], but not all AD patients have *FLG* mutations. Therefore, one or more other genetic factors can be expected to be associated with the pathogenesis. We had hypothesized that AD patients without *FLG* mutations have serine proteases-related gene variants such as *SPINK5* and aberrant protease activity, but our analyses revealed that there is no significant association between these mutations and the serine protease activity in the SC. On the contrary, there was a tendency for the AD patients with *FLG* mutations to have higher serine protease activity compared to the patients without *FLG* mutations. Further analyses might clarify the association between the increase in serine protease activity and genetic factors in AD patients.

In conclusion, the results of our present analyses demonstrated for the first time that epidermal serine protease activity is increased even in non-lesions of AD patients and this activity is associated with biomarkers of AD. In addition, p.D386N and p.E420K of *SPINK5* and *FLG* mutations did not affect the serine protease activity of the SC in Japanese individuals with AD. Further investigations of epidermal serine protease activity might enable the design of new therapeutic and prophylactic drugs for the treatment of AD.

4. Subjects and Methods

4.1. Human Samples

The SC samples and blood samples were collected with written informed consent from normal healthy volunteers and patients with AD at Okayama University Hospital and its affiliated hospitals. This study was approved by the Ethics Committee of Okayama University (approval nos. 1511-012, 1605-027 and 1809-015).

4.2. Collection of the Stratum Corneum

Samples of the SC of healthy individuals were obtained from the forearms of normal healthy volunteers ($n = 46$; ages 35.0 ± 8.8 years). The SC of patients who had been diagnosed with AD based on the diagnostic criteria of Hanifin and Rajka were obtained from the upper extremities (lesions and non-lesions) ($n = 63$; ages 38.2 ± 12.8 years). Cellotape™ (Nichiban, Tokyo) was used to collect the SC samples. The 10-cm-long tape was put on and peeled from the surface of the extremities (approx. 10–20 times) until the adhesion disappeared. The tape was then stored at $-20\,^{\circ}$C until the following treatment with hexane.

The tape was soaked in 5 mL of hexane and then shaken to detach the SC from the tape's adhesive film. After the insoluble tape was removed, the solution was centrifuged at 3000 rpm for 15 min. A supernatant was subtracted and 1 mL of hexane was added. A solution was transferred to a 1.5-mL microtube and centrifuged at 15,000 rpm for 15 min. A supernatant was subtracted again and the recovered samples were air-dried. The weight was measured. The dried SC samples were mixed with 200 µL of 10 mmol/L Tris-HCl (pH 7.8) and incubated at $37\,^{\circ}$C for 1 h on a shaker and then used in the protease assays.

4.3. Protease Assays

For the measurement of protease activity in the SC samples, 100 µL of sample solution was mixed with 100 µL of a substrate that is specific for trypsin-like serine proteases (Boc-Phe-Ser-Arg-MCA; Peptide Institute, Osaka, Japan) or chymotrypsin-like serine proteases (Suc-Leu-Leu-Val-Tyr-MCA; Peptide Institute) in 10 mmol/L Tris-HCl (pH 7.8). The final concentration of each substrate was 0.4 mmol/L. The mixture was incubated at $37\,^{\circ}$C for 24 h and the fluorescence (excitation/emission = 380/460 nm) was then measured by a FlexStation 3 Multi-Mode Microplate Reader (Molecular Devices, Sunnyvale, CA) at the Central Research Laboratory, Okayama University Medical School. For the correction of the differences in the SC sample amounts, the value of measured fluorescence (AU) was divided by dried weight of the SC sample (mg).

4.4. Blood Examinations and Medical Treatment Histories

The patients' laboratory data were extracted from their medical records. The serum total IgE level, serum TARC level and peripheral blood eosinophil count that had been obtained at the time point closest to the patient's tape stripping were selected. We also collected the medical treatment histories of the patients such as their use of topical corticosteroid and topical tacrolimus, oral antihistamine, oral corticosteroid and oral cyclosporine.

4.5. Analysis of the SPINK5 Gene and the FLG Gene

Genomic DNA was extracted from whole blood using the Wizard Genomic DNA Purification Kit (Promega, Madison, WI, USA). For exon 13 of SPINK5, the 453-bp DNA was amplified with two specific primers (SPINK5-E13-FW: 5′-TTCCTATCTCTTGGCATATGATGT-3′ and SPINK5-E13-RV: 5′-TGTCTCCAATCAGACAGTTTCTC-3′). For exon 14 of SPINK5, the 294-bp DNA was amplified with two specific primers (SPINK5-E14-FW: 5′-CAGGGTTAGGCACATCACATTC-3′ and SPINK5-E14-RV: 5′-TAAGGAATGCACGTGTTCCCTG-3′).

The polymerase chain reaction (PCR) products were purified using exonuclease I and shrimp alkaline phosphatase (USB, Cleveland, OH, USA) and sequenced using a BigDye Terminator v3.1 Cycle Sequencing Kit (Applied Biosystems, Foster City, CA, USA) and an ABI3100 DNA sequencer (Applied Biosystems) at the Central Research Laboratory, Okayama University Medical School.

Real-time PCR-based genotyping of *FLG* mutations was performed. In the present *FLG* mutation screening, we investigated the 10 *FLG* mutations as described [30]. Briefly, real-time PCR-based genotyping of the *FLG* mutations was performed with a TaqMan probe genotyping assay. Real-time PCR-based genotyping of the *FLG* mutations was performed with a TaqMan probe genotyping assay according to the manufacturer's instructions (Roche Diagnostics, Basel, Switzerland). To detect an allele of each mutation, a set of two TaqMan probes labeled with a fluorescent dye (FAM or CAL Fluor Orange 560) and a quencher dye (BHQ-1), in addition to sequence-specific forward and reverse primers, were synthesized by Biosearch Technologies (Novato, CA, USA). The sequence of assay probes/primers was as provided [30]. The real-time PCR was performed with a LightCycler 480 system II 384 plate (Roche Diagnostics) in a final volume of 5 µL. Genotyping was then performed using the endpoint genotyping analysis of the LightCycler 480 software.

4.6. Statistical Analyses

All statistical analyses were conducted with GraphPad Prism 4 ver. 4.03 software (GraphPad Software, La Jolla, CA, USA). Student's *t*-test was used to determine the significance of differences between pairs of groups. The correlation between serine protease activity and the blood examination results was analyzed by Spearman's rank correlation coefficient. Values of $p < 0.05$ were considered significant.

Author Contributions: Experimental design and interpretation of results: H.N., M.A., M.K. (Michihiro Kono), T.T. and S.M. Performing the experiments: H.N., Y.I., K.S., and M.S. Writing the manuscript: H.N. Review and editing the manuscript: H.N., M.K. (Mina Kobashi), S.S., A.K., T.M., Y.H., O.Y. and S.M. All authors have read and agreed to the published version of the manuscript.

Abbreviations

AD	Atopic dermatitis
D	Domain
FLG	Filaggrin
IgE	Immunoglobulin E
IL	Interleukin
KLK	Kallikrein-related peptidase
LEKTI	Lympho-epithelial Kazal-type-related inhibitor
SC	Stratum corneum
SLPI	Secretory leukocyte protease inhibitor
SPINK5	Serine protease inhibitor Kazal type 5
TARC	Thymus and activation-regulated chemokine
Th	T-helper lymphocytes

References

1. Eichenfield, L.F.; Tom, W.L.; Chamlin, S.L.; Feldman, S.R.; Hanifin, J.M.; Simpson, E.L.; Berger, T.G.; Bergman, J.N.; Cohen, D.E.; Cooper, K.D.; et al. Guidelines of care for the management of atopic dermatitis: Section 1. Diagnosis and assessment of atopic dermatitis. *J. Am. Acad. Dermatol.* **2014**, *70*, 338–351. [CrossRef]
2. Chavanas, S.; Bodemer, C.; Rochat, A.; Hamel-Teillac, D.; Ali, M.; Irvine, A.D.; Bonafe, J.L.; Wilkinson, J.; Taieb, A.; Barrandon, Y.; et al. Mutations in SPINK5, encoding a serine protease inhibitor, cause Netherton syndrome. *Nat. Genet.* **2000**, *25*, 141–142. [CrossRef]

3. Descargues, P.; Deraison, C.; Bonnart, C.; Kreft, M.; Kishibe, M.; Ishida-Yamamoto, A.; Elias, P.; Barrandon, Y.; Zambruno, G.; Sonnenberg, A.; et al. Spink5-Deficient mice mimic Netherton syndrome through degradation of desmoglein 1 by epidermal protease hyperactivity. *Nat. Genet.* **2005**, *37*, 56–65. [CrossRef]

4. Komatsu, N.; Saijoh, K.; Jayakumar, A.; Clayman, G.L.; Tohyama, M.; Suga, Y.; Mizuno, Y.; Tsukamoto, K.; Taniuchi, K.; Takehara, K.; et al. Correlation between SPINK5 gene mutations and clinical manifestations in Netherton syndrome patients. *J. Investig. Dermatol.* **2008**, *128*, 1148–1159. [CrossRef] [PubMed]

5. Komatsu, N.; Saijoh, K.; Kuk, C.; Liu, A.C.; Khan, S.; Shirasaki, F.; Takehara, K.; Diamandis, E.P. Human tissue kallikrein expression in the stratum corneum and serum of atopic dermatitis patients. *Exp. Dermatol.* **2007**, *16*, 513–519. [CrossRef] [PubMed]

6. Komatsu, N.; Saijoh, K.; Kuk, C.; Shirasaki, F.; Takehara, K.; Diamandis, E.P. Aberrant human tissue kallikrein levels in the stratum corneum and serum of patients with psoriasis: Dependence on phenotype, severity and therapy. *Br. J. Dermatol.* **2007**, *156*, 875–883. [CrossRef] [PubMed]

7. Yamasaki, K.; Di Nardo, A.; Bardan, A.; Murakami, M.; Ohtake, T.; Coda, A.; Dorschner, R.A.; Bonnart, C.; Descargues, P.; Hovnanian, A.; et al. Increased serine protease activity and cathelicidin promotes skin inflammation in rosacea. *Nat. Med.* **2007**, *13*, 975–980. [CrossRef]

8. Voegeli, R.; Rawlings, A.V.; Breternitz, M.; Doppler, S.; Schreier, T.; Fluhr, J.W. Increased stratum corneum serine protease activity in acute eczematous atopic skin. *Br. J. Dermatol.* **2009**, *161*, 70–77. [CrossRef]

9. Sotiropoulou, G.; Pampalakis, G.; Diamandis, E.P. Functional roles of human kallikrein-related peptidases. *J. Biol. Chem.* **2009**, *284*, 32989–32994. [CrossRef]

10. Caubet, C.; Jonca, N.; Brattsand, M.; Guerrin, M.; Bernard, D.; Schmidt, R.; Egelrud, T.; Simon, M.; Serre, G. Degradation of corneodesmosome proteins by two serine proteases of the kallikrein family, SCTE/KLK5/hK5 and SCCE/KLK7/hK7. *J. Investig. Dermatol.* **2004**, *122*, 1235–1244. [CrossRef]

11. Morizane, S. The role of kallikrein-related peptidases in atopic dermatitis. *Acta Med. Okayama* **2019**, *73*, 1–6. [CrossRef] [PubMed]

12. Briot, A.; Deraison, C.; Lacroix, M.; Bonnart, C.; Robin, A.; Besson, C.; Dubus, P.; Hovnanian, A. Kallikrein 5 induces atopic dermatitis-like lesions through PAR2-mediated thymic stromal lymphopoietin expression in Netherton syndrome. *J. Exp. Med.* **2009**, *206*, 1135–1147. [CrossRef] [PubMed]

13. Furio, L.; de Veer, S.; Jaillet, M.; Briot, A.; Robin, A.; Deraison, C.; Hovnanian, A. Transgenic kallikrein 5 mice reproduce major cutaneous and systemic hallmarks of Netherton syndrome. *J. Exp. Med.* **2014**, *211*, 499–513. [CrossRef] [PubMed]

14. Hansson, L.; Backman, A.; Ny, A.; Edlund, M.; Ekholm, E.; Ekstrand-Hammarstrom, B.; Tornell, J.; Wallbrandt, P.; Wennbo, H.; Egelrud, T. Epidermal overexpression of stratum corneum chymotryptic enzyme in mice: A model for chronic itchy dermatitis. *J. Investig. Dermatol.* **2002**, *118*, 444–449. [CrossRef]

15. Morizane, S.; Yamasaki, K.; Kajita, A.; Ikeda, K.; Zhan, M.; Aoyama, Y.; Gallo, R.L.; Iwatsuki, K. TH2 cytokines increase kallikrein 7 expression and function in patients with atopic dermatitis. *J. Allergy Clin. Immunol.* **2012**, *130*, 259–261. [CrossRef]

16. Meyer-Hoffert, U. Reddish, scaly, and itchy: How proteases and their inhibitors contribute to inflammatory skin diseases. *Arch. Immunol. Ther. Exp.* **2009**, *57*, 345–354. [CrossRef]

17. Deraison, C.; Bonnart, C.; Lopez, F.; Besson, C.; Robinson, R.; Jayakumar, A.; Wagberg, F.; Brattsand, M.; Hachem, J.P.; Leonardsson, G.; et al. LEKTI fragments specifically inhibit KLK5, KLK7, and KLK14 and control desquamation through a pH-dependent interaction. *Mol. Biol. Cell* **2007**, *18*, 3607–3619. [CrossRef]

18. Magert, H.J.; Standker, L.; Kreutzmann, P.; Zucht, H.D.; Reinecke, M.; Sommerhoff, C.P.; Fritz, H.; Forssmann, W.G. LEKTI, a novel 15-domain type of human serine proteinase inhibitor. *J. Biol. Chem.* **1999**, *274*, 21499–21502. [CrossRef]

19. Hovnanian, A. Netherton syndrome: Skin inflammation and allergy by loss of protease inhibition. *Cell Tissue Res.* **2013**, *351*, 289–300. [CrossRef]

20. Fortugno, P.; Furio, L.; Teson, M.; Berretti, M.; El Hachem, M.; Zambruno, G.; Hovnanian, A.; D'Alessio, M. The 420K LEKTI variant alters LEKTI proteolytic activation and results in protease deregulation: Implications for atopic dermatitis. *Hum. Mol. Genet.* **2012**, *21*, 4187–4200. [CrossRef]

21. Kato, A.; Fukai, K.; Oiso, N.; Hosomi, N.; Murakami, T.; Ishii, M. Association of SPINK5 gene polymorphisms with atopic dermatitis in the Japanese population. *Br. J. Dermatol.* **2003**, *148*, 665–669. [CrossRef] [PubMed]

22. Kusunoki, T.; Okafuji, I.; Yoshioka, T.; Saito, M.; Nishikomori, R.; Heike, T.; Sugai, M.; Shimizu, A.; Nakahata, T. SPINK5 polymorphism is associated with disease severity and food allergy in children with atopic dermatitis. *J. Allergy Clin. Immunol.* **2005**, *115*, 636–638. [CrossRef] [PubMed]

23. Nishio, Y.; Noguchi, E.; Shibasaki, M.; Kamioka, M.; Ichikawa, E.; Ichikawa, K.; Umebayashi, Y.; Otsuka, F.; Arinami, T. Association between polymorphisms in the SPINK5 gene and atopic dermatitis in the Japanese. *Genes Immun.* **2003**, *4*, 515–517. [CrossRef] [PubMed]

24. Walley, A.J.; Chavanas, S.; Moffatt, M.F.; Esnouf, R.M.; Ubhi, B.; Lawrence, R.; Wong, K.; Abecasis, G.R.; Jones, E.Y.; Harper, J.I.; et al. Gene polymorphism in Netherton and common atopic disease. *Nat. Genet.* **2001**, *29*, 175–178. [CrossRef]

25. Ramesh, K.; Matta, S.A.; Chew, F.T.; Mok, Y.K. Exonic mutations associated with atopic dermatitis disrupt lympho-epithelial Kazal-type related inhibitor action and enhance its degradation. *Allergy* **2019**. [CrossRef]

26. Brown, S.J.; McLean, W.H. One remarkable molecule: Filaggrin. *J. Investig. Dermatol.* **2012**, *132*, 751–762. [CrossRef]

27. Smith, F.J.; Irvine, A.D.; Terron-Kwiatkowski, A.; Sandilands, A.; Campbell, L.E.; Zhao, Y.; Liao, H.; Evans, A.T.; Goudie, D.R.; Lewis-Jones, S.; et al. Loss-of-function mutations in the gene encoding filaggrin cause ichthyosis vulgaris. *Nat. Genet.* **2006**, *38*, 337–342. [CrossRef]

28. Palmer, C.N.; Irvine, A.D.; Terron-Kwiatkowski, A.; Zhao, Y.; Liao, H.; Lee, S.P.; Goudie, D.R.; Sandilands, A.; Campbell, L.E.; Smith, F.J.; et al. Common loss-of-function variants of the epidermal barrier protein filaggrin are a major predisposing factor for atopic dermatitis. *Nat. Genet.* **2006**, *38*, 441–446. [CrossRef]

29. Nemoto-Hasebe, I.; Akiyama, M.; Nomura, T.; Sandilands, A.; McLean, W.H.; Shimizu, H. FLG mutation p.Lys4021X in the C-terminal imperfect filaggrin repeat in Japanese patients with atopic eczema. *Br. J. Dermatol.* **2009**, *161*, 1387–1390. [CrossRef]

30. Kono, M.; Nomura, T.; Ohguchi, Y.; Mizuno, O.; Suzuki, S.; Tsujiuchi, H.; Hamajima, N.; McLean, W.H.; Shimizu, H.; Akiyama, M. Comprehensive screening for a complete set of Japanese-population-specific filaggrin gene mutations. *Allergy* **2014**, *69*, 537–540. [CrossRef]

31. Bieber, T.; D'Erme, A.M.; Akdis, C.A.; Traidl-Hoffmann, C.; Lauener, R.; Schappi, G.; Schmid-Grendelmeier, P. Clinical phenotypes and endophenotypes of atopic dermatitis: Where are we, and where should we go? *J. Allergy Clin. Immunol.* **2017**, *139*, S58–S64. [CrossRef] [PubMed]

32. Kuperstock, J.E.; Brook, C.D.; Ryan, M.W.; Platt, M.P. Correlation between the number of allergen sensitizations and immunoglobulin E: Monosensitization vs. polysensitization. *Int. Forum Allergy Rhinol.* **2017**, *7*, 385–388. [CrossRef] [PubMed]

33. Kataoka, Y. Thymus and activation-regulated chemokine as a clinical biomarker in atopic dermatitis. *J. Dermatol.* **2014**, *41*, 221–229. [CrossRef] [PubMed]

34. Simon, D.; Braathen, L.R.; Simon, H.U. Eosinophils and atopic dermatitis. *Allergy* **2004**, *59*, 561–570. [CrossRef] [PubMed]

10

Efficacy and Safety of Biologics for Psoriasis and Psoriatic Arthritis and their Impact on Comorbidities

Masahiro Kamata and Yayoi Tada *

Department of Dermatology, Teikyo University School of Medicine, 2-11-1 Kaga, Itabashi-ku, Tokyo 173-8605, Japan; mkamata-tky@umin.ac.jp
* Correspondence: ytada-tky@umin.ac.jp

Abstract: Psoriasis is a chronic inflammatory skin disease characterized by scaly indurated erythema. It impairs patients' quality of life enormously. It has been recognized not only as a skin disease but as a systemic disease, since it also causes arthritis (psoriatic arthritis) and mental disorders. Furthermore, an association with cardiovascular events is indicated. With the advent of biologics, treatment of psoriasis dramatically changed due to its high efficacy and tolerable safety. A variety of biologic agents are available for the treatment of psoriasis nowadays. However, characteristics such as rapidity of onset, long-term efficacy, safety profile, and effects on comorbidities are different. Better understanding of those characteristic leads to the right choice for individual patients, resulting in higher persistence, longer drug survival, higher patient satisfaction, and minimizing the disease impact of psoriasis. In this paper, we focus on the efficacy and safety profile of biologics in psoriasis patients, including plaque psoriasis and psoriatic arthritis. In addition, we discuss the impact of biologics on comorbidities caused by psoriasis.

Keywords: biologics; psoriasis; psoriatic arthritis; tumor necrosis factor-α; inteleukin-23; interluekin-17

1. Introduction

Psoriasis is a chronic inflammatory skin disease characterized by scaly indurated erythema. The prevalence of psoriasis in children ranges from 0% (Taiwan) to 2.1% (Italy), and in adults it varies from 0.91% (United States) to 8.5% (Norway) [1]. It impairs patients' quality of life enormously. It has been recognized not only as a skin disease but as a systemic disease, since it also causes arthritis (psoriatic arthritis; PsA) and mental disorders. Furthermore, an association with cardiovascular events is indicated [2]. With the advent of biologics, treatment of psoriasis dramatically changed due to its high efficacy and tolerable safety. In addition, the efficacy of biologics helps us to understand the pathogenesis of psoriasis. Whereas biologics have shown dramatically excellent efficacy, their safety has been a concern. To date, data on their efficacy and safety have been accumulated. In this paper, we focus on the efficacy and safety profile of biologics in psoriasis patients, including plaque psoriasis and PsA. In addition, we discuss the impact of biologics on comorbidities caused by psoriasis.

2. Efficacy and Safety of Biologics

Although approved biologic agents differ by countries, biologic agents commonly used for the treatment of psoriasis are categorized into three groups, tumor necrosis factor (TNF)-α inhibitors, interleukin (IL)-23 inhibitors, and IL-17 inhibitors, as shown in Table 1. Infliximab, adalimumab, etanercept, certolizumab-pegol, and golimumab are TNF-α inhibitors. Golimumab is used only for PsA. Ustekinumab is an anti-IL-12/23p40 antibody. Guselkumab, risankizumab, tildrakizumab, and mirikizumab are anti-IL-23p19 antibodies. Secukinumab, and ixekizumab are anti-IL-17A antibodies. Brodalumab is an anti-IL-17RA antibody. Bimekizumab is an anti-IL-17A/F antibody, which blocks both IL-17A and IL-17F. Many randomized controlled trials (RCTs) were conducted, and they demonstrated that the drugs are efficacious for moderate-to-severe plaque psoriasis. Recently, network meta-analyses enabled indirect comparison among those agents.

Table 1. Target of biologics.

Target of biologics	Drug
TNF-α inhibitors	Infliximab Adalimumab Golimumab (for psoriatic arthritis) Certolizumab-pegol Etanercept
IL-12/23 inhibitor	Ustekinumab
IL-23 inhibitors	Guselkumab Risankizumab Tildrakizumab (not approved yet) Mirikizumab (not approved yet)
IL-17 inhibitors	Secukinumab Ixekizumab Brodalumab Bimekizumab (not approved yet)
CTLA4-Ig	Abatacept (for psoriatic arthritis)

2.1. Plaque Psoriasis

Since previous review articles have illustrated the pathogenesis of psoriasis, we do not refer to the details [3,4]. Briefly, various triggers activate plasmacytoid dendritic cells, which are important in early-phase psoriasis. Meanwhile, TNF-α/iNOS-producing dendritic cells (TIP-DCs) play a pivotal role in maintaining psoriasis. TIP-DC activated by TNF-α secrete TNF-α, which activate themselves in an autocrine way. TIP-DCs also produce IL-23, which maintains and proliferates Th-17 cells. IL-23-stimulated Th17 cells are pathogenic and produce excessive IL-17A, F, and IL-22. Those cytokines drive keratinocytes to abnormal differentiation and proliferation, which forms psoriasis plaque. Activated keratinocytes also work as immune cells. They produce anti-microbial peptides and TNF-α, which activate dendritic cells including TIP-DC. This vicious inflammatory cycle makes the plaque remain and deteriorate. Activated keratinocytes secrete IL-17C, which activates keratinocytes in an autocrine way. Recently, the contribution of resident memory T cells [5–8], epidermal dendritic cells [9] in the epidermis, and type 3 innate lymphoid cells [8,10] to the development of psoriasis and recurrent plaque has attracted attention.

New biologic agents such as risankizumab [11], guselkumab [12–16], ixekizumab [17–23], and brodalumab [24,25] demonstrated high efficacy for patients with moderate-to-severe psoriasis. The percentage of patients who achieved more than a 90% reduction in the Psoriasis Area Severity Index (PASI) score at 16 weeks after initiating each treatment (PASI 90) was about 70%–80%, and that at 52 weeks was about 80%–90% in respective clinical trials. PASI 100 was about 50%–60% at 52 weeks. Those biologic agents showed high efficacy.

Ellis et al. appraised two network-meta analyses that assessed systemic therapies for moderate-to-severe psoriasis [26]. They concluded that newer biologics targeting theIL-12/23 and IL-17 axes appear to be more effective than older biologics and oral agents.

Sawyer et al. analyzed 17 studies reporting outcomes at 40-64 weeks in order to evaluate long-term efficacy [27]. Four 52-week RCTs revealed that brodalumab was significantly more efficacious than secukinumab, ustekinumab, and etanercept. Secukinumab was also more efficacious than ustekinumab, and both outperformed etanercept. Evidence from 13 additional studies and four further therapies (adalimumab, apremilast, infliximab and ixekizumab) revealed that brodalumab was most effective, followed by ixekizumab and secukinumab, then ustekinumab, infliximab and adalimumab. Etanercept had the lowest expected long-term efficacy. They concluded that brodalumab is associated with a higher likelihood of sustained PASI response, including complete clearance, at week 52 than comparators.

Sawyer et al. performed a network meta-analysis including 77 trials (34,816 patients) [28]. They revealed the superiority of brodalumab, ixekizumab, secukinumab, guselkumab and risankizumab to tildrakizumab, ustekinumab, all TNF-α inhibitors, and non-biologic systemic treatments in efficacy for plaque psoriasis. Furthermore, brodalumab, ixekizumab, and risankizumab showed higher efficacy than secukinumab, but did not significantly compared with guselkumab. In terms of PASI 90 and PASI 100 response, brodalumab, ixekizumab, guselkumab, and risankizumab demonstrated the greatest benefits.

According to the meta-analysis of 140 studies reported by Shidian et al. [29], in terms of the percentage of patients who attained PASI 90, infliximab, ixekizumab, secukinumab, bimekizumab, brodalumab, risankizumab, and guselkumab showed higher efficacy than ustekinumab, adalimumab, certolizumab, and etanercept. Moreover, adalimumab and ustekinumab were more efficacious than certolizumab and etanercept. No significant difference was observed between any of the interventions and the placebo for the risk of severe adverse events.

Generally, we can expect a rapid onset of efficacy on IL-17 inhibitors, especially brodalumab [30,31] and ixekizumab [32–34]. IL-17 inhibitors and IL-23 inhibitors, especially brodalumab, ixekizumab, and risankizumab showed high efficacy in the long-term [28,29].

2.2. Psoriatic Arthritis

A systematic review revealed 14.0%–22.7% of psoriasis patients having arthritis PsA in psoriasis patients [35]. PsA is characterized by enthesitis and arthritis in peripheral and axial involvement with bone proliferation and erosion [36,37]. PsA patients show distal interphalangeal joint involvement, which is usually asymmetric. In the pathogenesis of PsA, it is advocated that inflammation occurs in entheses in the early phase, and that the progression of enthesitis results in accompaniment with synovitis. In the initiation phase of enthesitis, innate immune cells are thought to play a key role. Thereafter, once certain entheseal cells are stimulated with IL-23, they secrete inflammatory cytokines such as IL-17A, IL-22 and TNF-α, consequently augmenting inflammation [36]. Focusing on enthesitis which is characteristic of PsA, Araujo et al. reported that ustekinumab, an anti-IL-12/IL-23p40 antibody, was superior to TNF-α inhibitors in the clearance of enthesitis [38], which underscores the importance of IL-23 in enthesitis. With regard to the contributions of TNF-α to the development of PsA [39,40], TNF-α increases the number of osteoclast precursor cells. TNF-α promotes differentiation into osteoclasts through RANKL-dependent pathways and promotes bone resorption. TNF-α inhibits Wnt signaling and induces apoptosis of osteoblasts, thereby reducing bone repair capacity. Recently, IL-23-independent IL-17-producing cells have drawn attention, especially in the pathogenesis of axial involvement of PsA. PsA and ankylosing spondylitis (AS) are recognized as one of spondyloarthritis (SpA) characterized by enthesitis, peripheral and axial arthritis, and negative laboratory results of rheumatoid factor and anti-cyclic citrullinated peptide antibody [41]. It indicates that the responsiveness of a certain drug for AS reflects its responsiveness for axial involvement of PsA. Anti-IL-17 antibodies, secukinumab [42] and ixekizumab [43], demonstrated efficacy for AS, but anti-IL-23 antibody, risankizumab [44], did not. Those results of clinical trials suggest the importance of IL-23-independent IL-17-producing cells in the axial involvement of PsA. iNKT and $\gamma\delta$-T cells are candidates of IL-23-independent IL-17-producing cells in SpA joints. Venken et al. reported that iNKT and $\gamma\delta$-T cells were a major source of T-cell-derived IL-17 in SpA joints and that those cells produced abundant IL-17 with anti-CD3 antibody/anti-CD28 antibody stimulation even in the absence of IL-23 [45]. Those data suggest that PsA patients with axial involvement would be better to be treated with IL-17 inhibitors such as ixekizumab and secukinumab, or TNF-α inhibitors, instead of anti-IL-23 antibodies such as risankizumab. Although the prevalence of having axial involvement in PsA patients differs by diagnosis criteria, it is reported to be from 23.6% to 55.4% [46,47]. In treating PsA patients, we should consider the considerable percentage of PsA patients having axial involvement and choose the right biologic agent. Mease et al. found the clinical characteristics of 192 PsA patients with axial involvement by comparing them with 1338 PsA patients without it [48]. Axial involvement was defined as physician-reported presence of spinal involvement at enrollment, and/or radiograph or MRI showing sacroiliitis. Patients with axial involvement showed a higher likelihood of moderate-to-severe psoriasis(body surface area ≥ 3%, 42.5% vs. 31.5%), lower prevalence of minimal disease activity (30.1% vs. 46.2%), higher nail psoriasis scores (visual analog scale; VAS 11.4 vs. 6.5), enthesitis counts (5.1 vs. 3.4), serum C-reactive protein levels (4.1 vs. 2.4 mg/L), and scores for physical function (Health Assessment Questionnaire, 0.9 vs. 0.6), pain (VAS, 47.7 vs. 36.2), and fatigue (VAS, 50.2 vs. 38.6) than patients without axial involvement. The American College of Rheumatology (ACR) and the National Psoriasis Foundation (NPF) published guidelines for PsA in 2019 [49], although nearly all recommendations were conditional since the quality of evidence was most often low or very low, and occasionally moderate.

Kawalec et al. conducted the network meta-analysis with eight eligible RCTs for efficacy (ACR 20 and ACR 50, PASI 75) and safety outcomes [50]. RCTs for abatacept, apremilast, secukinumab, or ustekinumab in adults with moderate-to-severe PsA were included. There were significant differences in the ACR20 response rate between secukinumab 150 mg and apremilast 20 mg, and between secukinumab 300 mg and apremilast 20 or 30 mg. Any adverse events occurred more often in apremilast 20 and 30 mg compared with the placebo and compared with secukinumab 150 mg. No significant differences were revealed for severe adverse events among biologics and between biologics and the placebo. In the overall population, as well as in the anti-TNF-α-naive subpopulation, secukinumab at a dose of 300 and 150 mg was ranked the highest for the ACR20 endpoint, while in the anti-TNF-α-experienced subpopulation, secukinumab 300 mg and apremilast 30 mg revealed the highest rank. For severe adverse events, the safest was ustekinumab 90 mg.

Dressler et al. also conducted a systematic review of approved systemic treatments for PsA [51]. Data were extracted from 20 trials for ACR 20, ACR 50, and adverse events after 16–24 weeks. Results for ACR 20 were infliximab + methotrexate vs. methotrexate: relative risk (RR) 1.40 (95% CI 1.07–1.84), very low-quality evidence; ixekizumab Q2W vs. adalimumab Q2W: RR 1.08 (95% CI 0.86–1.36), very low quality. In three placebo-controlled comparisons, leflunomide, methotrexate (MTX), and sulfasalazine failed to show statistical superiority for ACR. Besides the established treatment of anti-TNF antibodies and ustekinumab for psoriatic arthritis, the newer treatment options of anti-IL-17 antibodies and apremilast are also effective for the treatment of PsA. Based on just one comparative trial and one drug each, the new class of anti-IL 17 antibodies appears to be equally effective compared to the group of anti-TNF antibodies; for apremilast, this is yet unclear.

Lu et al., RCTs evaluated the efficacy and safety of targeted synthetic disease modifying anti-rheumatic drugs (DMARDs: tofacitinib, apremilast), as well as biological DMARDs (guselkumab, ustekinumab, secukinumab, ixekizumab, brodalumab, abatacept, adalimumab, etanercept, infliximab, certolizumab, and golimumab) for active PsA by a systemic literature review of 29 RCTs, including 10,204 participants and 17 treatments [52]. All treatments showed efficacy in ACR 20 and PASI 75 at 12–16 weeks in comparison with a placebo. As for safety, tofacitinib, apremilast, and ixekizumab 80 mg every 2 weeks demonstrated a higher rate of adverse events; however, in severe adverse events no significant difference was observed among all treatments. Network meta-analysis revealed that infliximab, golimumab, etanercept, adalimumab, guselkumab, and secukinumab 300 mg showed superiority to other drugs in both ACR 20 and PASI 75. Focusing on biologic-naïve patients, the results were similar to those above. Among biologic-experienced/failed patients, ustekinumab, secukinumab (300 mg and 150 mg), ixekizumab, abatacept, certolizumab pegol, tofacitinib, and apremilast still demonstrated higher ACR 20 then placebo, whereas only ustekinumab, secukinumab (300 mg), ixekizumab and tofacitinib were still associated with higher PASI 75.

In interpreting these systematic reviews, we should be aware that most clinical trials only assessed peripheral arthritis and did not assess enthesitis, dactylitis, or even axial involvement. As written above, it would be better to treat PsA with axial involvement with TNF-α inhibitors or IL-17 inhibitors instead of IL-23 inhibitors. When deciding on a treatment for PsA, we should not focus only on efficacy for arthritis, but also take skin manifestation into consideration. The safety profile should be also considered.

2.3. Safety Concerns of Biologics

As written above, biologic agents demonstrated tolerable safety profiles in the clinical trials. However, accumulating evidence revealed drug-specific concerns. We have already discussed the safety concerns of biologics in the previous literature [53]. Therefore, we refer to this issue in brief. It has been reported that TNF-α inhibitors are associated with serious infection (slightly increased risk), tuberculosis, paradoxical reaction, lupus, and infusion reaction (only infliximab). IL-17 inhibitors are associated with candidiasis, neutropenia, and inflammatory bowel disease. As of now, there have never been IL-23 inhibitor-specific adverse events reported. Safety concerns common in biologics include hepatitis B virus reactivation and interstitial pneumonia. Those concerns were raised during use of TNF-α inhibitors. Evidence of newer drugs such as IL-17 inhibitors and IL-23 inhibitors are insufficient. Accumulation of evidence is needed. Regarding immunogenicity, generally, predispositions of higher immunogenicity are observed in humanized monoclonal antibodies rather than in human monoclonal antibodies. The effect of immunogenicity on efficacy and safety seems limited in new biologic agents. However, since psoriasis is a chronic disease and some patients need to receive biologics for a long period of time, it might affect effectiveness and safety in the long-term. Longer observation is necessary to clarify this. With respect to malignancy, its rates are higher in psoriasis patients than the adult general population, but these treatments do not appear to increase malignancy risk.

Kaushik and Lebwohl focus on pregnant and pediatric patients with moderate-to-severe psoriasis, and those with chronic infections, such as hepatitis, HIV, and latent tuberculosis, and describe appropriate systematic treatment for them [54].

3. Impact of Biologics on Comorbidities

Psoriasis imposes a psychological burden on patients. The prevalence of having depression or anxiety is higher in psoriasis patients than in controls [55–57]. A systematic review and meta-analysis investigating 18 studies including a total of 1,767,583 participants, of whom 330,207 had psoriasis, reported that patients with psoriasis had a significantly higher likelihood of suicidal ideation, suicide attempts, and completed suicides [58]. Strober et al. evaluated the effect of biologic therapy (ustekinumab, infliximab, etanercept, and adalimumab) on depression in psoriasis patients utilizing Psoriasis Longitudinal Assessment and Registry (PSOLAR). The incidence rates of depressive symptoms were 3.01 (95% CI, 2.73–3.32), 5.85 (95% CI, 4.29–7.97), and 5.70 (95% CI, 4.58–7.10) per 100 patient-years for biologics, phototherapy, and conventional therapy, respectively. Compared with conventional therapy, biologics reduced the risk for depressive symptoms (hazard ratio, 0.76; 95% CI, 0.59–0.98), whereas phototherapy did not (hazard ratio, 1.05; 95% CI, 0.71–1.54) [59].

Cohen et al. investigated 12,502 psoriasis patients aged 20 years and above and 24,287 age- and sex-matched controls utilizing Clalit Health Services, the largest healthcare provider organization in Israel, and revealed that psoriasis was associated with Crohn's disease (CD; odds ratio, 2.49; 95% CI, 1.71–3.62) as well as ulcerative colitis (UC; odds ratio, 1.64; 95% CI, 1.15–2.33) [60]. Focusing on the effect of biologics, randomized control trials for CD with secukinumab and brodalumab resulted in a disproportionate number of cases of worsening and no evidence of efficacy [61,62]. In addition, exacerbations of inflammatory disease have been reported in psoriasis patients receiving IL-17 inhibitors [22,25,60]. Lee et al. found that IL-17A-dependent regulation of the tight junction protein occludin in the intestinal mucosa during epithelial injury limits excessive permeability and maintains barrier integrity, and revealed that IL-23-independent IL-17 production by $\gamma\delta$ T cells was important for the maintenance and protection of epithelial barriers in the intestinal mucosa. Whereas IL-17 inhibition exacerbates inflammatory bowel disease, TNF-α inhibitors are approved for the treatment of CD and UC, and IL-23 inhibitors demonstrated clinical improvement [63,64].

Recently, "psoriatic march", the concept of a causal link between psoriasis and cardiovascular disease, has been widely recognized. Systemic inflammation may cause insulin resistance, which in turn triggers endothelial cell dysfunction, leading to atherosclerosis and finally myocardial infarction or stroke [65,66]. Systematic review and meta-analysis analyzing 14 papers, including a total of 25,042 patients with psoriasis, revealed the association of psoriasis with metabolic syndrome. They reported that metabolic syndrome was present in 31.4% of patients with psoriasis (odds ratio, 1.42; 95% CI, 1.28–1.65) [67]. Other articles indicated that obesity is associated with the onset, exacerbation, and intractability of psoriasis [68–72]. As for hyperglycemia, Ikumi et al. revealed that hyperglycemia is highly associated with psoriasis, mainly through IL-17. In patients, the severity of psoriasis correlated with high blood glucose levels, and anti-IL-17A monoclonal antibody therapy reduced HbA1c levels significantly in these patients. In imiquimod-induced psoriasiform dermatitis, treatment with anti-IL-17A monoclonal antibody decreased fasting blood glucose levels [73]. Concerning endothelial cell dysfunction, flow-mediated dilation (FMD) is a marker that reflects endothelial cell dysfunction. Avgerinou et al. investigated FMD in 14 psoriasis patients before and 12 weeks after treatment with adalimumab, and reported that it improved after treatment with adalimumab [74]. von Stebut et al. conducted a 52-week, randomized, double-blind, placebo-controlled, exploratory trial in patients with moderate-to-severe plaque psoriasis without clinical cardiovascular disease, named Evaluation of Cardiovascular Risk Markers in Psoriasis Patients Treated with Secukinumab (CARIMA) [75]. Although a statistical difference was not observed in the baseline-adjusted mean FMD between patients receiving secukinumab and those receiving placebo at week 12, FMD was significantly higher than baseline in patients receiving the label dose of 300 mg secukinumab for 52 weeks. Regarding atherosclerosis, Hjuler et al. examined calcified coronary plaque, utilizing cardiac computed tomography angiography in severe psoriasis patients, severe atopic dermatitis patients, and retrospectively matched controls [76]. They demonstrated that psoriasis patients showed an increased prevalence of severe coronary stenosis (stenosis >70%) (psoriasis 14.6%, controls 0%; $p = 0.02$) and 3-vessel coronary affection or left main artery disease (psoriasis 20%, controls 3%; $p = 0.02$), whereas AD patients showed an increased prevalence of mild single-vessel affection (AD 40.7%, controls 9.1%; $p = 0.005$). Elnabawi et al. conducted a prospective, observational study in order to investigate the effect of biologic therapy on coronary artery plaque [77]. Analysis of 121 participants who were biologics-naïve at baseline and received biologic therapy for one year revealed that biologic therapy was associated with a 6% reduction in non-calcified plaque burden ($p = 0.005$) reduction in necrotic core ($p = 0.03$), with no effect on fibrous burden ($p = 0.71$), indicating that biologic therapy in severe psoriasis was associated with favorable modulation of coronary plaque indices. After one-year of biologic therapy, non-calcified plaque burden decreased by 5% in patients treated with TNF-α inhibitors ($p = 0.06$), by 2% in patients treated with anti-IL12/23 antibody ($p = 0.36$), and by 12% in patients treated with IL-17 inhibitors ($p < 0.001$). Patients treated with IL-17 inhibitors demonstrated a significantly greater reduction in non-calcified coronary plaque burden compared with those treated with anti-IL12/23 antibody and those with no biologic treatment. Patients treated with TNF-α inhibitors showed a significantly greater reduction in non-calcified coronary plaque burden only compared those with non-biologic treatment ($p < 0.01$). Regarding cardiovascular events, a systemic review and meta-analysis demonstrated that mild and severe psoriasis are associated with an increased risk of myocardial infarction and stroke, and that severe psoriasis is also associated with an increased risk of cardiovascular mortality [78]. Yang et al. conducted a meta-analysis on the effect of TNF-α inhibitors on cardiovascular events in psoriasis and psoriatic arthritis, analyzing five studies (49,795 patients). Compared with topical/photo treatment, TNF-α inhibitors were associated with a significant lower risk of cardiovascular events (RR, 0.58; 95% confidence interval; CI, 0.43 to 0.77; $p < 0.001$). Additionally, compared with MTX treatment, risk of cardiovascular events was also markedly decreased in the

TNF-α inhibitor group (RR, 0.67; 95% CI, 0.52 to 0.88; $p = 0.003$). Wu et al. also examined patients receiving TNF-α inhibitors ($n = 9148$) and patients receiving MTX ($n = 8581$). Psoriasis patients receiving TNF-α inhibitors had a lower major cardiovascular event risk compared to those receiving MTX (Kaplan–Meier rates: 1.45% vs. 4.09%: $p < 0.01$. Hazard ratio = 0.55; $p < 0.01$) [79]. The direct effect of IL-17 inhibitors or IL-23 inhibitors on cardiovascular events has not been reported yet.

Kaushik and Lebwohl also described specific comorbidities and insights to choose the appropriate systemic treatment in patients with moderate-to-severe psoriasis [80]. The choice of appropriate biologic therapy for a patient is often determined by the presence of comorbidities.

4. Conclusions

Evidence of new drugs on long-term efficacy, safety, and impacts on comorbidities is relatively low. Further accumulation is needed to clarify them. Currently, a variety of biologic agents are available for the treatment of psoriasis. However, characteristics such as rapidity of onset, long-term efficacy, safety profile, and effects on comorbidities are different. Better understanding those characteristics leads to the right choice for individual patients, resulting in higher persistence, longer drug survival, higher patient satisfaction, and minimizing the disease impact of psoriasis.

References

1. Parisi, R.; Symmons, D.P.; Griffiths, C.E.; Ashcroft, D.M. Global epidemiology of psoriasis: a systematic review of incidence and prevalence. *J. Invest. Dermatol.* **2013**, *133*, 377–385. [CrossRef] [PubMed]
2. Takeshita, J.; Grewal, S.; Langan, S.M.; Mehta, N.N.; Ogdie, A.; Van Voorhees, A.S.; Gelfand, J.M. Psoriasis and comorbid diseases: Epidemiology. *J. Am. Acad. Dermatol.* **2017**, *76*, 377–390. [CrossRef] [PubMed]
3. Lynde, C.W.; Poulin, Y.; Vender, R.; Bourcier, M.; Khalil, S. Interleukin 17A: toward a new understanding of psoriasis pathogenesis. *J. Am. Acad. Dermatol.* **2014**, *71*, 141–150. [CrossRef] [PubMed]
4. Ogawa, E.; Sato, Y.; Minagawa, A.; Okuyama, R. Pathogenesis of psoriasis and development of treatment. *J. Dermatol.* **2018**, *45*, 264–272. [CrossRef]
5. Cheuk, S.; Wiken, M.; Blomqvist, L.; Nylen, S.; Talme, T.; Stahle, M.; Eidsmo, L. Epidermal Th22 and Tc17 cells form a localized disease memory in clinically healed psoriasis. *J. Immunol.* **2014**, *192*, 3111–3120. [CrossRef]
6. Cheuk, S.; Schlums, H.; Gallais Serezal, I.; Martini, E.; Chiang, S.C.; Marquardt, N.; Gibbs, A.; Detlofsson, E.; Introini, A.; Forkel, M.; et al. CD49a Expression Defines Tissue-Resident CD8(+) T Cells Poised for Cytotoxic Function in Human Skin. *Immunity* **2017**, *46*, 287–300. [CrossRef]
7. Gallais Serezal, I.; Classon, C.; Cheuk, S.; Barrientos-Somarribas, M.; Wadman, E.; Martini, E.; Chang, D.; Xu Landen, N.; Ehrstrom, M.; Nylen, S.; et al. Resident T Cells in Resolved Psoriasis Steer Tissue Responses that Stratify Clinical Outcome. *J. Invest. Dermatol.* **2018**, *138*, 1754–1763. [CrossRef]
8. Villanova, F.; Flutter, B.; Tosi, I.; Grys, K.; Sreeneebus, H.; Perera, G.K.; Chapman, A.; Smith, C.H.; Di Meglio, P.; Nestle, F.O. Characterization of innate lymphoid cells in human skin and blood demonstrates increase of NKp44+ ILC3 in psoriasis. *J. Invest. Dermatol.* **2014**, *134*, 984–991. [CrossRef]
9. Martini, E.; Wiken, M.; Cheuk, S.; Gallais Serezal, I.; Baharom, F.; Stahle, M.; Smed-Sorensen, A.; Eidsmo, L. Dynamic Changes in Resident and Infiltrating Epidermal Dendritic Cells in Active and Resolved Psoriasis. *J. Invest. Dermatol.* **2017**, *137*, 865–873. [CrossRef]
10. Dyring-Andersen, B.; Geisler, C.; Agerbeck, C.; Lauritsen, J.P.; Gudjonsdottir, S.D.; Skov, L.; Bonefeld, C.M. Increased number and frequency of group 3 innate lymphoid cells in nonlesional psoriatic skin. *Br. J. Dermatol.* **2014**, *170*, 609–616. [CrossRef]
11. Gordon, K.B.; Strober, B.; Lebwohl, M.; Augustin, M.; Blauvelt, A.; Poulin, Y.; Papp, K.A.; Sofen, H.; Puig, L.; Foley, P.; et al. Efficacy and safety of risankizumab in moderate-to-severe plaque psoriasis (UltIMMa-1 and UltIMMa-2): results from two double-blind, randomised, placebo-controlled and ustekinumab-controlled phase 3 trials. *Lancet* **2018**, *392*, 650–661. [CrossRef]
12. Reich, K.; Griffiths, C.E.M.; Gordon, K.B.; Papp, K.A.; Song, M.; Randazzo, B.; Li, S.; Shen, Y.K.; Han, C.; Kimball, A.B.; et al. Maintenance of clinical response and consistent safety profile with up to 3 years of continuous treatment with guselkumab: Results from the VOYAGE 1 and VOYAGE 2 trials. *J. Am. Acad. Dermatol.* **2019**. [CrossRef] [PubMed]

13. Reich, K.; Armstrong, A.W.; Langley, R.G.; Flavin, S.; Randazzo, B.; Li, S.; Hsu, M.C.; Branigan, P.; Blauvelt, A. Guselkumab versus secukinumab for the treatment of moderate-to-severe psoriasis (ECLIPSE): results from a phase 3, randomised controlled trial. *Lancet* **2019**, *394*, 831–839. [CrossRef]

14. Blauvelt, A.; Papp, K.A.; Griffiths, C.E.; Randazzo, B.; Wasfi, Y.; Shen, Y.K.; Li, S.; Kimball, A.B. Efficacy and safety of guselkumab, an anti-interleukin-23 monoclonal antibody, compared with adalimumab for the continuous treatment of patients with moderate to severe psoriasis: Results from the phase III, double-blinded, placebo- and active comparator-controlled VOYAGE 1 trial. *J. Am. Acad. Dermatol.* **2017**, *76*, 405–417.

15. Gordon, K.B.; Blauvelt, A.; Foley, P.; Song, M.; Wasfi, Y.; Randazzo, B.; Shen, Y.K.; You, Y.; Griffiths, C.E.M. Efficacy of guselkumab in subpopulations of patients with moderate-to-severe plaque psoriasis: A pooled analysis of the phase III VOYAGE 1 and VOYAGE 2 studies. *Br. J. Dermatol.* **2018**, *178*, 132–139. [CrossRef]

16. Foley, P.; Gordon, K.; Griffiths, C.E.M.; Wasfi, Y.; Randazzo, B.; Song, M.; Li, S.; Shen, Y.K.; Blauvelt, A. Efficacy of Guselkumab Compared With Adalimumab and Placebo for Psoriasis in Specific Body Regions: A Secondary Analysis of 2 Randomized Clinical Trials. *JAMA Dermatol* **2018**, *154*, 676–683. [CrossRef]

17. Paul, C.; Griffiths, C.E.M.; van de Kerkhof, P.C.M.; Puig, L.; Dutronc, Y.; Henneges, C.; Dossenbach, M.; Hollister, K.; Reich, K. Ixekizumab provides superior efficacy compared with ustekinumab over 52 weeks of treatment: Results from IXORA-S, a phase 3 study. *J. Am. Acad. Dermatol.* **2019**, *80*, 70–79. [CrossRef]

18. Blauvelt, A.; Gooderham, M.; Iversen, L.; Ball, S.; Zhang, L.; Agada, N.O.; Reich, K. Efficacy and safety of ixekizumab for the treatment of moderate-to-severe plaque psoriasis: Results through 108 weeks of a randomized, controlled phase 3 clinical trial (UNCOVER-3). *J. Am. Acad. Dermatol.* **2017**, *77*, 855–862. [CrossRef]

19. Imafuku, S.; Torisu-Itakura, H.; Nishikawa, A.; Zhao, F.; Cameron, G.S. Efficacy and safety of ixekizumab treatment in Japanese patients with moderate-to-severe plaque psoriasis: Subgroup analysis of a placebo-controlled, phase 3 study (UNCOVER-1). *J. Dermatol.* **2017**, *44*, 1285–1290. [CrossRef]

20. Nash, P.; Kirkham, B.; Okada, M.; Rahman, P.; Combe, B.; Burmester, G.R.; Adams, D.H.; Kerr, L.; Lee, C.; Shuler, C.L.; et al. Ixekizumab for the treatment of patients with active psoriatic arthritis and an inadequate response to tumour necrosis factor inhibitors: results from the 24-week randomised, double-blind, placebo-controlled period of the SPIRIT-P2 phase 3 trial. *Lancet* **2017**, *389*, 2317–2327. [CrossRef]

21. Saeki, H.; Nakagawa, H.; Nakajo, K.; Ishii, T.; Morisaki, Y.; Aoki, T.; Cameron, G.S.; Osuntokun, O.O. Efficacy and safety of ixekizumab treatment for Japanese patients with moderate to severe plaque psoriasis, erythrodermic psoriasis and generalized pustular psoriasis: Results from a 52-week, open-label, phase 3 study (UNCOVER-J). *J. Dermatol.* **2017**, *44*, 355–362. [CrossRef] [PubMed]

22. Gordon, K.B.; Blauvelt, A.; Papp, K.A.; Langley, R.G.; Luger, T.; Ohtsuki, M.; Reich, K.; Amato, D.; Ball, S.G.; Braun, D.K.; et al. Phase 3 Trials of Ixekizumab in Moderate-to-Severe Plaque Psoriasis. *N. Engl. J. Med.* **2016**, *375*, 345–356. [CrossRef] [PubMed]

23. Griffiths, C.E.; Reich, K.; Lebwohl, M.; van de Kerkhof, P.; Paul, C.; Menter, A.; Cameron, G.S.; Erickson, J.; Zhang, L.; Secrest, R.J.; et al. Comparison of ixekizumab with etanercept or placebo in moderate-to-severe psoriasis (UNCOVER-2 and UNCOVER-3): results from two phase 3 randomised trials. *Lancet* **2015**, *386*, 541–551. [CrossRef]

24. Puig, L.; Lebwohl, M.; Bachelez, H.; Sobell, J.; Jacobson, A.A. Long-term efficacy and safety of brodalumab in the treatment of psoriasis: 120-week results from the randomized, double-blind, placebo- and active comparator-controlled phase 3 AMAGINE-2 trial. *J. Am. Acad. Dermatol.* **2020**, *82*, 352–359. [CrossRef]

25. Lebwohl, M.; Strober, B.; Menter, A.; Gordon, K.; Weglowska, J.; Puig, L.; Papp, K.; Spelman, L.; Toth, D.; Kerdel, F.; et al. Phase 3 Studies Comparing Brodalumab with Ustekinumab in Psoriasis. *N. Engl. J. Med.* **2015**, *373*, 1318–1328. [CrossRef]

26. Ellis, A.G.; Flohr, C.; Drucker, A.M. Network meta-analyses of systemic treatments for psoriasis: a critical appraisal: Original Articles: Jabbar-Lopez ZK, Yiu ZZN, Ward V et al. Quantitative evaluation of biologic therapy options for psoriasis: a systematic review and network meta-analysis. J Invest Dermatol 2017; 137:1646-54. Sbidian E, Chaimani A, Garcia-Doval I et al. Systemic pharmacological treatments for chronic plaque psoriasis: a network meta-analysis. Cochrane Database Syst Rev 2017; 12:CD011535. *Br. J. Dermatol.* **2019**, *180*, 282–288.

27. Sawyer, L.M.; Cornic, L.; Levin, L.A.; Gibbons, C.; Moller, A.H.; Jemec, G.B. Long-term efficacy of novel therapies in moderate-to-severe plaque psoriasis: a systematic review and network meta-analysis of PASI response. *J. Eur Acad Dermatol Venereol* **2019**, *33*, 355–366. [CrossRef]

28. Sawyer, L.M.; Malottki, K.; Sabry-Grant, C.; Yasmeen, N.; Wright, E.; Sohrt, A.; Borg, E.; Warren, R.B. Assessing the relative efficacy of interleukin-17 and interleukin-23 targeted treatments for moderate-to-severe plaque psoriasis: A systematic review and network meta-analysis of PASI response. *PLoS ONE* **2019**, *14*, e0220868-10. [CrossRef]

29. Sbidian, E.; Chaimani, A.; Afach, S.; Doney, L.; Dressler, C.; Hua, C.; Mazaud, C.; Phan, C.; Hughes, C.; Riddle, D.; et al. Systemic pharmacological treatments for chronic plaque psoriasis: a network meta-analysis. *Cochrane Database Syst. Rev.* **2020**, *1*, Cd011535-10. [CrossRef]

30. Papp, K.A.; Lebwohl, M.G. Onset of Action of Biologics in Patients with Moderate-to-Severe Psoriasis. *J. Drugs Dermatol.* **2017**, *17*, 247–250.

31. Yao, C.J.; Lebwohl, M.G. Onset of Action of Antipsoriatic Drugs for Moderate-to-Severe Plaque Psoriasis: An Update. *J. Drugs Dermatol.* **2019**, *18*, 229–233. [PubMed]

32. Blauvelt, A.; Papp, K.; Gottlieb, A.; Jarell, A.; Reich, K.; Maari, C.; Gordon, K.B.; Ferris, L.K.; Langley, R.G.; Tada, Y.; et al. A head-to-head comparison of ixekizumab vs. guselkumab in patients with moderate-to-severe plaque psoriasis: 12-week efficacy, safety and speed of response from a randomized, double-blinded trial. *Br. J. Dermatol.* **2019**. [CrossRef] [PubMed]

33. Khattri, S.; Goldblum, O.; Solotkin, K.; Amir, Y.; Min, M.S.; Ridenour, T.; Yang, F.E.; Lebwohl, M. Early Onset of Clinical Improvement with Ixekizumab in a Randomized, Open-label Study of Patients with Moderate-to-severe Plaque Psoriasis. *J. Clin. Aesthet Dermatol.* **2018**, *11*, 33–37. [PubMed]

34. Blauvelt, A.; Papp, K.A.; Lebwohl, M.G.; Green, L.J.; Hsu, S.; Bhatt, V.; Rastogi, S.; Pillai, R.; Israel, R. Rapid onset of action in patients with moderate-to-severe psoriasis treated with brodalumab: A pooled analysis of data from two phase 3 randomized clinical trials (AMAGINE-2 and AMAGINE-3). *J. Am. Acad. Dermatol.* **2017**, *77*, 372–374. [CrossRef]

35. Alinaghi, F.; Calov, M.; Kristensen, L.E.; Gladman, D.D.; Coates, L.C.; Jullien, D.; Gottlieb, A.B.; Gisondi, P.; Wu, J.J.; Thyssen, J.P.; et al. Prevalence of psoriatic arthritis in patients with psoriasis: A systematic review and meta-analysis of observational and clinical studies. *J. Am. Acad. Dermatol.* **2019**, *80*, 251–265. [CrossRef]

36. Schett, G.; Lories, R.J.; D'Agostino, M.A.; Elewaut, D.; Kirkham, B.; Soriano, E.R.; McGonagle, D. Enthesitis: from pathophysiology to treatment. *Nat. Rev. Rheumatol* **2017**, *13*, 731–741. [CrossRef]

37. Merola, J.F.; Espinoza, L.R.; Fleischmann, R. Distinguishing rheumatoid arthritis from psoriatic arthritis. *RMD Open* **2018**, *4*, e000656-10. [CrossRef]

38. Araujo, E.G.; Englbrecht, M.; Hoepken, S.; Finzel, S.; Kampylafka, E.; Kleyer, A.; Bayat, S.; Schoenau, V.; Hueber, A.; Rech, J.; et al. Effects of ustekinumab versus tumor necrosis factor inhibition on enthesitis: Results from the enthesial clearance in psoriatic arthritis (ECLIPSA) study. *Semin Arthritis Rheum* **2019**, *48*, 632–637. [CrossRef]

39. Ritchlin, C.T.; Colbert, R.A.; Gladman, D.D. Psoriatic Arthritis. *N. Engl. J. Med.* **2017**, *376*, 957–970. [CrossRef]

40. Heiland, G.R.; Zwerina, K.; Baum, W.; Kireva, T.; Distler, J.H.; Grisanti, M.; Asuncion, F.; Li, X.; Ominsky, M.; Richards, W.; et al. Neutralisation of Dkk-1 protects from systemic bone loss during inflammation and reduces sclerostin expression. *Ann. Rheum Dis.* **2010**, *69*, 2152–2159. [CrossRef]

41. van Tubergen, A.; Weber, U. Diagnosis and classification in spondyloarthritis: identifying a chameleon. *Nat. Rev. Rheumatol.* **2012**, *8*, 253–261. [CrossRef] [PubMed]

42. Baeten, D.; Sieper, J.; Braun, J.; Baraliakos, X.; Dougados, M.; Emery, P.; Deodhar, A.; Porter, B.; Martin, R.; Andersson, M.; et al. Secukinumab, an Interleukin-17A Inhibitor, in Ankylosing Spondylitis. *N. Engl. J. Med.* **2015**, *373*, 2534–2548. [CrossRef] [PubMed]

43. Dougados, M.; Wei, J.C.; Landewe, R.; Sieper, J.; Baraliakos, X.; Van den Bosch, F.; Maksymowych, W.P.; Ermann, J.; Walsh, J.A.; Tomita, T.; et al. Efficacy and safety of ixekizumab through 52 weeks in two phase 3, randomised, controlled clinical trials in patients with active radiographic axial spondyloarthritis (COAST-V and COAST-W). *Ann. Rheum Dis.* **2020**, *79*, 176–185. [CrossRef] [PubMed]

44. Baeten, D.; Ostergaard, M.; Wei, J.C.; Sieper, J.; Jarvinen, P.; Tam, L.S.; Salvarani, C.; Kim, T.H.; Solinger, A.; Datsenko, Y.; et al. Risankizumab, an IL-23 inhibitor, for ankylosing spondylitis: results of a randomised, double-blind, placebo-controlled, proof-of-concept, dose-finding phase 2 study. *Ann. Rheum Dis.* **2018**, *77*, 1295–1302. [CrossRef] [PubMed]

45. Venken, K.; Jacques, P.; Mortier, C.; Labadia, M.E.; Decruy, T.; Coudenys, J.; Hoyt, K.; Wayne, A.L.; Hughes, R.; Turner, M.; et al. RORgammat inhibition selectively targets IL-17 producing iNKT and gammadelta-T cells enriched in Spondyloarthritis patients. *Nat. Commun.* **2019**, *10*, 9–10. [CrossRef] [PubMed]

46. Hanly, J.G.; Russell, M.L.; Gladman, D.D. Psoriatic spondyloarthropathy: a long term prospective study. *Ann. Rheum Dis.* **1988**, *47*, 386–393. [CrossRef] [PubMed]

47. Battistone, M.J.; Manaster, B.J.; Reda, D.J.; Clegg, D.O. The prevalence of sacroilitis in psoriatic arthritis: new perspectives from a large, multicenter cohort. A Department of Veterans Affairs Cooperative Study. *Skeletal Radiol.* **1999**, *28*, 196–201. [CrossRef]

48. Mease, P.J.; Palmer, J.B.; Liu, M.; Kavanaugh, A.; Pandurengan, R.; Ritchlin, C.T.; Karki, C.; Greenberg, J.D. Influence of Axial Involvement on Clinical Characteristics of Psoriatic Arthritis: Analysis from the Corrona Psoriatic Arthritis/Spondyloarthritis Registry. *J. Rheumatol.* **2018**, *45*, 1389–1396. [CrossRef]

49. Singh, J.A.; Guyatt, G.; Ogdie, A.; Gladman, D.D.; Deal, C.; Deodhar, A.; Dubreuil, M.; Dunham, J.; Husni, M.E.; Kenny, S.; et al. Special Article: 2018 American College of Rheumatology/National Psoriasis Foundation Guideline for the Treatment of Psoriatic Arthritis. *Arthritis Rheumatol.* **2019**, *71*, 5–32. [CrossRef]

50. Kawalec, P.; Holko, P.; Mocko, P.; Pilc, A. Comparative effectiveness of abatacept, apremilast, secukinumab and ustekinumab treatment of psoriatic arthritis: a systematic review and network meta-analysis. *Rheumatol. Int.* **2018**, *38*, 189–201. [CrossRef]

51. Dressler, C.; Eisert, L.; Pham, P.A.; Nast, A. Efficacy and safety of systemic treatments in psoriatic arthritis: a systematic review, meta-analysis and GRADE evaluation. *J. Eur. Acad. Dermatol. Venereol.* **2019**, *33*, 1249–1260. [CrossRef] [PubMed]

52. Lu, C.; Wallace, B.I.; Waljee, A.K.; Fu, W.; Zhang, Q.; Liu, Y. Comparative efficacy and safety of targeted DMARDs for active psoriatic arthritis during induction therapy: A systematic review and network meta-analysis. *Semin Arthritis Rheum* **2019**, *49*, 381–388. [CrossRef] [PubMed]

53. Kamata, M.; Tada, Y. Safety of biologics in psoriasis. *J. Dermatol.* **2018**, *45*, 279–286. [CrossRef] [PubMed]

54. Kaushik, S.B.; Lebwohl, M.G. Psoriasis: Which therapy for which patient: Focus on special populations and chronic infections. *J. Am. Acad. Dermatol.* **2019**, *80*, 43–53. [CrossRef]

55. Dalgard, F.J.; Gieler, U.; Tomas-Aragones, L.; Lien, L.; Poot, F.; Jemec, G.B.E.; Misery, L.; Szabo, C.; Linder, D.; Sampogna, F.; et al. The psychological burden of skin diseases: a cross-sectional multicenter study among dermatological out-patients in 13 European countries. *J. Invest. Dermatol.* **2015**, *135*, 984–991. [CrossRef]

56. Kurd, S.K.; Troxel, A.B.; Crits-Christoph, P.; Gelfand, J.M. The risk of depression, anxiety, and suicidality in patients with psoriasis: a population-based cohort study. *Arch. Dermatol.* **2010**, *146*, 891–895.

57. Dowlatshahi, E.A.; Wakkee, M.; Arends, L.R.; Nijsten, T. The prevalence and odds of depressive symptoms and clinical depression in psoriasis patients: a systematic review and meta-analysis. *J. Invest. Dermatol.* **2014**, *134*, 1542–1551. [CrossRef]

58. Singh, S.; Taylor, C.; Kornmehl, H.; Armstrong, A.W. Psoriasis and suicidality: A systematic review and meta-analysis. *J. Am. Acad. Dermatol.* **2017**, *77*, 425–440. [CrossRef]

59. Strober, B.; Gooderham, M.; de Jong, E.; Kimball, A.B.; Langley, R.G.; Lakdawala, N.; Goyal, K.; Lawson, F.; Langholff, W.; Hopkins, L.; et al. Depressive symptoms, depression, and the effect of biologic therapy among patients in Psoriasis Longitudinal Assessment and Registry (PSOLAR). *J. Am. Acad. Dermatol.* **2018**, *78*, 70–80. [CrossRef]

60. Cohen, A.D.; Dreiher, J.; Birkenfeld, S. Psoriasis associated with ulcerative colitis and Crohn's disease. *J. Eur. Acad. Dermatol. Venereol.* **2009**, *23*, 561–565. [CrossRef]

61. Hueber, W.; Sands, B.E.; Lewitzky, S.; Vandemeulebroecke, M.; Reinisch, W.; Higgins, P.D.; Wehkamp, J.; Feagan, B.G.; Yao, M.D.; Karczewski, M.; et al. Secukinumab, a human anti-IL-17A monoclonal antibody, for moderate to severe Crohn's disease: unexpected results of a randomised, double-blind placebo-controlled trial. *Gut* **2012**, *61*, 1693–1700. [CrossRef] [PubMed]

62. Targan, S.R.; Feagan, B.; Vermeire, S.; Panaccione, R.; Melmed, G.Y.; Landers, C.; Li, D.; Russell, C.; Newmark, R.; Zhang, N.; et al. A Randomized, Double-Blind, Placebo-Controlled Phase 2 Study of Brodalumab in Patients With Moderate-to-Severe Crohn's Disease. *Am. J. Gastroenterol.* **2016**, *111*, 1599–1607. [CrossRef] [PubMed]

63. Feagan, B.G.; Sandborn, W.J.; Gasink, C.; Jacobstein, D.; Lang, Y.; Friedman, J.R.; Blank, M.A.; Johanns, J.; Gao, L.L.; Miao, Y.; et al. Ustekinumab as Induction and Maintenance Therapy for Crohn's Disease. *N. Engl. J. Med.* **2016**, *375*, 1946–1960. [CrossRef] [PubMed]

64. Sands, B.E.; Chen, J.; Feagan, B.G.; Penney, M.; Rees, W.A.; Danese, S.; Higgins, P.D.R.; Newbold, P.; Faggioni, R.; Patra, K.; et al. Efficacy and Safety of MEDI2070, an Antibody Against Interleukin 23, in Patients With Moderate to Severe Crohn's Disease: A Phase 2a Study. *Gastroenterology* **2017** *153*, 77–86. [CrossRef]

65. Boehncke, W.H.; Boehncke, S.; Tobin, A.M.; Kirby, B. The 'psoriatic march': a concept of how severe psoriasis may drive cardiovascular comorbidity. *Exp. Dermatol.* **2011**, *20*, 303–307. [CrossRef]

66. Furue, M.; Kadono, T. "Inflammatory skin march" in atopic dermatitis and psoriasis. *Inflamm. Res.* **2017**, *66*, 833–842. [CrossRef]

67. Rodriguez-Zuniga, M.J.M.; Garcia-Perdomo, H.A. Systematic review and meta-analysis of the association between psoriasis and metabolic syndrome. *J. Am. Acad. Dermatol.* **2017**, *77*, 657–666. [CrossRef]

68. Naldi, L.; Chatenoud, L.; Linder, D.; Belloni Fortina, A.; Peserico, A.; Virgili, A.R.; Bruni, P.L.; Ingordo, V.; Lo Scocco, G.; Solaroli, C.; et al. Cigarette smoking, body mass index, and stressful life events as risk factors for psoriasis: results from an Italian case-control study. *J. Invest. Dermatol.* **2005**, *125*, 61–67. [CrossRef]

69. Sterry, W.; Strober, B.E.; Menter, A. Obesity in psoriasis: the metabolic, clinical and therapeutic implications. Report of an interdisciplinary conference and review. *Br. J. Dermatol.* **2007**, *157*, 649–655. [CrossRef]

70. Naldi, L.; Addis, A.; Chimenti, S.; Giannetti, A.; Picardo, M.; Tomino, C.; Maccarone, M.; Chatenoud, L.; Bertuccio, P.; Caggese, E.; et al. Impact of body mass index and obesity on clinical response to systemic treatment for psoriasis. Evidence from the Psocare project. *Dermatology (Basel, Switzerland)* **2008**, *217*, 365–373. [CrossRef]

71. Tobin, A.M.; Hackett, C.B.; Rogers, S.; Collins, P.; Richards, H.L.; O'Shea, D.; Kirby, B. Body mass index, waist circumference and HOMA-IR correlate with the Psoriasis Area and Severity Index in patients with psoriasis receiving phototherapy. *Br. J. Dermatol.* **2014**, *171*, 436–438. [CrossRef] [PubMed]

72. Gisondi, P.; Del Giglio, M.; Di Francesco, V.; Zamboni, M.; Girolomoni, G. Weight loss improves the response of obese patients with moderate-to-severe chronic plaque psoriasis to low-dose cyclosporine therapy: a randomized, controlled, investigator-blinded clinical trial. *Am. J. Clin Nutr* **2008**, *88*, 1242–1247. [PubMed]

73. Ikumi, K.; Odanaka, M.; Shime, H.; Imai, M.; Osaga, S.; Taguchi, O.; Nishida, E.; Hemmi, H.; Kaisho, T.; Morita, A.; et al. Hyperglycemia Is Associated with Psoriatic Inflammation in Both Humans and Mice. *J. Invest. Dermatol.* **2019**, *139*, 1329–1338. [CrossRef] [PubMed]

74. Avgerinou, G.; Tousoulis, D.; Siasos, G.; Oikonomou, E.; Maniatis, K.; Papageorgiou, N.; Paraskevopoulos, T.; Miliou, A.; Koumaki, D.; Latsios, G.; et al. Anti-tumor necrosis factor alpha treatment with adalimumab improves significantly endothelial function and decreases inflammatory process in patients with chronic psoriasis. *Int. J. Cardiol.* **2011**, *151*, 382–383. [CrossRef]

75. von Stebut, E.; Reich, K.; Thaci, D.; Koenig, W.; Pinter, A.; Korber, A.; Rassaf, T.; Waisman, A.; Mani, V.; Yates, D.; et al. Impact of Secukinumab on Endothelial Dysfunction and Other Cardiovascular Disease Parameters in Psoriasis Patients over 52 Weeks. *J. Invest. Dermatol.* **2019**, *139*, 1054–1062. [CrossRef]

76. Hjuler, K.F.; Bottcher, M.; Vestergaard, C.; Deleuran, M.; Raaby, L.; Botker, H.E.; Iversen, L.; Kragballe, K. Increased Prevalence of Coronary Artery Disease in Severe Psoriasis and Severe Atopic Dermatitis. *Am. J. Med.* **2015**, *128*, 1325–1334. [CrossRef]

77. Elnabawi, Y.A.; Dey, A.K.; Goyal, A.; Groenendyk, J.W.; Chung, J.H.; Belur, A.D.; Rodante, J.; Harrington, C.L.; Teague, H.L.; Baumer, Y.; et al. Coronary artery plaque characteristics and treatment with biologic therapy in severe psoriasis: results from a prospective observational study. *Cardiovasc. Res.* **2019**, *115*, 721–728. [CrossRef]

78. Armstrong, E.J.; Harskamp, C.T.; Armstrong, A.W. Psoriasis and major adverse cardiovascular events: a systematic review and meta-analysis of observational studies. *J. Am. Heart Assoc.* **2013**, *2*, e000062-10. [CrossRef]

79. Wu, J.J.; Guerin, A.; Sundaram, M.; Dea, K.; Cloutier, M.; Mulani, P. Cardiovascular event risk assessment in psoriasis patients treated with tumor necrosis factor-alpha inhibitors versus methotrexate. *J. Am. Acad. Dermatol.* **2017**, *76*, 81–90. [CrossRef]

80. Kaushik, S.B.; Lebwohl, M.G. Psoriasis: Which therapy for which patient: Psoriasis comorbidities and preferred systemic agents. *J. Am. Acad. Dermatol.* **2019**, *80*, 27–40. [CrossRef]

11

Butyric Acid from Probiotic *Staphylococcus epidermidis* in the Skin Microbiome Down-Regulates the Ultraviolet-Induced Pro-Inflammatory IL-6 Cytokine via Short-Chain Fatty Acid Receptor

Sunita Keshari [1], Arun Balasubramaniam [2], Binderiya Myagmardoloonjin [2], Deron Raymond Herr [3], Indira Putri Negari [2] and Chun-Ming Huang [2,4,*]

[1] Department of Life Sciences, National Central University, Taoyuan 32001, Taiwan
[2] Department of Biomedical Sciences and Engineering, National Central University, Taoyuan 32001, Taiwan
[3] Department of Pharmacology, National University of Singapore, Singapore 117600, Singapore
[4] Department of Dermatology, School of Medicine, University of California, San Diego, CA 92093, USA
* Correspondence: chunming@ncu.edu.tw

Abstract: The glycerol fermentation of probiotic *Staphylococcus epidermidis* (*S. epidermidis*) in the skin microbiome produced butyric acid in vitro at concentrations in the millimolar range. The exposure of dorsal skin of mice to ultraviolet B (UVB) light provoked a significant increased production of pro-inflammatory interleukin (IL)-6 cytokine. Topical application of butyric acid alone or *S. epidermidis* with glycerol remarkably ameliorated the UVB-induced IL-6 production. In vivo knockdown of short-chain fatty acid receptor 2 (FFAR2) in mouse skin considerably blocked the probiotic effect of *S. epidermidis* on suppression of UVB-induced IL-6 production. These results demonstrate that butyric acid in the metabolites of fermenting skin probiotic bacteria mediates FFAR2 to modulate the production of pro-inflammatory cytokines induced by UVB.

Keywords: butyric acid; microbiome; probiotic; *S. epidermidis*; UVB

1. Introduction

Skin is a fundamental component of the innate immune system, providing a protective barrier against the penetration of microorganisms and preventing environmental damage to the body. Exposure to UV is known to induce clustering of specific cell-surface receptors, resulting in the activation of signal transduction pathways [1]. Prolonged exposure of ultraviolet B (UVB) with a wavelength of 280–320 nm is a significant risk factor causing chronic inflammation, DNA damage, and lipid peroxidation in the epidermis [2]. Chronic exposure to this cellular stressor commonly results in skin pathologies such as epidermal hyperplasia, erythema, and edema [3]. Within the skin epidermis, keratinocytes have been found to play a critical role in the response to photo-damage to UVB by releasing key inflammatory mediators such as interleukin (IL)-1, -6, -8, -10 and tumor necrosis factor (TNF). Among these, keratinocyte-derived IL-1 and IL-6 seem to be of particular importance [4]. Many studies have demonstrated that both human and murine keratinocytes produce these cytokines because of UV exposure [5,6]. Continuous exposure to UV results in the generation of reactive oxygen species (ROS), exposing a variety of biomolecules to oxidative stress. This leads to damage of biological structures, contributes to cellular injury, and ultimately resulting in tissue destruction [7].

The skin microbiome consists of a complex community of organisms that mediates essential physiological and pathological processes. Among these organisms, *Staphylococcus epidermidis* (*S. epidermidis*) is the predominant commensal bacterial species that colonizes normal human skin [8]. Derangement of the bacterial milieu can alter epidermal function, and thus, disrupt the local ecology of the skin [9]. This interplay of microbe and host appears to be critical for establishing homeostasis. *S. epidermidis* has also been shown to benefit the skin immune function by diminishing inflammation after injury [10]. Study have shown that 6-*N*-hydroxyaminopurine, a metabolite from *S. epidermidis* could selectively inhibit UV induced skin tumors in mice [11]. Additionally, studies have provided evidence that peptides and other metabolites produced from *S. epidermidis*, might also act as antimicrobial agents and contribute to normal defense at the epidermal interface [12,13]. In the current study, we demonstrate that butyric acid, one of the major metabolites produced by *S. epidermidis* fermentation, attenuates the UVB-induced production of inflammatory cytokines by interacting with cognate receptors expressed by keratinocytes. This suggests that manipulation of the *S. epidermidis*-butyric acid-FFAR2 axis is a potential therapeutic target to protect against skin inflammatory diseases.

2. Results

2.1. S. epidermidis Mediates Glycerol Fermentation and Acetolactate Synthase (ALS) Activity

To investigate whether *S. epidermidis* (ATCC 12228) can ferment glycerol, *S. epidermidis* (10^7 colony-forming unit (CFU) were incubated with and without glycerol (2%) in rich media with phenol red for 12 h. Uninoculated rich media containing phenol red with glycerol served as controls. Phenol red was used as an indicator to monitor bacterial fermentation. In rich media incubated with bacteria, the color of phenol red changed from red to orange because of the bacterial replication during incubation. However, in agreement with earlier results, the rich media containing bacteria along with glycerol, the phenol red color changed from red to yellow indicating the use of glycerol as a carbon source for fermentation by *S. epidermidis* after 12 h culture (Figure 1a) [13–15]. The color change of phenol red was quantified by measuring the optical density at 560 nm (OD_{560}) (Figure 1b). Furthermore, OD_{560nm} in rich media with *S. epidermidis* and glycerol was significantly lower than that in rich media with *S. epidermidis* alone (Figure 1a). Next, to confirm the fermentation activity of *S. epidermidis* using glycerol as a carbon source, we added furfural, a potent fermentation inhibitor [16], in rich media containing *S. epidermidis* and glycerol. Media with and without *S. epidermidis*, glycerol and furfural were used as controls. We did not detect any color change in the media incubated with *S. epidermidis* with furfural in the presence or absence of glycerol (Figure 1a). Additionally, the OD_{560nm} was comparable to the control group containing media only, or media with furfural, or media with glycerol. This indicates that the fermentation or metabolic activity of *S. epidermidis* might have been inhibited by furfural (Figure 1b). Microbial enzymes are found to be the major source of bacterial fermentation by catalyzing the hydrolysis of starch or peptides. Moreover, a recent study reported that acetolactate synthase (ALS) is a crucial enzyme in *Staphylococcus aureus* (*S. aureus*) which converts pyruvate into α-acetolactate, promoting the production of branched-chain amino acids (BCAA) and playing an important role in the activation of the tricarboxylic acid (TCA) cycle [17]. It also promotes anaerobic fermentation in *Bacillius subtilis* (*B. subtilis*) by converting two molecules of pyruvate to form acetolactate, functioning as a key regulatory enzyme in fermentation [18]. Reports also demonstrated that furfural exerts its inhibitory effects on microbial fermentation via interfering with the activities of enzymes in the pathways of microbial fermentation [19]. We confirmed that the ALS enzyme activity of *S. epidermidis* is significantly reduced when it is incubated with furfural (inhibitor) (Figure 1c). Taken together, we confirmed that *S. epidermidis* induced glycerol fermentation, which required furfural-sensitive ALS activity.

Figure 1. *S. epidermidis* mediates glycerol fermentation by ALS (acetolactate synthase) enzyme activity. (**a**) *S. epidermidis* bacteria (B) (10^7 CFU/mL) were incubated in rich media (M) containing phenol red with or without 2% glycerol (G) and in the presence and absence of fermentation inhibitor furfural (F) for 12 h. Media with glycerol (M + G), bacteria (M + B), furfural (M + F), glycerol plus furfural (M + G + F), or bacteria plus furfural (M + B + F) were taken as controls. Bacterial fermentation was indicated by the color change of phenol red to yellow (arrow). (**b**) A graph showing the OD_{560} value in all the above groups. (**c**) ALS activity by furfural. The reaction mixture containing lysates of *S. epidermidis* bacteria (B) (10^7 CFU/mL) was incubated with and without furfural (F). The activity (U/mg) of ALS in *S. epidermidis* bacteria was quantified. Data shown represent the mean ± SE of experiment performed in triplicate. *** $p < 0.001$ (two-tailed *t*-test).

2.2. Butyric Acid, a Product in Fermented Media upon Glycerol Fermentation by S. epidermidis

Previous studies have detected the presence of multiple short-chain fatty acids (SCFAs) such as acetic acid, butyric acid, lactic acid, and succinic in fermented media of *S. epidermidis* from glycerol fermentation [13]. Butyric acid from *S. epidermidis* was found to exert growth suppressive effects on USA300, a community-associated methicillin-resistant *S. aureus* (MRSA). Moreover, it shows potent anti-inflammatory activity in skin keratinocytes by effectively inhibiting histone deacetylase (HDAC) [20,21]. In the current study, we have screened the supernatant following glycerol fermentation of *S. epidermidis* to quantify their butyric acid producing capacity by high-performance liquid chromatography-ultraviolet (HPLC-UV) analysis. Butyric acid was detected as a sharp specific peak in the HPLC chromatogram and was determined to be at a concentration of 6 mM in the fermented media by comparison to a butyric acid standard curve (Figure 2a,b).

Figure 2. High-performance liquid chromatography-ultraviolet (HPLC-UV) analysis of the butyric acid. The fermented media from glycerol (G) fermentation by *S. epidermidis* bacteria (B) analyzed by HPLC. (**a**) Chromatograph of only media (M), media with glycerol (M + G), media with bacteria (M + B), and media with bacteria plus glycerol (M + B + G). The x-axis is retention time in minutes, and the y-axis is the milli-absorbance unit at 210 nm. (**b**) The concentrations of BA (butyric acid) was quantified from the height of butyric acid standard (STD) peaks. Data shown represent the mean ± SE of experiment performed in triplicate. *** $p < 0.0001$ (two-tailed t-test).

2.3. Mixture of S. epidermidis and Glycerol or Butyric Acid alone Inhibited UVB Induced Skin Inflammation

Exposure to prolonged UVB radiation is deleterious to human skin, which may lead to expression and secretion of pro-inflammatory cytokines such as IL-6 in human keratinocytes [22]. Furthermore, chronic UVB is responsible for epidermal hyperplasia. The dorsal skin of the Institute of Cancer Research (ICR) mice were shaved and exposed to 12 doses of UVB (195 mJ/cm^2) over 4 weeks concurrent with 4 topical applications of a mixture of *S. epidermidis* (10^7) and glycerol (2%) in phosphate-buffered saline (PBS) over the same time period. Mice topically applied with mixture of *S. epidermidis* (10^7) and glycerol (2%) in PBS with no UVB exposure were included as control. The dorsal skin of mice was photographed to measure the wound healing from 0, 16, and 30 days. Mice from all groups were sacrificed on the 30th day and skin samples were lysed to extract total protein. In mice treated with either PBS, *S. epidermidis*, or glycerol alone, variable lesions were recorded which started from edema, redness, and ulceration of the UVB exposed area and ended with thickening of the skin. However, in mice that received topical applications of *S. epidermidis* and glycerol, a comparatively lower level of erythema and ulceration were observed on UVB-exposed skin on day 16. Further improvement was noticed on day 30, signifying maximum recovery from UVB damage (Figure 3a,b) compared to non-exposed groups (Figure S1a). Upregulated levels of IL-6 and noticeable epidermal hyperplasia (as quantified by epidermal thickness) were detected in mice skin topically applied with PBS, *S. epidermidis*, or glycerol alone following UVB exposure because of an increase in the number of keratinocytes and epidermal layers. By contrast, in the *S. epidermidis* plus glycerol treated group, IL-6 levels were significantly reduced (Figure 3c) compared to non-exposed groups (Figure S1b) and the skin remained almost completely intact, showing a marked attenuation of UVB-induced skin thickening

(Figure S3a,b). This indicates that metabolites from glycerol fermentation by *S. epidermidis* might induce anti-inflammatory activity against chronic UVB radiation. To further confirm the anti-inflammatory activity of *S. epidermidis* fermentation, another group of mice were topically applied with a mixture of *S. epidermidis* and glycerol along with fermentation inhibitor, furfural. UVB irradiation-induced skin lesions, elevation of IL-6, and epidermal hyperplasia were not ameliorated upon topical application of *S. epidermidis* plus glycerol and furfural compared to control group receiving water and furfural alone (Figure 3d and Figure S3c–f). However, significant recovery from inflammation was detected in mice topically applied with a mixture of *S. epidermidis* and glycerol. This was again accompanied by a downregulated level of IL-6 and decreased epidermal thickness, confirming that glycerol fermentation from *S. epidermidis* exerts anti-inflammatory activity. In the present study, we detected the production of butyric acid in significant amount as a metabolite in the fermentation of glycerol by *S. epidermidis*. Since butyric acid has been shown to be a potent anti-inflammatory agent in skin keratinocytes and has been tested for the attenuation of different inflammatory disorders [23,24], we first investigated its role against UVB induced inflammation in human keratinocytes (CCD 1106 KERTr). The human keratinocytes were irradiated with 195 mJ/cm^2 UVB and the IL-6 production was dramatically enhanced in water control group until 12 h after irradiation. However, the addition of BA (butyric acid, 4 mM), significantly reduced the upregulated level of IL-6 (Figure S2a). As studies mentioned, both IL-6 and IL-8 undoubtedly play pivotal roles in immunologic regulation in human skin and are involved in skin inflammation in response to UV radiation [25]. We have also detected the upregulated level of IL-8 in UVB exposed keratinocytes, which further rescued upon BA treatment (Figure S2b). Further, we detected effect of BA application upon UVB exposure in vivo. Our results show that topical application of 4 mM butyric acid ameliorated UVB-induced wound formation, and wound healing was mild to significant from day 16 to day 30 (Figure S3g,h). In a similar manner, IL-6 was downregulated and epidermal hyperplasia was diminished (Figure 3e and Figure S3i,j), which was consistent with the model that butyric acid is the active glycerol fermentation metabolite by which *S. epidermidis* can inhibit UV induced inflammation in the skin.

2.4. Knocking Down Free Fatty Acid Receptor 2 (FFAR2) Inhibited Butyric Acid Mediated Attenuation of Inflammation in Chronic UVB

Most beneficial roles of SCFAs in the gastrointestinal tract (GI) are mediated by directly activating its cognate G protein-coupled receptor, GPR43 (also known as FFAR2). For example, the chemoattractant and anti-inflammatory activities of butyrate in chondrocytes are completely mediated by its binding to GPR43 [26]. The activation of FFAR2 has emerged as a potentially important mechanism by which SCFAs could directly regulate the immune cells and the process of inflammatory diseases, thus drawing much attention in recent years [27,28]. Considering the key function of FFAR2 in inflammatory processes, blocking the signaling of this receptor by a selective inhibitor could be a useful approach to evaluate the role of butyric acid in the regulation of immune function in skin during chronic UVB exposure. In the present study, FFAR2 was inhibited by via gavage feeding of FFAR2 selective antagonist GLPG0974 (0.1–1 mg/kg) 20 min prior to topical application of butyric acid followed by UVB exposure. In addition, we have also blocked FFAR2 receptor via subcutaneous injection of FFAR2 siRNA (5 μM) into the dorsal skin of ICR mice 20 min prior to topical application of butyric acid followed by UVB exposure. In both conditions of blocking FFAR2, significant wound area and redness from UVB radiation was observed (Figure S4a,b,g,h) on mice dorsal skin, which further did not recover even after topical application of butyric acid. Inflammation, as detected by upregulation of IL-6 and epidermal hyperplasia, was increased in mice upon FFAR2 inhibition and further remained unchanged even on topical application of butyric acid compared to mice applied with butyric acid alone (Figure 4a,b and Figure S4c,d,i,j). We have also confirmed the FFAR2 inhibition or gene knockdown by measuring the protein expression level of FFAR2 by Western blot analysis and mRNA relative expression by RTPCR analysis (Figure S4e,f,k,l). Our overall results demonstrate an essential role of FFAR2/GPR43 in butyrate activity in UVB-induced chronic inflammation process. Butyrate reduced pro-inflammatory mediators IL-6, by binding to its FFAR2 receptor, which further inhibits the epidermal hyperplasia in chronic UVB exposure.

Figure 3. Attenuation of UVB induced inflammation by application of mixture of *S. epidermidis* and glycerol and its fermentation metabolite, butyric acid. (**a**) Skin morphology of ICR mice, topically applied with PBS, glycerol (G) (2%), *S. epidermidis* bacteria (B) (10^7 CFU/mL), or mixture of *S. epidermidis* bacteria plus glycerol (B + G) followed by exposure with UVB (195 mJ/cm^2) irradiation are shown at 0, 16, and 30 day. Skin lesions are indicated by red arrows. Scale bar = 5 mm. Graph (**b**) indicates percent wound area remaining of mice skin. The level of IL-6 in skin (**c**) from above all groups of ICR mice was quantified using a mouse IL-6 enzyme-linked immunosorbent assay (ELISA) kit (R&D Systems). (**d**) The IL-6 level in skin of ICR mice topically applied with H$_2$O, furfural (0.4%), *S. epidermidis* bacteria (B) (10^7 CFU/mL), glycerol (G) (2%) plus furfural (F) (0.4%), (B + G + F) or a mixture of *S. epidermidis* bacteria plus glycerol (B + G) followed by exposure with UVB (195 mJ/cm^2) irradiation is shown. (**e**) The IL-6 level in skin of ICR mice topically applied with H$_2$O and butyric acid (BA) (4 mM) followed by exposure with UVB (195 mJ/cm^2) irradiation is shown. Data are the means of three individual experiments using five mice per group. ns = non-significant. *** $p < 0.001$. (two-tailed t-tests).

Figure 4. Blocking FFAR2 prevents the butyric acid mediated amelioration of inflammation. (**a**) The level of IL-6 in the dorsal skin of ICR mice upon gavage feeding of FFAR2 antagonist GLPG0974 dissolved in dimethyl sulfoxide (DMSO) in saline (0.01%) and topically applied butyric acid (BA) (4 mM) and was measured by ELISA. Mice fed with DMSO in saline and topically applied with H_2O were included as control. (**b**) The level of IL-6 in the dorsal skin of ICR mice subcutaneously injected with FFAR2 siRNA 10 min prior to topical application with butyric acid (BA) (4 mM) was measured by ELISA. Mice injected with scrambled or negative control siRNA and topically applied with H_2O were included as control. Data are the means of three separate experiments using five mice per group. ns = non-significant. *** $p < 0.001$. (two-tailed t-tests).

3. Discussion

Skin and its constituent epidermal keratinocytes make-up the outer most protective covering of the body, and as such, are the primary targets for solar UVB radiation. Exposure to chronic UVB radiation alters the cutaneous and systemic immune systems by causing several pathological alteration in cell signaling resulting in sunburn, erythema, inflammation, and skin carcinogenesis [29]. It primarily activates various pro-inflammatory mediators such as tumor necrosis factor-alpha (TNF-α), cyclooxygenase-2 (COX-2), and IL-6, leading to the activation of nuclear factor kappa-light-chain-enhancer of activated B cells (NF-κB) [30]. The findings from the previous studies showed that *S. epidermidis*, a commensal bacteria from human skin, could ferment glycerol into butyric acid, one of the four SCFAs detected in fermented media [13,15]. Glycerol is a major component in stratum corneum (SC) hydration with varied amount in different parts of human skin (0.7 μg/cm^2 in the cheek and 0.1 μg/cm^2 in forearm and sole). Multiple diseases characterized by xerosis and impaired epidermal barrier function, such as atopic dermatitis were improved by topical application of glycerol. Although glycerol could not penetrate deeper in SC but the SCFAs generated from glycerol fermentation by skin commensal bacteria, may modulate physiological processes such as skin barrier homeostasis and inflammation [15,31,32]. In this study, we evaluated the role of butyric acid, a major SCFA from the fermentation of glycerol by *S. epidermidis*, on chronic UVB radiation induced inflammation on ICR mice skin. The fermentation of glycerol by *S. epidermidis* was detected by change in color of phenol red from red to yellow (more acidic), which was further validated quantitatively by a significant decrease in OD$_{560nm}$. In addition to SCFAs, furfural is another metabolite produced by bacterial fermentation, and its accumulation has been shown to inhibit fermentation by blocking the activities of multiple enzymes involved in bacterial fermentation pathway [19,33]. We did not detect fermentation by color change or by OD$_{560nm}$ quantification upon adding furfural to media containing *S. epidermidis* with glycerol. Furthermore, no bacterial growth was detected when furfural was added to media containing *S. epidermidis* alone, demonstrating the activity of furfural in suppressing bacterial fermentation activity. ALS is one of the major fermentation enzymes catalyzing the conversion of pyruvate to α-acetolactate which is further converted to isobutyrate and then ultimately to butyrate in subsequent pathways [34,35]. Our recent study showed, ALS activity in *S. epidermidis* was inhibited by a furfural derivative 5-methyl furfural (5MF) [14]. In the current study, we detected a significant reduction in ALS activity upon incubation of bacterial lysate with furfural. This demonstrates that ALS plays an essential role in *S. epidermidis* metabolism, triggering glycerol fermentation. We detected the production of butyric acid in fermented media by HPLC analysis on the basis of comparing the retention time and spectra with a butyric acid standard, confirming butyric acid as one of the most abundant metabolites produced from fermentation of 2% glycerol by *S. epidermidis*.

Metabolites from microbial fermentation have been under investigation as potential therapeutics against different infectious and inflammatory diseases [36]. For example, research suggested that ingestion of probiotic bacteria, *Lactobacillus johnsonii* (La1) could protect against the UVR-induced inflammation [37]. Furthermore, several lines of evidence suggest that metabolites from the fermentation of glycerol by *S. epidermidis* can inhibit the growth of pathogenic *Cutibacterium acnes* (*C. acnes*), thus, *S. epidermidis* may be an excellent probiotic for the treatment of chronic sinusitis [13,15,38]. Here we detected the probiotic effect of *S. epidermidis* in skin against UVB mediated chronic inflammation. Topical application of *S. epidermidis* or glycerol alone on ICR mice dorsal skin exposed to UVB showed noticeable erythema, ulceration, epidermal hyperplasia, and increased IL-6 levels. Following UVB exposure, increased infiltration of dermal inflammatory cells may lead to epidermal proliferation of keratinocytes and hyperplastic lesion [39,40]. A significant decrease in inflammation with attenuation of IL-6 and a reduction of epidermal thickness was observed in skin topically applied with mixture of *S. epidermidis* and glycerol, suggesting that the anti-inflammatory effect observed here is likely to be mediated through *S. epidermidis* fermentation using glycerol as a carbon source. Further, we confirmed that the anti-inflammatory activity was the result of *S. epidermidis* fermentation with the use of the fermentation inhibitor, furfural. Control mice topically applied with water or furfural alone followed by irradiation with UVB appeared to have significant ulceration, epidermal thickening, and increased IL-6. Importantly, there was no recovery from ulceration or inflammation in skin applied with a mixture of *S. epidermidis* and glycerol along with furfural. Based on these findings, we infer that a product from the fermentation of glycerol by *S. epidermidis* could inhibit inflammation from chronic UVB. Bacterial interference using live beneficial bacteria is a promising method of preventing or treating many infections. Because of the US Food and Drug Administration (FDA) restriction in use of live probiotic bacteria for cosmetics, the promotion of beneficial effects through the generation of fermentation metabolites from live probiotic bacteria has become a desirable alternative [28,29]. Consistent with a previous study [13], the current work used HPLC analysis to detect a substantial amount of butyric acid in the fermented media of *S. epidermidis* using glycerol as a carbon source. Anti-microbial, anti-inflammatory, and anti-cancer activity of butyric acid and its derivatives make it as a potential drug of choice [41,42]. It has been shown that application of both butyric acid and its co-drug could reportedly inhibit skin tumorigenesis and psoriasis-like skin inflammation [43,44]. In the current study, topical application of butyric acid markedly decreases skin ulceration and epidermal thickness from UVB exposure compared to the control mice skin applied with H_2O. In line with the anti-inflammatory activity of butyric acid, a significant reduction in IL-6 level was detected both in keratinocytes and in mice skin exposed to prolonged UVB, indicating its potential use as an agent to prevent inflammation in chronic UVB exposed skin. Reduction in level of IL-8 upon butyric acid treatment, provided new insight for the application of butyric acid against other upregulated cytokines against UVB induced inflammation.

Research demonstrated that butyrate can control immune/inflammatory reactions in the skin [42]. SCFAs exert their immunomodulatory effects via binding to its cognate receptor, GPR43 [45]. Exacerbated or unresolved inflammation was observed in GPR43-deficient ($Gpr43^{-/-}$) mice in models of colitis, arthritis, and asthma, demonstrating that SCFA-GPR43 interactions are obligatory for normal resolution of certain inflammatory responses [27]. Moreover, decreased expression of GPR43 by keratinocytes in psoriatic skin could be rescued by topical application of sodium butyrate, indicating that butyrate-GPR43 interactions might exert anti-inflammatory effects in psoriasis [46]. In our study, gavage feeding of mice with GLPG0974, an antagonist for FFAR2/GPR43 receptor, inhibited the anti-hyperplasic, anti-inflammatory effect of butyric acid. Further, topical application of butyric acid did not rescue the UVB induced skin damage and inflammatory level of IL-6 when FFAR2 receptor was knocked down by subcutaneous injection of FFAR2 siRNA. Overall, these results demonstrate that butyric acid interaction with the FFAR2 receptor is a crucial phenomenon during skin inflammation. Moreover, butyric acid-FFAR2 interactions could represent a central mechanism to account for the effect of probiotics on immune responses modulated by chronic UV radiation.

The skin microbiome plays an important role in preserving skin homeostasis. Thus, skin microbiome through fermentation activity might influence the skin immune system in a similar way to the gut under inflammatory disease conditions. A recent study demonstrated that topical application of antioxidants against UVB were found more effective than dietary supplementation because of the length of time needed to reach optimal concentrations in the skin [47]. In this current study, we determined that topical application of butyric acid, as a fermentation metabolite could act as a potent regulator of immune system during chronic UVB. Additionally, the dose of butyric acid is non-toxic to skin cells and thus may gain broad acceptance for not only therapeutics but also as an active ingredient in cosmetics with the ultimate aim of avoiding the strong effects from chronic UVB.

4. Materials and Methods

4.1. Ethics Statement

This research was conducted in strict accordance with an approved Institutional Animal Care and Use Committee (IACUC) protocol of the National Central University (NCU), Taiwan (NCU-106-016, 19 December 2017). ICR mice (8–9 week-old females; National Laboratory Animal Centre, Taipei, Taiwan) were sacrificed using dry ice in a closed box.

4.2. Chemicals

Butyric acid (Sigma), acetonitrile, H_3PO_4, ether anhydrous, formaldehyde, hydrochloric acid (HCl, 37%), sodium hydroxide (NaOH), Sodium dihydrogenphosphate (NaH_2PO_4), and phosphoric acid (H_3PO_4) were purchased from J.T.Baker, Avantor Performance Materials Taiwan Co. Ltd. DMSO and glycerol were purchased from Sigma. PBS was purchased from Gibco (Gaithersburg, MD, USA). GLPG0974 (FFAR2 inhibitor) was also obtained from Tocris Bioscience (Ellisville, MO, USA). Butyric acid was obtained from Sigma (St. Louis, MO, USA).

4.3. Bacterial Culture

S. epidermidis bacteria, from ATCC 12228 was cultured on 3% tryptic soy broth (TSB) (Sigma, St. Louis, MO, USA) agar plates overnight at 37 °C. A single colony was inoculated in 3% TSB medium (Difco, Becton Dickinson UK Ltd., Oxford, UK) and cultured at 37 °C until the logarithmic growth phase. Bacterial pellets were harvested by centrifugation at 5000× g for 10 min, washed with PBS, and suspended in PBS.

4.4. Fermentation of Bacteria

S. epidermidis (10^7 CFU/mL) were incubated in 10 mL rich media (10 g/L yeast extract (Biokar Diagnostics, Beauvais, France), 3 g/L TSB, 2.5 g/L K_2HPO_4, and 1.5 g/L KH_2PO_4) in the absence and presence of glycerol (2%) under aerobic conditions at 37 °C with shaking at 200 rpm. The rich media glycerol (2%) without bacteria were included as a control. The 0.002% (w/v) phenol red (Sigma) in rich media with glycerol (2%) acted as a fermentation indicator. A color change from red-orange to yellow indicated the occurrence of bacterial fermentation, which was detected as absorbance at 560 nm.

4.5. Inhibition of ALS Activity by Furfural

ALS (EC: 4.1. 3.18) is responsible for the conversion of pyruvate to acetolactate which can be eventually metabolized to diacetyl and 2,3-butanediol. The rate of reaction was monitored by the depletion of NADH at 340 nm during the conversion of pyruvate to 2,3-butanediol. The reaction mixture contained 70 mM sodium acetate buffer (pH 5.4), 0.17 mM thiamine pyrophosphate, and lysate (10 mg) of heat (100 °C) killed *S. epidermidis*. The reaction was started by addition of pyruvate [48] in the presence or absence of 0.4% furfural at 45 °C for 5 min. Absorbance was measured with a visible spectrophotometer at 340 nm. Values of ALS activity were expressed in enzyme as unit per mg (U/mg), in which one unit of ALS is defined as the amount of enzyme able to produce 0.1 absorbance unit per min.

4.6. Ultraviolet Light Exposure

ICR mice were exposed to chronic UVB with a ramping dose using an UV lamp (Model EB-280C, Spectronics Corp., Westbury, NY, USA). The UVB light source was set at a distance such that the dorsal surface of each mouse received 195 mJ/cm^2. Dorsal skin was exposed three times per week, followed by topical application with *S. epidermidis* (10^7) and glycerol (2%) in PBS one time per week. Whole UVB radiation and treatment was conducted for 4 weeks. Animals were photographed at 0, 16, and 30 day for measurement of wound from UVB and recovery from treatment. Animals were sacrificed 3 day following the last dose and whole skin samples, including epidermis and dermis were collected. Tissue samples (approximately 1 cm^2) were taken from similar dorso-caudal locations for histological examination. The remaining portions of the dorsal skin were used to prepare whole skin lysate for ELISA analyses. Hematoxylin and eosin (H&E) staining was performed by the Histopathology Shared Resources Core at Li-Tzung Biotechnology Inc. Quantitative measurements of skin thickness from H&E were made using ImageJ software.

4.7. Wound Measurement

To investigate the wound improvement of ICR hairless mice skin induced by UVB irradiation, the mice were transiently anesthetized using isoflurane, and the wound were measured by ImageJ software by calculating the percent of remaining wound area to the total area of skin exposed at 0, 16, and 30 day of UVB irradiation. Wounds were photographed using a USB digital microscope.

4.8. Histological Analysis

Histological analysis was performed to determine the epidermal thickness. Dorsal skin samples of the experimental groups were obtained after 4 weeks of UVB exposure, fixed with 10% formalin and embedded in paraffin. Sections were stained with H&E to examine epidermal thickness. Epidermal thickness was measured at 10× magnification using Olympus BX63 microscope (Olympus, Tokyo, Japan).

4.9. siRNA-Mediated Gene Silencing of GPR43/FFAR2

In order to silence GPR43 gene, we used the chemically-modified siRNA that targets GPR43 receptor and the siRNA negative control, which does not target any known sequence were obtained from GenePharma Co. (Shanghai, China). Their oligonucleotide sequences are siFFAR2: sense strand, 5'-CCGGUGCAGUACAAGUUAUTT-3'; anti-sense strand, 5'-AUAACUUGUACUGCACC GGTT-3'. SiControl: sense strand, 5'-UUCUCCGAACGUGUCACGUTT; anti-sense strand, 5'-ACGUGACACGUUCGGAGAATT-3'. These chemically-modified siRNAs were delivered by intradermal injection in dorsal skin of mice using a microneedle [49,50].

4.10. Drug Treatment

Selective FFAR2 antagonist GLPG0974 (0.1 or 1 mg/kg ig) was administered to ICR mice by gavage feeding [51]. GLPG0974 was dissolved in DMSO (0.01% in saline) and DMSO (0.01% in saline) was used as the vehicle control. Butyric acid (4 mM) was topically applied on dorsal skin of mice. Butyric acid was dissolved in double distilled water.

4.11. ELISA

Skin samples from ICR mice were collected after 4 weeks of UVB exposure and were then lysed with T-PER™ Tissue Protein Extraction Reagent (ThermoFisher Scientific, Waltham, MA, USA) supplemented with an ethylenediaminetetraacetic acid (EDTA)-free protease inhibitor cocktail (Sigma-Aldrich, St Louis, MO, USA). Supernatant was collected from UVB irradiated and non-irradiated human keratinocytes (CCD 1106 KERTr) with and without BA treatment. IL-6 concentration in mice skin and IL-6 and IL-8 concentration in supernatant from human keratinocytes were determined by mouse or human IL-6 and IL-8 ELISA assay kit (R&D Systems, Minneapolis, MN, USA) following previous published protocol [52].

4.12. HPLC

Media samples were vortexed and equilibrated at room temperature for 5 min. Thereafter 100 μL of concentrated HCl was added per mL of each sample, followed by a vortex-mixing step of 15 s. The samples were extracted for 20 min (by gently rolling) using 5 mL of diethyl ether. After centrifugation (5 min, 3500 rpm), the supernatant was transferred to another Pyrex extraction tube and 500 μL of a 1 M solution of NaOH was added. The samples were extracted again for 20 min, followed by a centrifugation step. The aqueous phase was transferred to an auto sampler vial and 100 μL of concentrated HCl was added. After vortex mixing, 10 μL was injected onto the HPLC–UV apparatus. The mobile phase consisted of 20 mM of NaH_2PO_4 in HPLC water (pH adjusted to 2.2 using phosphoric acid) (A) and acetonitrile (B). The UV detector was set at a wavelength of 210 nm for detection of butyric acid in sample.

4.13. Statistical Analysis

Data analysis was performed by unpaired t-test or by one-way ANOVA using GraphPad Prism® software. The p-values of <0.05 (*), <0.01 (**), and <0.001 (***) were considered significant. The mean ± standard error (SE) for at least three independent experiments was calculated.

Author Contributions: S.K., A.B., B.M., and I.P.N. performed the experiments. C.-M.H. designed all experiments. S.K. wrote the manuscript. S.K., C.-M.H., and D.R.H. reviewed and edited the manuscript.

Acknowledgments: We wish to thank Yu-Fen Huang, Department of Biomedical Engineering and Environmental Sciences, National Tsing Hua University, Taiwan for providing HPLC-UV analysis facility and Postdoctoral Scholar Irving Po-Jung Lai, National Central University, Taiwan for skillful help during HPLC-UV analysis.

References

1. Lopez-Camarillo, C.; Ocampo, E.A.; Casamichana, M.L.; Perez-Plasencia, C.; Alvarez-Sanchez, E.; Marchat, L.A. Protein kinases and transcription factors activation in response to UV-radiation of skin: Implications for carcinogenesis. *Int. J. Mol. Sci.* **2012**, *13*, 142–172. [CrossRef] [PubMed]

2. Armstrong, B.K.; Kricker, A. The epidemiology of UV induced skin cancer. *J. Photochem. Photobiol. B* **2001**, *63* 8–18. [CrossRef]

3. De Fabo, E.C.; Noonan, F.P. Mechanism of immune suppression by ultraviolet irradiation in vivo. I. Evidence for the existence of a unique photoreceptor in skin and its role in photoimmunology. *J. Exp. Med.* **1983**, *158* 84–98. [CrossRef] [PubMed]

4. Ishida, T.; Sakaguchi, I. Protection of human keratinocytes from UVB-induced inflammation using root extract of Lithospermum erythrorhizon. *Biol. Pharm. Bull.* **2007**, *30*, 928–934. [CrossRef] [PubMed]

5. Ansel, J.C.; Luger, T.A.; Green, I. The effect of in vitro and in vivo UV irradiation on the production of ETAF activity by human and murine keratinocytes. *J. Investig. Dermatol.* **1983**, *81*, 519–523. [CrossRef] [PubMed]

6. Kirnbauer, R.; Kock, A.; Neuner, P.; Forster, E.; Krutmann, J.; Urbanski, A.; Schauer, E.; Ansel, J.C.; Schwarz, T.; Luger, T.A. Regulation of epidermal cell interleukin-6 production by UV light and corticosteroids. *J. Investig. Dermatol.* **1991**, *96*, 484–489. [CrossRef]

7. Acker, T.; Fandrey, J.; Acker, H. The good, the bad and the ugly in oxygen-sensing: ROS, cytochromes and prolyl-hydroxylases. *Cardiovasc. Res.* **2006**, *71*, 195–207. [CrossRef] [PubMed]

8. Kloos, W.E.; Musselwhite, M.S. Distribution and persistence of Staphylococcus and Micrococcus species and other aerobic bacteria on human skin. *Appl. Microbiol.* **1975**, *30*, 381–385. [PubMed]

9. Sanford, J.A.; Gallo, R.L. Functions of the skin microbiota in health and disease. *Semin. Immunol.* **2013**, *25*, 370–377. [CrossRef] [PubMed]

10. Lai, Y.; Di Nardo, A.; Nakatsuji, T.; Leichtle, A.; Yang, Y.; Cogen, A.L.; Wu, Z.R.; Hooper, L.V.; Schmidt, R.R.; von Aulock, S.; et al. Commensal bacteria regulate Toll-like receptor 3-dependent inflammation after skin injury. *Nat. Med.* **2009**, *15*, 1377–1382. [CrossRef]

11. Nakatsuji, T.; Chen, T.H.; Butcher, A.M.; Trzoss, L.L.; Nam, S.-J.; Shirakawa, K.T.; Zhou, W.; Oh, J.; Otto, M.; Fenical, W.; et al. A commensal strain of *Staphylococcus epidermidis* protects against skin neoplasia. *Sci. Adv.* **2018**, *4*. [CrossRef] [PubMed]

12. Cogen, A.L.; Yamasaki, K.; Sanchez, K.M.; Dorschner, R.A.; Lai, Y.; MacLeod, D.T.; Torpey, J.W.; Otto, M.; Nizet, V.; Kim, J.E.; et al. Selective Antimicrobial Action Is Provided by Phenol-Soluble Modulins Derived from Staphylococcus epidermidis, a Normal Resident of the Skin. *J. Investig. Dermatol.* **2010**, *130*, 192–200. [CrossRef] [PubMed]

13. Wang, Y.; Kuo, S.; Shu, M.; Yu, J.; Huang, S.; Dai, A.; Two, A.; Gallo, R.L.; Huang, C.M. Staphylococcus epidermidis in the human skin microbiome mediates fermentation to inhibit the growth of Propionibacterium acnes: Implications of probiotics in acne vulgaris. *Appl. Microbiol. Biotechnol.* **2014**, *98*, 411–424. [CrossRef] [PubMed]

14. Kumar, M.; Myagmardoloonjin, B.; Keshari, S.; Negari, I.P.; Huang, C.M. 5-Methyl Furfural Reduces the Production of Malodors by Inhibiting Sodium l-Lactate Fermentation of Staphylococcus epidermidis: Implication for Deodorants Targeting the Fermenting Skin Microbiome. *Microorganisms* **2019**, *7*, 239. [CrossRef] [PubMed]

15. Yang, A.J.; Marito, S.; Yang, J.J.; Keshari, S.; Chew, C.H.; Chen, C.C.; Huang, C.M. A Microtube Array Membrane (MTAM) Encapsulated Live Fermenting Staphylococcus epidermidis as a Skin Probiotic Patch against Cutibacterium acnes. *Int. J. Mol. Sci.* **2018**, *20*, 14. [CrossRef] [PubMed]

16. Malav, M.K.; Prasad, S.; Kharia, S.K.; Kumar, S.; Sheetal, K.; Kannojiya, S. Furfural and 5-HMF: Potent fermentation inhibitors and their removal techniques. *Int. J. Curr. Microbiol. Appl. Sci.* **2017**, *6*, 2060–2066. [CrossRef]

17. Carvalho, S.M.; de Jong, A.; Kloosterman, T.G.; Kuipers, O.P.; Saraiva, L.M. The Staphylococcus aureus α-Acetolactate Synthase ALS Confers Resistance to Nitrosative Stress. *Front. Microbiol.* **2017**, *8*, 1273. [CrossRef] [PubMed]

18. Härtig, E.; Jahn, D. Regulation of the Anaerobic Metabolism in Bacillus subtilis. *Adv. Microb. Physiol.* **2012**, *61*, 195–216. [CrossRef]

19. Palmqvist, E.; Hahn-Hägerdal, B. Fermentation of lignocellulosic hydrolysates. II: Inhibitors and mechanisms of inhibition. *Bioresour. Technol.* **2000**, *33*, 25–33. [CrossRef]

20. Meijer, K.; de Vos, P.; Priebe, M.G. Butyrate and other short-chain fatty acids as modulators of immunity: What relevance for health? *Curr. Opin. Clin. Nutr. Metab. Care* **2010**, *13*, 715–721. [CrossRef] [PubMed]

21. Kao, M.S.; Huang, S.; Chang, W.L.; Hsieh, M.F.; Huang, C.J.; Gallo, R.L.; Huang, C.M. Microbiome precision editing: Using PEG as a selective fermentation initiator against methicillin-resistant Staphylococcus aureus. *Biotechnol. J.* **2017**, *12*. [CrossRef] [PubMed]

22. Xia, J.; Song, X.; Bi, Z.; Chu, W.; Wan, Y. UV-induced NF-kappaB activation and expression of IL-6 is attenuated by (-)-epigallocatechin-3-gallate in cultured human keratinocytes in vitro. *Int. J. Mol. Med.* **2005**, *16*, 943–950. [PubMed]

23. Smerdon, M.J.; Lan, S.Y.; Calza, R.E.; Reeves, R. Sodium butyrate stimulates DNA repair in UV-irradiated normal and xeroderma pigmentosum human fibroblasts. *J. Biol. Chem.* **1982**, *257*, 13441–13447. [PubMed]

24. Xiong, F.; Mou, Y.Z.; Xiang, X.Y. Inhibition of mouse B16 melanoma by sodium butyrate correlated to tumor associated macrophages differentiation suppression. *Int. J. Clin. Exp. Med.* **2015**, *8*, 4170–4174. [PubMed]

25. Yoshizumi, M.; Nakamura, T.; Kato, M.; Ishioka, T.; Kozawa, K.; Wakamatsu, K.; Kimura, H. Release of cytokines/chemokines and cell death in UVB-irradiated human keratinocytes, HaCaT. *Cell Biol. Int.* **2008**, *32*, 1405–1411. [CrossRef]

26. Pirozzi, C.; Francisco, V.; Guida, F.D.; Gomez, R.; Lago, F.; Pino, J.; Meli, R.; Gualillo, O. Butyrate Modulates Inflammation in Chondrocytes via GPR43 Receptor. *Cell Physiol. Biochem.* **2018**, *51*, 228–243. [CrossRef] [PubMed]

27. Maslowski, K.M.; Vieira, A.T.; Ng, A.; Kranich, J.; Sierro, F.; Yu, D.; Schilter, H.C.; Rolph, M.S.; Mackay, F.; Artis, D.; et al. Regulation of inflammatory responses by gut microbiota and chemoattractant receptor GPR43. *Nature* **2009**, *461*, 1282–1286. [CrossRef]

28. Masui, R.; Sasaki, M.; Funaki, Y.; Ogasawara, N.; Mizuno, M.; Iida, A.; Izawa, S.; Kondo, Y.; Ito, Y.; Tamura, Y.; et al. G protein-coupled receptor 43 moderates gut inflammation through cytokine regulation from mononuclear cells. *Inflamm. Bowel Dis.* **2013**, *19*, 2848–2856. [CrossRef] [PubMed]

29. Bode, A.M.; Dong, Z. Mitogen-activated protein kinase activation in UV-induced signal transduction. *Sci. STKE* **2003**, *2003*. [CrossRef] [PubMed]

30. Choi, K.-S.; Kundu, J.K.; Chun, K.-S.; Na, H.-K.; Surh, Y.-J. Rutin inhibits UVB radiation-induced expression of COX-2 and iNOS in hairless mouse skin: p38 MAP kinase and JNK as potential targets. *Arch. Biochem. Biophys.* **2014**, *559*, 38–45. [CrossRef] [PubMed]

31. Fluhr, J.W.; Darlenski, R.; Surber, C. Glycerol and the skin: Holistic approach to its origin and functions. *Br. J. Dermatol.* **2008**, *159*, 23–34. [CrossRef] [PubMed]

32. Lin, T.K.; Zhong, L.; Santiago, J.L. Anti-Inflammatory and Skin Barrier Repair Effects of Topical Application of Some Plant Oils. *Int. J. Mol. Sci.* **2017**, *19*, 70. [CrossRef] [PubMed]

33. Thomsen, M.H.; Thygesen, A.; Thomsen, A.B. Identification and characterization of fermentation inhibitors formed during hydrothermal treatment and following SSF of wheat straw. *Appl. Microbiol. Biotechnol.* **2009**, *83*, 447–455. [CrossRef] [PubMed]

34. Perrine, S.P.; Dover, G.H.; Daftari, P.; Walsh, C.T.; Jin, Y.; Mays, A.; Faller, D.V. Isobutyramide, an orally bioavailable butyrate analogue, stimulates fetal globin gene expression in vitro and in vivo. *Br. J. Haematol.* **1994**, *88*, 555–561. [CrossRef]

35. Vassilev, I.; Hernandez, P.A.; Batlle-Vilanova, P.; Freguia, S.; Krömer, J.O.; Keller, J.; Ledezma, P.; Virdis, B. Microbial Electrosynthesis of Isobutyric, Butyric, Caproic Acids, and Corresponding Alcohols from Carbon Dioxide. *ACS Sustain. Chem. Eng.* **2018**, *6*, 8485–8493. [CrossRef]

36. Kober, M.-M.; Bowe, W.P. The effect of probiotics on immune regulation, acne, and photoaging. *Int. J. Women's Dermatol.* **2015**, *1*, 85–89. [CrossRef]

37. Guéniche, A.; Benyacoub, J.; Buetler, T.M.; Smola, H.; Blum, S. Supplementation with oral probiotic bacteria maintains cutaneous immune homeostasis after UV exposure. *Eur. J. Dermatol.* **2006**, *16*, 511–517.

38. Cope, E.K.; Lynch, S.V. Novel microbiome-based therapeutics for chronic rhinosinusitis. *Curr. Allergy Asthma Rep.* **2015**, *15*, 9. [CrossRef]

39. Agarwal, R.; Katiyar, S.K.; Khan, S.G.; Mukhtar, H. Protection against ultraviolet B radiation-induced effects in the skin of SKH-1 hairless mice by a polyphenolic fraction isolated from green tea. *Photochem. Photobiol.* **1993**, *58*, 695–700. [CrossRef]

40. Wilgus, T.A.; Ross, M.S.; Parrett, M.L.; Oberyszyn, T.M. Topical application of a selective cyclooxygenase inhibitor suppresses UVB mediated cutaneous inflammation. *Prostaglandins Other Lipid Mediat.* **2000**, *62*, 367–384. [CrossRef]

41. Borycka-Kiciak, K.; Banasiewicz, T.; Rydzewska, G. Butyric acid—A well-known molecule revisited. *Prz. Gastroenterol.* **2017**, *12*, 83–89. [CrossRef] [PubMed]

42. Schwarz, A.; Bruhs, A.; Schwarz, T. The Short-Chain Fatty Acid Sodium Butyrate Functions as a Regulator of the Skin Immune System. *J. Investig. Dermatol.* **2017**, *137*, 855–864. [CrossRef] [PubMed]

43. Gupta, K.P.; Mehrotra, N.K. Differential effects of butyric acid on mouse skin tumorigenesis. *Biomed. Env. Sci.* **1997**, *10*, 436–441.

44. Bruhs, A.; Schwarz, T.; Schwarz, A. 325 The short chain fatty acid sodium butyrate attenuates imiquimod-induced psoriasis-like skin inflammation. *J. Investig. Dermatol.* **2017**, *137*, S248. [CrossRef]

45. Karaki, S.; Mitsui, R.; Hayashi, H.; Kato, I.; Sugiya, H.; Iwanaga, T.; Furness, J.B.; Kuwahara, A. Short-chain fatty acid receptor, GPR43, is expressed by enteroendocrine cells and mucosal mast cells in rat intestine. *Cell Tissue Res.* **2006**, *324*, 353–360. [CrossRef] [PubMed]

46. Krejner, A.; Bruhs, A.; Mrowietz, U.; Wehkamp, U.; Schwarz, T.; Schwarz, A. Decreased expression of G-protein-coupled receptors GPR43 and GPR109a in psoriatic skin can be restored by topical application of sodium butyrate. *Arch. Dermatol. Res.* **2018**, *310*, 751–758. [CrossRef] [PubMed]

47. Jurkiewicz, B.A. The Role of Free Radicals, Iron, and Antioxidants in Ultraviolet Radiation-Induced Skin Damage. Available online: https://www.healthcare.uiowa.edu/CoreFacilities/esr/education/theses/pdf/Jurkiewicz-PhD-1995.pdf (accessed on 11 August 2019).

48. Cogan, T.M.; Fitzgerald, R.J.; Doonan, S. Acetolactate synthase of Leuconostoc lactis and its regulation of acetoin production. *J. Dairy Res.* **2009**, *51*, 597–604. [CrossRef]

49. Pan, J.; Ruan, W.; Qin, M.; Long, Y.; Wan, T.; Yu, K.; Zhai, Y.; Wu, C.; Xu, Y. Intradermal delivery of STAT3 siRNA to treat melanoma via dissolving microneedles. *Sci. Rep.* **2018**, *8*, 1117. [CrossRef]

50. Dou, S.; Yao, Y.-D.; Yang, X.-Z.; Sun, T.-M.; Mao, C.-Q.; Song, E.-W.; Wang, J. Anti-Her2 single-chain antibody mediated DNMTs-siRNA delivery for targeted breast cancer therapy. *J. Control. Release* **2012**, *161*, 875–883. [CrossRef]

51. Pizzonero, M.; Dupont, S.; Babel, M.; Beaumont, S.; Bienvenu, N.; Blanque, R.; Cherel, L.; Christophe, T.; Crescenzi, B.; De Lemos, E.; et al. Discovery and optimization of an azetidine chemical series as a free fatty acid receptor 2 (FFA2) antagonist: From hit to clinic. *J. Med. Chem.* **2014**, *57*, 10044–10057. [CrossRef]

52. Keshari, S.; Sipayung, A.D.; Hsieh, C.C.; Su, L.J.; Chiang, Y.R.; Chang, H.C.; Yang, W.C.; Chuang, T.H.; Chen, C.L.; Huang, C.M. The IL-6/p-BTK/p-ERK signaling mediates the calcium phosphate-induced pruritus. *FASEB J.* **2019**. [CrossRef] [PubMed]

12

The Role of Th17-Related Cytokines in Atopic Dermatitis

Makoto Sugaya

Department of Dermatology, International University of Health and Welfare, Ichikawa Hospital, 6-1-14, Kounodai, Ichikawa, Chiba 272-0827, Japan; sugayamder@iuhw.ac.jp

Abstract: T helper-17 (Th17) cells, which mainly produce IL-17, are associated with development of various autoimmune diseases such as rheumatoid arthritis, inflammatory bowel diseases, multiple sclerosis, and psoriasis. IL-17 and related cytokines are therapeutic targets of these diseases. In atopic dermatitis (AD), Th2 cytokines such as IL-4 and IL-13 are regarded to be the main player of the disease; however, Th17 cytokines are also expressed in AD skin lesions. Expression of IL-22 rather than IL-17 is predominant in AD skin, which is contrary to cytokine expression in psoriasis skin. Relatively low IL-17 expression in AD skin can induce relatively low antimicrobial peptide expression, which may be a reason why bacterial infection is frequently seen in AD patients. Failure of clinical trials for investigating the efficacy of anti-IL-12/23 p40 in AD has suggested that IL-17 expressed in skin lesions should not be the main player but a bystander responding to barrier dysfunction.

Keywords: IL-22; IL-26; subtypes of atopic dermatitis; ustekinumab; wound healing; antimicrobial peptides

1. Introduction

Atopic dermatitis (AD) is a chronic skin disease characterized by relapsing eczema with pruritus as a primary lesion. Most patients with AD have atopic diathesis such as family history of allergic diseases or past history of asthma, rhinitis, or conjunctivitis [1]. In Japan, AD is not a rare skin disease, whose frequency is about 10–15% until the age of forty [2]. Age-related remission is achieved in a certain proportion of patients with AD, especially when the onset is younger or the symptoms are milder [3,4]. Although some patients develop AD in their adulthood, onset of AD in elderly people is very rare. Other skin diseases such as cutaneous T-cell lymphoma (CTCL), drug eruption, and bullous diseases should be considered as a possible diagnosis. Most of all, CTCL should not be misdiagnosed with AD because immunosuppressive drugs such as cyclosporine and anti-tumor necrosis factor (TNF)-α antibody can exacerbate disease activity of CTCL [5–7]. When the diagnosis is not clear, topical steroid or ultraviolet phototherapy should be applied.

AD has significant negative social and economic impacts, substantially decreasing the quality of life of the patients and their families [8,9]. Skin conditions of AD children influence quality of life of both children and their caregivers. Pruritus, emotional distress, and sleep disturbance are big problems for them, which should be paid more attention to. It is important to induce long-term remission. Remission can be achieved by conventional treatment for mild or moderate AD, while it is very difficult for severe AD patients [3,4]. Treatment strategies consist of drug therapy with topical agents such as steroid or tacrolimus, skin care with moisturizers for dry skin, and investigation and elimination of exacerbating factors [1]. The pathogenesis of AD can be explained from the perspectives of the skin barrier, allergic inflammation, and neuroendocrine dysfunction represented by severe pruritus [10]. With regards to allergic immune responses, cytokines expressed by T helper (Th) 2 cells and group 2 innate lymphoid cells such as interleukin (IL)-4, IL-5, and IL-13 have been assumed as main players of AD [11–13]. It was also reported that Th1 cytokines like interferon (IFN)-γ were expressed in AD lesional skin [14,15]. In recent years, Th17 cytokines such as IL-17 and IL-22 were reported to be expressed in AD lesional skin [16–20]. In this review, the importance of Th17-related cytokines in pathogenesis and treatment of AD will be discussed.

2. Th17 Cells in Pathogenesis of Psoriasis

CD4+ helper T cells, upon activation, develop into different T helper cell subsets. Th17 cells, which are different from Th1 or Th2 cells, produce IL-17, IL-17F, and IL-22 as well as IL-21 [21]. Th17 cells are essential in clearing pathogens during host defense reactions. IL-17 and IL-22 are also important for chronic autoinflammatory diseases such as rheumatoid arthritis, inflammatory bowel diseases including Chron's disease and ulcerative colitis, multiple sclerosis, and psoriasis. While transforming growth factor-β and IL-6 are important for differentiation of the subset, IL-23 produced by dendritic cells activated by TNF-α is essential for its maintenance and activation. It is widely accepted that a vicious circle among TNF-α, IL-23, and IL-17 is established in psoriasis. Monoclonal antibodies against TNF-α, IL-12/23p40 subunit, IL-23p19, and IL-17 are clinically used and very effective [22–25].

IL-17 has multiple physiological functions. It activates macrophages to express TNF-α and IL-1β [26] and fibroblasts to produce IL-6, IL-8, and matrix metalloproteinases [27]. These cytokines are important for inflammatory process and tissue remodeling. It also stimulates blood endothelial cells to produce chemoattractants and express VCAM-1 and ICAM-1 in a p38 MAPK-dependent manner, which helps immune cells evade from blood to tissues [28]. Epithelial cells stimulated by IL-17 express IL-8 and granulocyte colony-stimulating factor, inducing migration and activation of neutrophils [29]. In addition, IL-17 was found to synergistically enhance TNF-α-induced production of these cytokines. IL-17 also increases production of antimicrobial peptides (AMPs), which are part of the innate immune response and are found among all classes of life [30,31]. These peptides kill bacteria, mycobacteria, enveloped viruses, and fungi. Skin-resident commensal microbes produce their own AMPs, act to enhance the normal production of AMPs by keratinocytes, and are beneficial to maintaining inflammatory homeostasis by suppressing excess cytokine release after minor epidermal injury [32]. IL-22, which is another cytokine expressed by Th17, enhances AMP production together with IL-17 [31]. This cytokine induces epidermal proliferation [33]. IL-26, an antimicrobial protein that has the ability to directly kill extracellular bacteria, is also secreted by Th17 [34]. IL-26 was more strongly expressed in lesions from the self-limited tuberculoid leprosy compared with expression in progressive lepromatous patients. IL-26 directly bound to *Mycobacterium leprae* in axenic culture and reduced bacteria viability. Thus, Th17 is important for neutrophilic infiltration, epidermal proliferation called acanthosis, and innate immune responses including enhanced production of AMPs, which are main histological findings characteristic to psoriasis.

3. Involvement of Th17-Related Cytokines in AD

3.1. Th17-Related Cytokine Expression in AD

Possible involvement of Th17 in the pathogenesis of AD has been reported by some researchers [16–20]. The percentage of IL-17-poducing CD4+ T cells in peripheral blood from AD patients was increased and associated with severity of AD [16]. There was a significant correlation between the percentages of IL-17+ and IFN-γ+ cells, although the percentage of Th17 cells was not closely related to Th1/Th2 balance. Immunohistochemically, IL-17+ cells infiltrated in the papillary dermis of AD lesional skin. There was another study showing that more IL-17-producing cells infiltrated into the site of an atopy patch test than in healthy skin [17]. IL-17 secretion was not enhanced by IL-23, IL-1β, or IL-6, but was enhanced by the *Staphylococcus aureus*-derived superantigen staphylococcal enterotoxin B. Another group, however, showed that the number of Th1 and Th17 subsets in peripheral blood from AD patients was significantly decreased, but that of the Th2 subset was similar to that of normal controls [35]. The frequency of Th17 cells showed a significant, negative correlation with serum thymus and activation-regulated chemokine (TARC) and IgE levels and the number of eosinophils. It was recently reported that the frequency of IL-13+ cells, which was correlated with IgE levels and SCORing AD (SCORAD) score, was associated with IL-22-producing T cells in severe AD patients [36]. When examining skin samples from AD, psoriasis, and healthy controls, IL-17 expression level was increased in AD skin compared to normal skin, although it was much lower than that in psoriasis skin [18]. By contrast, Th2 cells were significantly elevated in AD. Distinct IL-22-producing CD4+ and CD8+ T-cell populations were significantly increased in AD skin compared with psoriasis. IL-22-producing CD8+ T-cell frequency correlated with AD disease severity. Taken together, IL-22 rather than IL-17 is dominant in AD skin, while IL-17 is dominant in psoriasis skin.

It is a recent trend to divide various diseases into subgroups by cytokine production. Two subgroups of asthma, intrinsic and extrinsic, have been proposed [37]. Extrinsic asthma is triggered by allergens and is characterized by enhanced Th2 cytokine production. Intrinsic asthma is characterized by later onset in life, female predominance, higher degree of severity, and more frequent association to nasosinusal polyposis. This nonallergic asthma characterized by Th1 production can be objectively distinguished from allergic asthma based on negative skin tests to usual aeroallergens. Similar subgroups have been proposed for AD: intrinsic AD and extrinsic AD [38,39]. Extrinsic or allergic AD shows high total serum IgE levels and the presence of specific IgE for environmental and food allergens, whereas intrinsic or nonallergic AD exhibits normal total IgE values and the absence of specific IgE [38]. Extrinsic AD is much more common than intrinsic AD, which is approximately 20% with female predominance. The clinical features of intrinsic AD include relative late onset, milder severity, a higher frequency of metal allergy, and Dennie–Morgan folds, but no ichthyosis vulgaris or palmar hyperlinearity. The skin barrier dysfunction and filaggrin gene mutations are not a feature of intrinsic AD. The intrinsic type is characterized by the lower expression of IL-4, IL-5, and IL-13, and the higher expression of IFN-γ. In patients with intrinsic AD, Th17-related cytokines are highly expressed [39]. Positive correlations between Th17-related molecules and SCORAD scores were only found in patients with intrinsic AD, whereas only patients with extrinsic AD showed positive correlations between SCORAD scores and Th2 cytokine levels and negative correlations with keratinocyte differentiation markers such as loricrin and periplakin. Another classification of AD was proposed: Asian type and European American type. A principal component analysis using real-time PCR data clustered the Asian AD phenotype between the European American AD and psoriasis phenotypes [19]. Significantly higher Th17 and lower Th1 gene induction typified AD skin in Asian patients. Moreover, AD lesional skin in pediatric patients was reported to contain more Th17-related cytokines and AMPs than that in adult patients [20]. Taken together, it may be safely said that IL-17 expression in lesional skin of a certain group of AD patients is higher than that in normal skin. It is yet to be elucidated whether IL-17 plays a critical role in AD as it does in psoriasis.

With regards to serum levels of cytokines, it was reported that IL-22 in AD patients significantly correlated with disease activity, while IL-17 did not reflect disease burden [35].

IL-26 is another cytokine produced by Th17 cells. It was recently reported that IL-26 mRNA expression levels were elevated in AD lesional skin compared with healthy controls and that IL-26-producing cells were increased in AD lesional skin by immunohistochemistry [40]. IL-26 may play an important role for bridging between Th17 and Th2 responses, resulting in the development of AD.

3.2. AD Mouse Models and Th17-Related Cytokines

With regards to basic research, IL-17 was reported to regulate Th2 responses in the mouse AD model [41]. IL-17 triggered the production of IL-4 by Th2 cells. The lack of IL-17A reduced dermatitis and IL-4 production as well as IgE production. It is also known that IL-17 promotes the differentiation of B cells to IgE-producing plasma cells [42]. A murine epicutaneous infection model showed that *Malassezia*, which has been reported to exacerbate AD skin conditions, selectively induced IL-17-related cytokines [43]. This process is important for preventing fungal infection through the skin. Under skin barrier dysfunction mimicking AD, the presence of *Malassezia* aggravated cutaneous inflammation, which was dependent on IL-23 and IL-17. A CCR6+ Th17 subset of memory T cells specific to *Malassezia* was more frequently detected in AD skin than in healthy skin. Thus, the *Malassezia*-induced Th17 response is important not only in antifungal immunity but also in worsening skin inflammatory conditions. TNF-like weak inducer of apoptosis (TWEAK) and its receptor fibroblast growth factor (FGF) inducible 14 are highly expressed in AD skin lesions. BALB/c mice deficient in this molecule showed attenuated skin inflammation in an AD model, accompanied by less infiltration of inflammatory cells and lower local levels of proinflammatory cytokines, including TWEAK, TNF-α, and IL-17 [44]. Thus, IL-17 may be an important mediator of TWEAK-induced AD-like inflammation. The numbers of ILC3, expressing IL-17, in the skin of AD-induced mice were increased, and that neutralizing IL-17A delayed development of AD in the mouse model [45]. ILC3 induced IL-33 production by keratinocytes and fibroblasts. IL-26, another Th17 cytokine, promoted production of various cytokines such as IL-8, IL-1β, CCL20, IL-33, and β-defensin 2 by keratinocytes through phosphorylation of signal transducer and activator of transcription 1 and signal transducer and activator of transcription 3 [37]. JAK inhibitors, which are promising drugs for AD, blocked IL-26-induced cytokine production in keratinocytes. Injection of IL-26 exacerbated an oxazolone-induced AD mouse model and upregulated Th2 and Th17 cytokine expression in vivo. Thus, basic research findings also support the idea that IL-17 and its related cytokines are important in AD pathogenesis.

4. Expression of Th17 Cytokines in Other Skin Diseases

Some reports have suggested importance of IL-17 in various skin diseases other than psoriasis and AD. For example, IL-17 expression is reported to be increased in sera or lesional skin of systemic lupus erythematosus [46]. IL-17A expression was significantly increased in the involved skin and sera of systemic sclerosis patients, suggesting possible roles in the development of the disease [47,48]. Our group reported that lesional skin of mycosis fungoides (MF) and Sezary syndrome (SS), representative diseases of CTCL, contained a high amount of IL-17 and IL-22, the latter of which was dominant [49]. Serum IL-22 levels were significantly positively associated with disease activity in MF/SS. There are many clinical similarities between MF/SS and AD. Both diseases are characterized by persistent erythematous lesions with severe itch, sometimes developing to erythroderma. Bacterial, fungal, and viral infections such as impetigo contagiosum, phlegmone, tinea corporis, and herpes simplex are frequently accompanied. The number of eosinophils in peripheral blood is often increased and serum TARC level is elevated. Dominancy of IL-22 over IL-17 is seen in both diseases, which may explain clinical pictures of these diseases. Taken together, Th17 cytokine expression is widely seen in various skin diseases.

5. Clinical Trial for AD Targeting Th17 Cytokines

5.1. Clinical Effect of Ustekinumab on AD

Ustekinumab is a recombinant human IgG1 monoclonal antibody against p40, which is a common subunit of IL-12 and IL-23 [25]. This drug is used for psoriasis vulgaris and psoriatic arthritis. A previous report about four male patients with severe AD between 23 and 29 years old, whose skin eruption had been refractory to oral corticosteroids, phototherapy, and to at least two systemic drugs, showed improvement of SCORAD and itch score after treatment with 45 mg of ustekinumab injection at 0, 4 weeks, and every 12 weeks afterwards [50]. A 16-year-old woman with over a 13-year history of severe AD was also reported to show clearance of severe itch after one injection of ustekinumab 45 mg, although it had been resistant to phototherapy and systemic agents such as cyclosporine and azathioprine [51]. Complete remission was achieved with ustekinumab at the fourth week and every 12 weeks afterwards. There are, however, other reports denying efficacy of ustekinumab [52–54]. A 21-year-old man with a 7-year history of severe psoriasis refractory to conventional systemic treatments and childhood AD history was treated with ustekinumab [52]. The patient was without major respiratory symptoms and AD lesions within a period of five years before the date of starting the treatment. After an eight-month interval, ustekinumab was restarted and severe AD appeared on the neck and lower limbs. Peripheral blood eosinophilia and abnormal increase in serum IgE were also noted. The eczema lasted during 12 months of follow up after the final dose of ustekinumab, supporting the diagnosis of AD. Another group reported two psoriatic patients with high serum IgE levels, in whom ustekinumab completely improved psoriasis but paradoxically provoked or exacerbated AD-like symptoms [54]. Recently, the possibility of ustekinumab for AD was tested in clinical trials all over the world [55,56]. In the randomized, placebo-controlled, phase II study in Japan, 79 patients aged between 20 and 65 years with severe or very severe AD entered a 12-week, double-blind treatment period during which they received (1:1:1) ustekinumab 45 mg, 90 mg, or placebo subcutaneous injections at weeks 0 and 4, with follow-up until week 24 [55]. There was no significant improvement with ustekinumab treatment in least-squares mean change from baseline Eczema Area and Severity Index score at week 12. In another phase II, double-blind, placebo-controlled study, 33 patients with moderate-to-severe AD were randomly assigned to either ustekinumab ($n = 16$) or placebo ($n = 17$), with subsequent crossover at 16 weeks and last dose at 32 weeks [56]. Background therapy with mild topical steroids was allowed. Study endpoints included clinical and biopsy-based measures of tissue structure and inflammation, using protein and gene expression studies. The ustekinumab group achieved higher clinical responses at 12, 16 (the primary endpoint), and 20 weeks compared to placebo, but the difference between groups was not significant. The AD molecular profile/transcriptome showed early robust gene modulation, with sustained further improvements until 32 weeks in the initial ustekinumab group. It is still possible that a certain subset of patients with AD may particularly benefit from ustekinumab. However, it may be safely said that ustekinumab is much more effective in psoriasis than in AD.

5.2. Other Biologics and AD

There have been anecdotal case reports showing exacerbation of AD-like dermatitis after treatment with anti-IL17 antibody for psoriasis [57–59]. A 31-year-old man with severe psoriasis treated with ixekizumab presented with a one-month history of pruritic lesions [57]. The patient had no personal or family history of allergy, AD, or eczema. Treatment with ixekizumab, started 14 months before the episode, achieved an almost complete response of his skin disease. The patient developed the palms exudative erythematous plaques on the hands, the trunk, and the medial aspects of the limbs. Histologically, epidermal spongiosis with vesicle formation with dermal edema and lymphocytic perivascular infiltrate with some eosinophils were seen. Ixekizumab may suppress the expression of keratinocyte-derived AMPs, increasing the risk of bacterial and fungal infection, which can lead to the eczematous phenotype. Another group reported a 70-year-old woman with intractable psoriasis vulgaris treated with 300 mg of secukinumab [58]. Six months after the first dose of secukinumab was administered, psoriasis lesions were cleared. Blepharitis, cheilitis, and dermatitis around the nose, however, developed four days after every secukinumab injection. A common skin-resident fungus *Malassezia* may account for these skin lesions, which might be more adequately named seborrheic dermatitis-like lesions instead of AD-like eczema. Fezakinumab, an anti-IL-22 antibody, has been recently tried for treatment of AD. A randomized, double-blind, placebo-controlled trial with intravenous fezakinumab monotherapy every 2 weeks for 10 weeks, with follow-up assessments until 20 weeks, was performed for adult patients with moderate-to-severe AD [60]. At 12 weeks, the mean declines in SCORAD for the entire study population were not different between the fezakinumab arm and the placebo arm. In the severe AD patient subset, SCORAD decline was significantly stronger in the drug-treated patients than placebo-treated patients at 12 weeks. Common adverse events were upper respiratory tract infections. Although this drug significantly downregulated gene expression of multiple immune pathways including Th1, Th2, and Th17, it was clinically effective only in patients with severe AD expressing a high level of IL-22 at the baseline [61]. Taken together, biologics targeting Th17-related cytokines are not promising for the treatment of AD, except for anti-IL-22 antibody.

6. Th2 Cytokines Are Key Players in AD

If antibodies against Th17 cytokines are not useful for AD, what is the best therapeutic target? Th2-type immune responses induced by allergens such as mites and pollen are associated with worsening of AD skin conditions. Th2 immune responses including increased IL-4/IL-13 expression induce the production of IgE and TARC [62]. Serum TARC levels are useful as a marker of the disease activity of AD, which are more sensitive than serum IgE levels, lactate dehydrogenaselevels, and peripheral blood eosinophil counts [63]. Recently, thymic stromal lymphopoietin (TSLP) and periostin have been discovered to be key cytokines in Th2-dominant microenvironment [64,65]. TSLP-activated dendritic cells primed naïve T cells to produce IL-4, IL-5, IL-13, and TNF-α, while down-regulating IL-10 and IFN-γ [64]. TSLP was highly expressed by epithelial cells, especially keratinocytes from AD patients. Th2 cytokines IL-4 and IL-13 stimulated fibroblasts to produce periostin, which interacted with a functional periostin receptor on keratinocytes [65]. It induces production of proinflammatory cytokines, which consequently accelerated Th2-type immune responses. It was recently reported that the TSLP receptor was expressed by some T cell subsets from patients with Th2-dominant diseases and that TSLP directly enhanced IL-4/IL-13 production by T cells [66,67]. Taken together, these Th2-related cytokines, IL-4/IL-13, TSLP, and periostin are driving factors of a vicious circle in AD and can be good candidates for therapeutic targets. Indeed, dupilumab, a monoclonal antibody against the IL-4 receptor, is very effective for severe AD [68].

7. The Importance of Th17 Cytokines in the Skin

Skin is a border between the outer world and the body. It is important to block invasion of foreign materials such as poison and parasites. Trauma and loss of skin barrier function in diseased skin, such as in AD and psoriasis, causes a high risk of the invasion. In both conditions, mechanical stimulation can be the cause of onset. It is called the Kobner phenomenon in psoriasis. High proliferation of epidermal cells and rapid keratinization are seen in both skin conditions. Expression of K6 and K16 is increased and that of K1 and K10 is decreased [69,70]. Increased expression of cathepsin D, which modulates expression of involucrin, loricrin, and filaggrin, has been reported [71].

Cytokine expression and cellular infiltration in psoriasis lesional skin is also very similar to what is seen in cases of trauma. IL-17A, which is expressed both in wounded skin and psoriasis skin, plays important roles in wound healing, tissue regeneration, and carcinogenesis [72]. The cytokine mediates activation of EGFR, which is critical for the expansion and migration of Lrig1+ stem cells, promoting wound healing [73]. FGF2 or IL-17 deficiency resulted in impaired epithelial proliferation, increased pro-inflammatory microbiota outgrowth, and consequently worse pathology in a mouse colitis model [74]. The dysregulated microbiota in the model induced transforming growth factor-β1 expression, which in turn induced FGF2 expression mainly in regulatory T cells. Thus, microbiota-driven FGF2 and IL-17 cooperate to repair the damaged intestinal epithelium. Injury of the mucosa causes fast expansion of Th17 cells and their induction [75]. Th17 cells produce various cytokines, such as TNF-α, IL-17, and IL-22, which can promote cell survival and proliferation, and thus tissue regeneration, in several organs including the skin [72]. IL-17 promoted macrophage infiltration into wounded skin and scar formation through an indirect mechanism [76]. Depletion of macrophages with clodronate liposomes abrogated the effect of IL-17. Levels of monocyte chemotactic protein (MCP) 1, MCP2, and MCP3 were increased by IL-17 stimulation. IL-17 induced the infiltration of a specific subtype of macrophages to aggravate fibrosis through an MCP-dependent mechanism. On the other hand, Th17 cells are potentially pathogenic if not tightly controlled. Failure of these control mechanisms can result in chronic inflammatory conditions such as psoriasis.

Infiltration of neutrophils and macrophages is commonly seen, and AMP expression is increased both in wounded skin and in psoriasis skin. Vascular formation is prominent in the dermis. Taken together, it may be safely said that psoriasis is a hyperreaction to traumatic stimuli with the background of genetics, circumstances, and metabolic status (Figure 1).

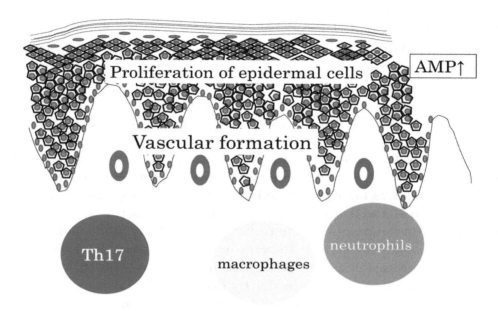

Figure 1. Proliferation of epidermal cells, AMP expression, vascular formation, and infiltration of Th17, neutrophils, and macrophages, commonly seen in wounded skin and in psoriasis skin. We sometimes experience fungal infection in patients treated with anit-IL7A or anti-IL17 receptor A antibody. Considering that Th17 cytokines are expressed in various skin diseases with barrier dysfunction and that antibodies against IL-12/IL-23p40 or IL-17A are not effective for AD, IL-17 and its related cytokine expression can be regarded as a common defense mechanism in the skin. Relatively low AMP expression leads to a higher risk of infection seen in AD and CTCL [77,78]. Targeting the Th17 cytokine has been successful for psoriasis, but may not be always the case in other skin diseases.

8. Ideal Biologics for Psoriasis, AD, and CTCL

Clinical effects of biologics are remarkable, and many diseases including skin diseases are currently treated with them. The cost of developing these agents, however, is huge and it is important to predict which molecule is promising or not. First of all, the molecule should be highly expressed in lesional skin compared to normal skin. Second, the expression of the target should be highest in the disease among various skin diseases. It is important not to block bystander cytokines. IL-22 is highly expressed in psoriasis, but its expression is lower in AD. IL-17 expression in AD is not as high as that in psoriasis. Anti-IL-22 antibody is not effective in psoriasis, and anti-IL12/23p40 or anti-IL-17A antibodies are not promising as treatment for AD. Only the anti-IL-22 antibody may be beneficial for a certain group of AD patients (Table 1). Blocking cytokines uniquely expressed in the disease is important to stop a vicious circle. Third, it would be safer to block interactions between cytokines and their receptors than targeting surface molecules. Exclusion of a certain cell type by antibody-dependent cellular cytotoxicity induced by biologics may cause unexpected severe effects. This kind of strategy targeting surface molecules should be adopted for the treatment of malignancy [79,80].

Table 1. Antibodies against Th17 and Th2-related cytokines for atopic dermatitis (AD).

Cytokines	Clinical Response	References
IL-17A	Worsening of dermatitis	[57–59]
IL-12/23p40	No effect in clinical trial	[55,56]
IL-22	Effective for some patients	[60,61]
IL-4/13	Very effective	[68]

9. Conclusions

It is true that Th17 cells infiltrate into lesional skin of AD, and Th17-related cytokines are expressed there. These cytokines have some roles in the inflammatory process of the disease. It is, however, also true that IL-17 in AD is not as important as it is in psoriasis. Expression of IL-17 and other Th17-related cytokines is widely seen in many skin diseases. My current assumption is that IL-17 expression in the skin is a defense mechanism against foreign materials invading the body.

Abbreviations

AD	atopic dermatitis
CTCL	cutaneous T-cell lymphoma
TNF	tumor necrosis factor
Th	T helper
IL	interleukin
IFN	interferon
AMPs	antimicrobial peptides
TARC	thymus and activation-regulated chemokine
SCORAD	SCORing AD
TWEAK	TNF-like weak inducer of apoptosis
FGF	fibroblast growth factor
MF	mycosis fungoides
SS	Sezary syndrome
TSLP	thymic stromal lymphopoietin
MCP	monocyte chemotactic protein

References

1. Saeki, H.; Nakahara, T.; Tanaka, A.; Kabashima, K.; Sugaya, M.; Murota, H.; Ebihara, T.; Kataoka, Y.; Aihara, M.; Etoh, T.; et al. Clinical practice guidelines for the management of atopic dermatitis. *J. Dermatol.* **2016**, *43*, 1117–1145. [CrossRef] [PubMed]
2. Saeki, H.; Oiso, N.; Honma, M.; Iizuka, H.; Kawada, A.; Tamaki, K. Prevalence of atopic dermatitis in Japanese adults and community validation of the U.K. diagnostic criteria. *J. Dermatol. Sci.* **2009**, *55*, 140–141. [CrossRef] [PubMed]
3. Williams, H.C.; Strachan, D.P. The natural history of childhood eczema: Observations from the British 1958 birth cohort study. *Br. J. Dermatol.* **1998**, *139*, 834–839. [CrossRef] [PubMed]
4. Fukiwake, N.; Furusyo, N.; Kubo, N.; Takeoka, H.; Toyoda, K.; Morita, K.; Shibata, S.; Nakahara, T.; Kido, M.; Hayashida, S.; et al. Incidence of atopic dermatitis in nursery school children—A follow-up study from 2001 to 2004, Kyushu University Ishigaki Atopic Dermatitis Study (KIDS). *Eur. J. Dermatol.* **2006**, *16*, 416–419. [PubMed]
5. Zackheim, H.S.; Koo, J.; LeBoit, P.E.; McCalmont, T.H.; Bowman, P.H.; Kashani-Sabet, M.; Jones, C.; Zehnder, J. Psoriasiform mycosis fungoides with fatal outcome after treatment with cyclosporine. *J. Am. Acad. Dermatol.* **2002**, *47*, 155–157. [CrossRef] [PubMed]
6. Miyagaki, T.; Sugaya, M. Erythrodermic cutaneous T-cell lymphoma: How to differentiate this rare disease from atopic dermatitis. *J. Dermatol. Sci.* **2011**, *64*, 1–6. [CrossRef]
7. Suga, H.; Sugaya, M.; Toyama, T.; Sumida, H.; Fujita, H.; Kogure, A.; Igarashi, A.; Sato, S. A case of mycosis fungoides with large cell transformation associated with infliximab treatment. *Acta. Derm. Venereol.* **2014**, *94*, 233–234. [CrossRef]
8. Xu, X.; van Galen, L.S.; Koh, M.J.A.; Bajpai, R.; Thng, S.; Yew, Y.W.; Ho, V.P.Y.; Alagappan, U.; Järbrink, K.S.A.; Car, J. Factors influencing quality of life in children with atopic dermatitis and their caregivers: A cross-sectional study. *Sci. Rep.* **2019**, *9*, 15990. [CrossRef]

9. Ražnatović Đurović, M.; Janković, J.; Tomić Spirić, V.; Relić, M.; Sojević Timotijević, Z.; Ćirković, A.; Đurić, S.; Janković, S. Does age influence the quality of life in children with atopic dermatitis? *PLoS ONE* **2019**, *14*, e0224618. [CrossRef]

10. Kabashima, K. New concept of the pathogenesis of atopic dermatitis: Interplay among the barrier, allergy, and pruritus as a trinity. *J. Dermatol. Sci.* **2013**, *70*, 3–11. [CrossRef]

11. Salimi, M.; Barlow, J.L.; Saunders, S.P.; Xue, L.; Gutowska-Owsiak, D.; Wang, X.; Huang, L.C.; Johnson, D.; Scanlon, S.T.; McKenzie, A.N.; et al. A role for IL-25 and IL-33-driven type-2 innate lymphoid cells in atopic dermatitis. *J. Exp. Med.* **2013**, *210*, 2939–2950. [CrossRef] [PubMed]

12. Imai, Y.; Yasuda, K.; Sakaguchi, Y.; Haneda, T.; Mizutani, H.; Yoshimoto, T.; Nakanishi, K.; Yamanishi, K. Skin-specific expression of IL-33 activates group 2 innate lymphoid cells and elicits atopic dermatitis-like inflammation in mice. *Proc. Natl. Acad. Sci. USA* **2013**, *110*, 13921–13926. [CrossRef] [PubMed]

13. Van de Veen, W.; Akdis, M. The use of biologics for immune modulation in allergic disease. *J. Clin. Invest.* **2019**, *130*, 1452–1462. [CrossRef] [PubMed]

14. Grewe, M.; Gyufko, K.; Schöpf, E.; Krutmann, J. Lesional expression of interferon-gamma in atopic eczema. *Lancet* **1994**, *343*, 25–26. [CrossRef]

15. Czarnowicki, T.; He, H.; Canter, T.; Han, J.; Lefferdink, R.; Erickson, T.; Rangel, S.; Kameyama, N.; Kim, H.J.; Pavel, A.B.; et al. Evolution of pathologic T-cell subsets in atopic dermatitis from infancy to adulthood. *J. Allergy Clin. Immunol.* **2020**, *145*, 215–228. [CrossRef] [PubMed]

16. Koga, C.; Kabashima, K.; Shiraishi, N.; Kobayashi, M.; Tokura, Y. Possible pathogenic role of Th17 cells for atopic dermatitis. *J. Invest. Dermatol.* **2008**, *128*, 2625–2630. [CrossRef] [PubMed]

17. Eyerich, K.; Pennino, D.; Scarponi, C.; Foerster, S.; Nasorri, F.; Behrendt, H.; Ring, J.; Traidl-Hoffmann, C.; Albanesi, C.; Cavani, A. IL-17 in atopic eczema: Linking allergen-specific adaptive and microbial-triggered innate immune response. *J. Allergy. Clin. Immunol.* **2009**, *123*, 59–66. [CrossRef]

18. Nograles, K.E.; Zaba, L.C.; Shemer, A.; Fuentes-Duculan, J.; Cardinale, I.; Kikuchi, T.; Ramon, M.; Bergman, R.; Krueger, J.G.; Guttman-Yassky, E. IL-22-producing "T22" T cells account for upregulated IL-22 in atopic dermatitis despite reduced IL-17-producing TH17 T cells. *J. Allergy. Clin. Immunol.* **2009**, *123*, 1244–1252. [CrossRef]

19. Noda, S.; Suárez-Fariñas, M.; Ungar, B.; Kim, S.J.; de Guzman Strong, C.; Xu, H.; Peng, X.; Estrada, Y.D.; Nakajima, S.; Honda, T.; et al. The Asian atopic dermatitis phenotype combines features of atopic dermatitis and psoriasis with increased TH17 polarization. *J. Allergy. Clin. Immunol.* **2015**, *136*, 1254–1264. [CrossRef]

20. Esaki, H.; Brunner, P.M.; Renert-Yuval, Y.; Czarnowicki, T.; Huynh, T.; Tran, G.; Lyon, S.; Rodriguez, G.; Immaneni, S.; Johnson, D.B.; et al. Early-onset pediatric atopic dermatitis is Th2 but also Th17 polarized in skin. *J. Allergy. Clin. Immunol.* **2016**, *138*, 1639–1651. [CrossRef] [PubMed]

21. Korn, T.; Bettelli, E.; Oukka, M.; Kuchroo, V.K. IL-17 and Th17 cells. *Annu. Rev. Immunol.* **2009**, *27*, 485–517. [CrossRef] [PubMed]

22. Chaudhari, U.; Romano, P.; Mulcahy, L.D.; Dooley, L.T.; Baker, D.G.; Gottlieb, A.B. Efficacy and safety of infliximab monotherapy for plaque-type psoriasis: A randomised trial. *Lancet* **2001**, *357*, 1842–1847. [CrossRef]

23. Leonardi, C.L.; Kimball, A.B.; Papp, K.A.; Yeilding, N.; Guzzo, C.; Wang, Y.; Li, S.; Dooley, L.T.; Gordon, K.B.; PHOENIX 1 study investigators. Efficacy and safety of ustekinumab, a human interleukin-12/23 monoclonal antibody, in patients with psoriasis: 76-week results from a randomised, double-blind, placebo-controlled trial (PHOENIX 1). *Lancet* **2008**, *371*, 1665–1674. [CrossRef]

24. Leonardi, C.; Matheson, R.; Zachariae, C.; Cameron, G.; Li, L.; Edson-Heredia, E.; Braun, D.; Banerjee, S. Anti-interleukin-17 monoclonal antibody ixekizumab in chronic plaque psoriasis. *N. Engl. J. Med.* **2012**, *366*, 1190–1199. [CrossRef] [PubMed]

25. Gordon, K.B.; Duffin, K.C.; Bissonnette, R.; Prinz, J.C.; Wasfi, Y.; Li, S.; Shen, Y.K.; Szapary, P.; Randazzo, B.; Reich, K. A phase 2 trial of guselkumab versus adalimumab for plaque psoriasis. *N. Engl. J. Med.* **2015**, *373*, 136–144. [CrossRef] [PubMed]

26. Jovanovic, D.V.; Di Battista, J.A.; Martel-Pelletier, J.; Jolicoeur, F.C.; He, Y.; Zhang, M.; Mineau, F.; Pelletier, J.P. IL-17 stimulates the production and expression of proinflammatory cytokines, IL-beta and TNF-alpha, by human macrophages. *J. Immunol.* **1998**, *160*, 3513–3521. [PubMed]

27. Shibata, M.; Shintaku, Y.; Matsuzaki, K.; Uematsu, S. The effect of IL-17 on the production of proinflammatory cytokines and matrix metalloproteinase-1 by human periodontal ligament fibroblasts. *Orthod. Craniofac. Res.* **2014**, *17*, 60–68. [CrossRef]

28. Roussel, L.; Houle, F.; Chan, C.; Yao, Y.; Bérubé, J.; Olivenstein, R.; Martin, J.G.; Huot, J.; Hamid, Q.; Ferri, L.; et al. IL-17 promotes p38 MAPK-dependent endothelial activation enhancing neutrophil recruitment to sites of inflammation. *J. Immunol.* **2010**, *184*, 4531–4537. [CrossRef]

29. Jones, C.E.; Chan, K. Interleukin-17stimulates the expression of interleukin-8, growth-related oncogene-alpha, and granulocyte-colony-stimulating factor by human airway epithelial cells. *Am. J. Respir. Cell. Mol. Biol.* **2002**, *26*, 748–753. [CrossRef]

30. Ganz, T. Defensins: Antimicrobial peptides of innate immunity. *Nat. Rev. Immunol.* **2003**, *3*, 710–720. [CrossRef]

31. Sonnenberg, G.F.; Fouser, L.A.; Artis, D. Border patrol: Regulation of immunity, inflammation and tissue homeostasis at barrier surfaces by IL-22. *Nat. Immunol.* **2011**, *12*, 383–390. [CrossRef] [PubMed]

32. Gallo, R.L.; Nakatsuji, T. Microbial symbiosis with the innate immune defense system of the skin. *J. Invest. Dermatol.* **2011**, *131*, 1974–1980. [CrossRef] [PubMed]

33. Boniface, K.; Bernard, F.X.; Garcia, M.; Gurney, A.L.; Lecron, J.C.; Morel, F. IL-22 inhibits epidermal differentiation and induces proinflammatory gene expression and migration of human keratinocytes. *J. Immunol.* **2005**, *174*, 3695–3702. [CrossRef] [PubMed]

34. Dang, A.T.; Teles, R.M.; Weiss, D.I.; Parvatiyar, K.; Sarno, E.N.; Ochoa, M.T.; Cheng, G.; Gilliet, M.; Bloom, B.R.; Modlin, R.L. IL-26 contributes to host defense against intracellular bacteria. *J. Clin. Investg.* **2019**, *129*, 1926–1939. [CrossRef] [PubMed]

35. Hayashida, S.; Uchi, H.; Moroi, Y.; Furue, M. Decrease in circulating Th17 cells correlates with increased levels of CCL17, IgE and eosinophils in atopic dermatitis. *J. Dermatol. Sci.* **2011**, *61*, 180–186. [CrossRef] [PubMed]

36. Czarnowicki, T.; Gonzalez, J.; Shemer, A.; Malajian, D.; Xu, H.; Zheng, X.; Khattri, S.; Gilleaudeau, P.; Sullivan-Whalen, M.; Suárez-Fariñas, M.; et al. Severe atopic dermatitis is characterized by selective expansion of circulating TH2/TC2 and TH22/TC22, but not TH17/TC17, cells within the skin-homing T-cell population. *J. Allergy. Clin. Immunol.* **2015**, *136*, 104–115. [CrossRef]

37. Romanet-Manent, S.; Charpin, D.; Magnan, A.; Lanteaume, A.; Vervloet, D.; EGEA Cooperative Group. Allergic vs nonallergic asthma: What makes the difference? *Allergy* **2002**, *57*, 607–613. [CrossRef]

38. Tokura, Y. Extrinsic and intrinsic types of atopic dermatitis. *J. Dermatol. Sci.* **2010**, *58*, 1–7. [CrossRef]

39. Suárez-Fariñas, M.; Dhingra, N.; Gittler, J.; Shemer, A.; Cardinale, I.; de Guzman Strong, C.; Krueger, J.G.; Guttman-Yassky, E. Intrinsic atopic dermatitis shows similar TH2 and higher TH17 immune activation compared with extrinsic atopic dermatitis. *J. Allergy. Clin. Immunol.* **2013**, *132*, 361–370. [CrossRef]

40. Kamijo, H.; Miyagaki, T.; Hayashi, Y.; Akatsuka, T.; Watanabe-Otobe, S.; Oka, T.; Shishido-Takahashi, N.; Suga, H.; Sugaya, M.; Sato, S. Increased IL-26 expression promotes T helper type 17- and T helper type 2-associated cytokine production by keratinocytes in atopic dermatitis. *J. Invest. Dermatol.* **2019**, in press. [CrossRef]

41. Nakajima, S.; Kitoh, A.; Egawa, G.; Natsuaki, Y.; Nakamizo, S.; Moniaga, C.S.; Otsuka, A.; Honda, T.; Hanakawa, S.; Amano, W.; et al. IL-17A as an inducer for Th2 immune responses in murine atopic dermatitis models. *J. Invest. Dermatol.* **2014**, *134*, 2122–2130. [CrossRef] [PubMed]

42. Milovanovic, M.; Drozdenko, G.; Weise, C.; Babina, M.; Worm, M. Interleukin-17A promotes IgE production in human B cells. *J. Invest. Dermatol.* **2010**, *130*, 2621–2628. [CrossRef] [PubMed]

43. Sparber, F.; De Gregorio, C.; Steckholzer, S.; Ferreira, F.M.; Dolowschiak, T.; Ruchti, F.; Kirchner, F.R.; Mertens, S.; Prinz, I.; Joller, N.; et al. The skin commensal yeast Malassezia triggers a type 17 response that coordinates anti-fungal immunity and exacerbates skin inflammation. *Cell. Host. Microbe.* **2019**, *25*, 389–403. [CrossRef] [PubMed]

44. Liu, Q.; Wang, H.; Wang, X.; Lu, M.; Tan, X.; Peng, L.; Tan, F.; Xiao, T.; Xiao, S.; Xia, Y. Experimental atopic dermatitis is dependent on the TWEAK/Fn14 signaling pathway. *Clin. Exp. Immunol.* **2020**, *199*, 56–67. [CrossRef]

45. Kim, M.H.; Jin, S.P.; Jang, S.; Choi, J.Y.; Chung, D.H.; Lee, D.H.; Kim, K.H.; Kim, H.Y. IL-17A-producing innate lymphoid cells promote skin inflammation by inducing IL-33-driven type 2 immune responses. *J. Investg. Dermatol.* **2019**, in press. [CrossRef]

46. Shen, H.H.; Fan, Y.; Wang, Y.N.; Zhao, C.N.; Zhang, Z.K.; Pan, H.F.; Wu, G.C. Elevated Circulating Interleukin-17 levels in patients with systemic lupus erythematosus: A meta-analysis. *Immunol. Invest.* **2019**, in press. [CrossRef]

47. Nakashima, T.; Jinnin, M.; Yamane, K.; Honda, N.; Kajihara, I.; Makino, T.; Masuguchi, S.; Fukushima, S.; Okamoto, Y.; Hasegawa, M.; et al. Impaired IL-17 signaling pathway contributes to the increased collagen expression in scleroderma fibroblasts. *J. Immunol.* **2012**, *188*, 3573–3583. [CrossRef]

48. Ahmed, S.; Misra, D.P.; Agarwal, V. Interleukin-17 pathways in systemic sclerosis-associated fibrosis. *Rheumatol. Int.* **2019**, *39*, 1135–1143. [CrossRef]

49. Miyagaki, T.; Sugaya, M.; Suga, H.; Kamata, M.; Ohmatsu, H.; Fujita, H.; Asano, Y.; Tada, Y.; Kadono, T.; Sato, S. IL-22, but not IL-17, dominant environment in cutaneous T-cell lymphoma. *Clin. Cancer Res.* **2011**, *17*, 7529–7538. [CrossRef]

50. Fernández-Antón Martínez, M.C.; Alfageme Roldán, F.; Ciudad Blanco, C.; Suárez Fernández, R. Ustekinumab in the treatment of severe atopic dermatitis: A preliminary report of our experience with 4 patients. *Actas Dermosifiliogr.* **2014**, *105*, 312–313. [CrossRef]

51. Agusti-Mejias, A.; Messeguer, F.; García, R.; Febrer, I. Severe refractory atopic dermatitis in an adolescent patient successfully treated with ustekinumab. *Ann. Dermatol.* **2013**, *25*, 368–370. [CrossRef] [PubMed]

52. Lis-Święty, A.; Skrzypek-Salamon, A.; Arasiewicz, H.; Brzezińska-Wcisło, L. Atopic dermatitis exacerbated with ustekinumab in a psoriatic patient with childhood history of atopy. *Allergol. Int.* **2015**, *64*, 382–383. [CrossRef] [PubMed]

53. Samorano, L.P.; Hanifin, J.M.; Simpson, E.L.; Leshem, Y.A. Inadequate response to ustekinumab in atopic dermatitis - a report of two patients. *J. Eur. Acad. Dermatol. Venereol.* **2016**, *30*, 522–523. [CrossRef] [PubMed]

54. Ishiuji, Y.; Umezawa, Y.; Asahina, A.; Fukuta, H.; Aizawa, N.; Yanaba, K.; Nakagawa, H. Exacerbation of atopic dermatitis symptoms by ustekinumab in psoriatic patients with elevated serum immunoglobulin E levels: Report of two cases. *J. Dermatol.* **2018**, *45*, 732–734. [CrossRef] [PubMed]

55. Saeki, H.; Kabashima, K.; Tokura, Y.; Murata, Y.; Shiraishi, A.; Tamamura, R.; Randazzo, B.; Imanaka, K. Efficacy and safety of ustekinumab in Japanese patients with severe atopic dermatitis: A randomized, double-blind, placebo-controlled, phase II study. *Br. J. Dermatol.* **2017**, *177*, 419–427. [CrossRef]

56. Khattri, S.; Brunner, P.M.; Garcet, S.; Finney, R.; Cohen, S.R.; Oliva, M.; Dutt, R.; Fuentes-Duculan, J.; Zheng, X.; Li, X.; et al. Efficacy and safety of ustekinumab treatment in adults with moderate-to-severe atopic dermatitis. *Exp. Dermatol.* **2017**, *26*, 28–35. [CrossRef]

57. Munera-Campos, M.; Ballesca, F.; Richarz, N.; Ferrandiz, C.; Carrascosa, J.M. Paradoxical eczematous reaction to ixekizumab. *J. Eur. Acad. Dermatol. Venereol.* **2019**, *33*, e40–e42.

58. Burlando, M.; Cozzani, E.; Russo, R.; Parodi, A. Atopic-like dermatitis after secukinumab injection: A case report. *Dermatol. Ther.* **2019**, *32*, e12751. [CrossRef]

59. Napolitano, M.; Gallo, L.; Patruno, C.; Fabbrocini, G.; Megna, M. Eczematous reaction to ixekizumab successfully treated with dupilumab. *Dermatol. Ther.* **2020**, in press. [CrossRef]

60. Guttman-Yassky, E.; Brunner, P.M.; Neumann, A.U.; Khattri, S.; Pavel, A.B.; Malik, K.; Singer, G.K.; Baum, D.; Gilleaudeau, P.; Sullivan-Whalen, M.; et al. Efficacy and safety of fezakinumab (an IL-22 monoclonal antibody) in adults with moderate-to-severe atopic dermatitis inadequately controlled by conventional treatments: A randomized, double-blind, phase 2a trial. *J. Am. Acad. Dermatol.* **2018**, *78*, 872–881. [CrossRef]

61. Brunner, P.M.; Pavel, A.B.; Khattri, S.; Leonard, A.; Malik, K.; Rose, S.; Jim On, S.; Vekaria, A.S.; Traidl-Hoffmann, C.; Singer, G.K.; et al. Baseline IL-22 expression in patients with atopic dermatitis stratifies tissue responses to fezakinumab. *J. Allergy. Clin. Immunol.* **2019**, *143*, 142–154. [CrossRef] [PubMed]

62. Furue, M.; Ulzii, D.; Vu, Y.H.; Tsuji, G.; Kido-Nakahara, M.; Nakahara, T. Pathogenesis of atopic dermatitis: CurrentpParadigm. *Iran. J. Immunol.* **2019**, *16*, 97–107. [PubMed]

63. Kakinuma, T.; Nakamura, K.; Wakugawa, M.; Mitsui, H.; Tada, Y.; Saeki, H.; Torii, H.; Asahina, A.; Onai, N.; Matsushima, K.; et al. Thymus and activation-regulated chemokine in atopic dermatitis: Serum thymus and activation-regulated chemokine level is closely related with disease activity. *J. Allergy. Clin. Immunol.* **2001**, *107*, 535–541. [CrossRef] [PubMed]

64. Soumelis, V.; Reche, P.A.; Kanzler, H.; Yuan, W.; Edward, G.; Homey, B.; Gilliet, M.; Ho, S.; Antonenko, S.; Lauerma, A.; et al. Human epithelial cells trigger dendritic cell mediated allergic inflammation by producing TSLP. *Nat. Immunol.* **2002**, *3*, 673–680. [CrossRef]

65. Masuoka, M.; Shiraishi, H.; Ohta, S.; Suzuki, S.; Arima, K.; Aoki, S.; Toda, S.; Inagaki, N.; Kurihara, Y.; Hayashida, S.; et al. Periostin promotes chronic allergic inflammation in response to Th2 cytokines. *J. Clin. Invest.* **2012**, *122*, 2590–2600. [CrossRef]

66. Tatsuno, K.; Fujiyama, T.; Yamaguchi, H.; Waki, M.; Tokura, Y. TSLP directly interacts with skin-homing Th2 Cells highly expressing its receptor to enhance IL-4 production in atopic dermatitis. *J. Investg. Dermatol.* **2015**, *135*, 3017–3024. [CrossRef]

67. Takahashi, N.; Sugaya, M.; Suga, H.; Oka, T.; Kawaguchi, M.; Miyagaki, T.; Fujita, H.; Sato, S. Thymic stromal chemokine TSLP acts through Th2 cytokine production to induce cutaneous T-cell lymphoma. *Cancer Res.* **2016**, *76*, 6241–6252. [CrossRef]

68. Blauvelt, A.; de Bruin-Weller, M.; Gooderham, M.; Cather, J.C.; Weisman, J.; Pariser, D.; Simpson, E.L.; Papp, K.A.; Hong, H.C.; Rubel, D.; et al. Long-term management of moderate-to-severe atopic dermatitis with dupilumab and concomitant topical corticosteroids (LIBERTY AD CHRONOS): A 1-year, randomised, double-blinded, placebo-controlled, phase 3 trial. *Lancet* **2017**, *389*, 2287–2303. [CrossRef]

69. Thewes, M.; Stadler, R.; Korge, B.; Mischke, D. Normal psoriatic epidermis expression of hyperproliferation-associated keratins. *Arch. Derm. Res.* **1991**, *283*, 465–471. [CrossRef]

70. Zhang, X.; Yin, M.; Zhang, L.J. Keratin 6, 16 and 17-Critical Barrier Alarmin Molecules in Skin Wounds and Psoriasis. *Cells* **2019**, *8*, E807. [CrossRef]

71. Egberts, F.; Heinrich, M.; Jensen, J.M.; Winoto-Morbach, S.; Pfeiffer, S.; Wickel, M.; Schunck, M.; Steude, J.; Saftig, P.; Proksch, E.; et al. Cathepsin D is involved in the regulation of transglutaminase 1 and epidermal differentiation. *J. Cell. Sci.* **2004**, *117*, 2295–2307. [CrossRef] [PubMed]

72. Brockmann, L.; Giannou, A.D.; Gagliani, N.; Huber, S. Regulation of Th17 cells and associated cytokines in wound healing, tissue regeneration, and carcinogenesis. *Int. J. Mol. Sci.* **2017**, *18*, E1033. [CrossRef] [PubMed]

73. Chen, X.; Cai, G.; Liu, C.; Zhao, J.; Gu, C.; Wu, L.; Hamilton, T.A.; Zhang, C.J.; Ko, J.; Zhu, L.; et al. IL-17R-EGFR axis links wound healing to tumorigenesis in Lrig1+ stem cells. *J. Exp. Med.* **2019**, *216*, 195–214.

74. Song, X.; Dai, D.; He, X.; Zhu, S.; Yao, Y.; Gao, H.; Wang, J.; Qu, F.; Qiu, J.; Wang, H.; et al. Growth factor FGF2 cooperates with interleukin-17 to repair intestinal epithelial damage. *Immunity* **2015**, *43*, 488–501. [CrossRef] [PubMed]

75. Khader, S.A.; Gaffen, S.L.; Kolls, J.K. Th17 cells at the crossroads of innate and adaptive immunity against infectious diseases at the mucosa. *Mucosal. Immunol.* **2009**, *2*, 403–411.

76. Zhang, J.; Qiao, Q.; Liu, M.; He, T.; Shi, J.; Bai, X.; Zhang, Y.; Li, Y.; Cai, W.; Han, S.; et al. IL-17 promotes scar formation by inducing macrophage infiltration. *Am. J. Pathol.* **2018**, *188*, 1693–1702. [CrossRef] [PubMed]

77. Suga, H.; Sugaya, M.; Miyagaki, T.; Ohmatsu, H.; Kawaguchi, M.; Takahashi, N.; Fujita, H.; Asano, Y.; Tada, Y.; Kadono, T.; et al. Skin barrier dysfunction and low antimicrobial peptide expression in cutaneous T-cell lymphoma. *Clin. Cancer Res.* **2014**, *20*, 4339–4348. [CrossRef]

78. Miyagaki, T.; Sugaya, M. Recent advances in atopic dermatitis and psoriasis: Genetic background, barrier function, and therapeutic targets. *J. Dermatol. Sci.* **2015**, *78*, 89–94. [CrossRef]

79. Prince, H.M.; Kim, Y.H.; Horwitz, S.M.; Dummer, R.; Scarisbrick, J.; Quaglino, P.; Zinzani, P.L.; Wolter, P.; Sanches, J.A.; Ortiz-Romero, P.L.; et al. ALCANZA study group. Brentuximab vedotin or physician's choice in CD30-positive cutaneous T-cell lymphoma (ALCANZA): An international, open-label, randomised, phase 3, multicentre trial. *Lancet* **2017**, *390*, 555–566. [CrossRef]

80. Kim, Y.H.; Bagot, M.; Pinter-Brown, L.; Rook, A.H.; Porcu, P.; Horwitz, S.M.; Whittaker, S.; Tokura, Y.; Vermeer, M.; Zinzani, P.L.; et al. MAVORIC Investigators. Mogamulizumab versus vorinostat in previously treated cutaneous T-cell lymphoma (MAVORIC): An international, open-label, randomised, controlled phase 3 trial. *Lancet Oncol.* **2018**, *19*, 1192–1204. [CrossRef]

13

IL-4 Augments IL-31/IL-31 Receptor Alpha Interaction Leading to Enhanced Ccl 17 and Ccl 22 Production in Dendritic Cells: Implications for Atopic Dermatitis

Sho Miake [1], Gaku Tsuji [1,2,*], Masaki Takemura [1], Akiko Hashimoto-Hachiya [1], Yen Hai Vu [1], Masutaka Furue [1,2,3] and Takeshi Nakahara [1,3]

[1]   Department of Dermatology, Graduate School of Medical Sciences, Kyushu University, Maidashi 3-1-1, Higashiku, Fukuoka 812-8582, Japan

[2]   Research and Clinical Center for Yusho and Dioxin, Kyushu University, Maidashi 3-1-1, Higashiku, Fukuoka 812-8582, Japan

[3]   Division of Skin Surface Sensing, Graduate School of Medical Sciences, Kyushu University, Maidashi 3-1-1, Higashiku, Fukuoka 812-8582, Japan

*   Correspondence: gakku@dermatol.med.kyushu-u.ac.jp

Abstract: Severe pruritus is a characteristic feature of atopic dermatitis (AD) and is closely related to its activity. Recent studies have shown that IL-31 is a key determinant of pruritus in AD. Anti-IL-31 receptor alpha (IL-31RA) antibody treatment has also been reported to improve pruritus clinically, subsequently contributing to the attenuation of AD disease activity. Therefore, IL-31 has been thought to be an important cytokine for regulating pruritus and AD disease activity; however, how IL-31 is involved in the immune response in AD has remained largely unknown. Epidermal Langerhans cells (LCs) and dermal dendritic cells (DCs) derived from bone marrow cells have been reported to play a critical role in AD pathogenesis. LCs and DCs produce Ccl 17 and Ccl 22, which chemoattract Th2 cells, leading to AD development. Therefore, we aimed to clarify how IL-31/IL-31RA interaction affects Ccl 17 and Ccl 22 production. To test this, we analyzed murine bone marrow-derived DCs (BMDCs) stimulated with IL-4, an important cytokine in AD development. We found that IL-31RA expression was upregulated by IL-4 stimulation in a dose-dependent manner in BMDCs. Furthermore, IL-31 upregulates Ccl 17 and Ccl 22 production in the presence of IL-4, whereas IL-31 stimulation alone did not produce Ccl 17 and Ccl 22. These findings suggest that IL-4 mediates IL-31RA expression and IL-31/IL-31RA interaction augments Ccl 17 and Ccl 22 production in BMDCs, which promotes Th2-deviated immune response in AD. Since we previously reported that soybean tar Glyteer, an aryl hydrocarbon receptor (AHR) ligand, impairs IL-4/Stat 6 signaling in BMDCs, we examined whether Glyteer affects IL-31RA expression induced by IL-4 stimulation. Glyteer inhibited upregulation of IL-31RA expression induced by IL-4 stimulation in a dose-dependent manner. Glyteer also inhibited Ccl 17 and Ccl 22 production induced by IL-4 and IL-31 stimulation. Taken together, these findings suggest that Glyteer treatment may improve AD disease activity by impairing IL-31/IL-31RA interaction in DCs.

Keywords: IL-31; IL-31 receptor alpha; Ccl 17; Ccl 22; dendritic cell; atopic dermatitis

1. Introduction

Interleukin (IL)-31 is a four-helix bundle cytokine closely related to the IL-6 cytokine family [1]. It is the only known ligand for IL-31 receptor alpha (IL-31RA), which belongs to the glycoprotein 130 receptor family [2]. IL-31/IL-31RA interaction initiates signal transduction resulting in the expression of several pro-inflammatory cytokines and chemokines, which play a crucial role in inflammatory diseases relating to Th2 cytokines including IL-4 and IL-13 [3,4].

Atopic dermatitis (AD) is a chronic or chronically relapsing, eczematous, and severely pruritic skin disorder. The lesional skin of AD exhibits Th2-deviated immune reactions such as those involving IL-4, IL-5, and IL-13, which contribute to the development of this disease [5]. It has been shown that the anti-IL-4 receptor alpha (IL-4RA) antibody dupilumab causes marked and rapid improvement in AD patients [6], indicating that IL-4 plays a critical role in AD development. A recent study has also shown that anti-IL-31 receptor alpha (IL-31RA) antibody treatment using nemolizumab produced clinical improvement of pruritus, subsequently contributing to the attenuation of AD disease activity [7]. The mechanism behind this is still not fully understood, but it has been shown that IL-31RA is expressed on sensory neurons and IL-31 derived from activated T cells under Th2-skewed conditions stimulates IL-31RA on sensory nerves, resulting in severe pruritus in AD [8]. Although IL-31/IL-31RA interaction has been identified as one of the key determinants of pruritus in AD, there are limited reports regarding the effect of IL-31/IL-31RA interaction on Th2-deviated immune conditions in AD [4,9]. It has been reported that transgenic mice overexpressing IL-31 develop AD-like skin lesions with severe pruritus [10]. In addition, the neutralization of IL-31 and genetic inhibition of EPAS1, a regulator of IL-31 induction in CD4+ T cells, have been reported to ameliorate AD-like skin lesions [11]. Therefore, IL-31/IL-31RA interaction is deeply involved in AD disease activity in addition to pruritus.

Given that (1) CCL 17 and CCL 22 chemoattract Th2 cells and maintain the Th2 immune response [12,13], (2) serum CCL 17 and CCL 22 levels are closely related to the disease activity of AD [14], and (3) Langerhans cells and dermal dendritic cells (DCs) produce prominent CCL 17 and CCL 22 in the skin of AD patients [12,15], we investigated whether IL-31/IL-31RA interaction affects CCL 17 and CCL 22 production in DCs during the development of AD. To test this, we analyzed murine bone marrow-derived DCs (BMDCs) treated with IL-4, which is thought to recapitulate the conditions of skin myeloid DCs in AD.

2. Results

2.1. IL-4 Stimulation Upregulated IL-31RA Expression in BMDCs

We first examined whether IL-4 stimulation upregulated IL-31RA expression in BMDCs. We analyzed BMDCs stimulated with IL-4 (0.1, 1, and 10 ng/mL) for 24 h. Quantitative reverse-transcription (qRT-PCR) analysis revealed that IL-4 stimulation upregulated IL-31RA expression at the mRNA level in a dose-dependent manner (Figure 1a). Flow cytometry analysis of BMDCs stimulated with IL-4 (10 ng/mL) for 24 h also showed that IL-4 stimulation upregulated IL-31RA expression at the protein level (Figure 1b). We also examined expression of OSMRβ, the other subunit of IL-31 receptor; however, it was not upregulated by IL-4 stimulation at the mRNA level (Figure 1c) in BMDCs stimulated with IL-4 (0.1, 1 and 10 ng/mL) for 24 h (Figure 1c).

Figure 1. IL-4 stimulation upregulated IL-31RA expression in bone marrow-derived dendritic cells (BMDCs). (**a,c**) Data are expressed as mean ± standard error of the mean (S.E.M.); $n = 3$ for each group; * $p < 0.05$. Expression of IL-31RA (**a**) and OSMRβ (**c**) mRNA in BMDCs stimulated with IL-4 (0.1, 1 and 10 ng/mL) for 24 h. mRNA levels normalized for ACTB are expressed as fold induction compared with that in the control group. ACTB was utilized as a housekeeping gene. (**b**) BMDCs were treated with or without IL-4 (10 ng/mL) for 24 h. IL-31RA expression was evaluated using anti-murine IL-31RA antibody. Data are representative of experiments repeated three times with similar results.

2.2. IL-31 Stimulation Enhanced IL-4-Induced Ccl 17 and Ccl 22 Production in BMDCs

In addition to our previous report [15] describing that IL-4 stimulation induced Ccl 17 and Ccl 22 production in BMDCs, we next examined how IL-31 stimulation affects Ccl 17 and Ccl 22 production. We analyzed Ccl 17 and Ccl 22 expression in BMDCs stimulated with or without IL-4 (10 ng/mL) and IL-31 (50 and 100 ng/mL) for 24 h. qRT-PCR analysis showed that IL-31 stimulation alone (50 and 100 ng/mL) did not induce upregulation of Ccl 17 and Ccl 22 mRNA expression. Alternatively, IL-31 (50 and 100 ng/mL) with IL-4 (10 ng/mL) stimulation enhanced expression of Ccl 17 and Ccl 22 rather than IL-4 alone at the mRNA level (Figure 2a,c). ELISA analysis of the culture medium of BMDCs stimulated with IL-31 (50 and 100 ng/mL) with IL-4 (10 ng/mL) for 48 h also showed that IL-31 (50 and 100 ng/mL) with IL-4 (10 ng/mL) stimulation enhanced production of Ccl 17 and Ccl 22 rather than IL-4 alone at the protein level (Figure 2b,d). These results suggest that IL-4-induced IL-31RA upregulation is functional through IL-31/IL-31RA interaction, which leads to the enhanced production of Ccl 17 and Ccl 22 in BMDCs. Since another previous report stimulation with a high concentration (250 ng/mL) of

IL-31 led to CCL22 production in human monocyte-derived DCs [16], we examined whether IL-31 stimulation (250 ng/mL) affects Ccl 22 expression. In our study, IL-31 stimulation alone (250 ng/mL) did not induce upregulation of Ccl 22 expression at the mRNA level (Figure S1a) and the protein level (Figure S1b), in BMDCs.

Figure 2. IL-31 stimulation enhanced IL-4-induced Ccl 17 and Ccl 22 production in BMDCs. (**a–d**) Data are expressed as mean ± standard error of the mean (S.E.M.); $n = 3$ for each group; * $p < 0.05$. Expression of Ccl 17 (a) and Ccl 22 (c) mRNA in BMDCs stimulated with or without IL-4 (10 ng/mL) and IL-31 (50 and 100 ng/mL) for 48 h and production of Ccl 17 (b) and Ccl 22 (d) in the culture supernatant were measured.

2.3. Glyteer Treatment Inhibited IL-4-Induced IL-31RA Expression in BMDCs

Since we previously reported that Glyteer treatment impairs the IL-4/STAT6 signaling pathway in BMDCs [15] and human keratinocytes [17], we examined whether Glyteer treatment also inhibits IL-31RA expression induced by IL-4 stimulation in BMDCs. We analyzed BMDCs stimulated with IL-4 (10 ng/mL) for 24 h in the presence or absence of Glyteer (10^{-5}, 10^{-6}, and 10^{-7}%). qRT-PCR analysis showed that Glyteer treatment inhibited IL-4-induced IL-31RA expression at the mRNA level in a dose-dependent manner (Figure 3a). Flow cytometry analysis of BMDCs stimulated with IL-4 (10 ng/mL) for 24 h in the presence or absence of Glyteer (10^{-5}%) also showed that IL-31RA-positive cells increased upon stimulation with IL-4 (10 ng/mL), compared with that in the control group, which was inhibited by Glyteer treatment (10^{-5}%) (around the area indicated by a white arrow).

Figure 3. Glyteer impaired IL-4-induced IL-31RA expression. (**a**) Data are expressed as mean ± standard error of the mean (S.E.M.); $n = 3$ for each group; * $p < 0.05$. Expression of IL-31RA mRNA in BMDCs stimulated with or without IL-4 (10 ng/mL) and Glyteer (10^{-7}, 10^{-6} and 10^{-5}%) for 24 h. (**b**) BMDCs were treated with or without IL-4 (10 ng/mL) and Glyteer (10^{-5}%) for 24 h. IL-31RA expression was evaluated using anti-murine IL-31RA antibody. IL-31RA-positive cells increased upon stimulation with IL-4 (10 ng/mL), compared with that in the control group, which was inhibited by Glyteer treatment (10–5%) (around the area indicated by a white arrow). Data is representative of experiments repeated three times with similar results.

2.4. Glyteer Treatment Inhibited IL-4- and IL-31-Induced Ccl 17 and Ccl 22 Production in BMDCs

To further confirm the inhibitory effects of Glyteer treatment, we examined whether the enhancement of Ccl 17 and Ccl 22 production by IL-31 with IL-4 stimulation was inhibited in BMDCs. We analyzed Ccl 17 and Ccl 22 expression in BMDCs stimulated with or without IL-4 (10 ng/mL) and IL-31 (50 and 100 ng/mL) for 24 h in the presence or absence of Glyteer (10^{-5}, 10^{-6} and 10^{-7}%). qRT-PCR analysis showed that Glyteer treatment inhibited the upregulation of Ccl 17 and Ccl 22 induced by IL-4 stimulation at the mRNA level (Figure 4a,c). ELISA analysis of the culture medium of BMDCs stimulated with or without IL-4 (10 ng/mL) and IL-31 (50 and 100 ng/mL) for 48 h in the presence or absence of Glyteer (10^{-5}, 10^{-6} and 10^{-7}%) also showed that Glyteer treatment inhibited the upregulation of Ccl 17 and Ccl 22 induced by IL-4 stimulation at the protein level (Figure 4b,d). These results are already proven in our previous report [15]. Furthermore, Glyteer treatment inhibited the upregulation of Ccl 17 and Ccl 22 by IL-31 with IL-4 stimulation at the mRNA level (Figure 4a,c) and the protein level (Figure 4b,d) in a dose-dependent manner.

Figure 4. Glyteer impaired IL-4 with IL-31-induced Ccl 17 and Ccl 22 production in BMDCs. (**a–d**) Data are expressed as mean ± standard error of the mean (S.E.M.); $n = 3$ for each group; * $p < 0.05$. Expression of Ccl 17 (**a**) and Ccl 22 (**c**) mRNA in BMDCs stimulated with or without IL-4 (10 ng/mL), IL-31 (100 ng/mL), and Glyteer (10^{-7}, 10^{-6} and 10^{-5}%) for 48 h and production of Ccl 17 (**b**) and Ccl 22 (**d**) in the culture supernatant were measured.

3. Discussion

Although it has been reported that the IFN-γ/STAT1 signal mediates IL-31RA expression in DCs [16], whether Th2 cytokines such as IL-4 and IL-13 can upregulate IL-31RA expression in DCs has not been examined. Since recent studies have shown that IL-31 and its interaction with IL-31RA play a crucial role in the development of AD [7,11], clarifying the regulatory mechanism of IL-31RA expression under Th2-deviated conditions is very useful for treating AD. The present study has shown for the first time that IL-4 stimulation is capable of upregulating IL-31RA in BMDCs, which is consistent with a previous report describing that either IL-4 or IL-13 can upregulate IL-31RA via Stat6 in murine macrophages [4].

To further determine whether the IL-4-induced IL-31RA is functional, we stimulated IL-4-treated BMDCs with IL-31. This IL-31 stimulation without IL-4 treatment did not induce Ccl 17 and Ccl 22 production, indicating that the upregulation of IL-31RA expression is required for Ccl 17 and Ccl 22 production induced by IL-31, which is partially consistent with a previous report describing that CCL 17 is not produced by IL-31-stimulated human DCs [16]. Nevertheless, the IL-31 stimulation with IL-4 treatment enhanced Ccl 17 and Ccl 22 production compared with IL-4 treatment alone. These findings suggest that a Th2-prone immune condition including IL-4 treatment augments IL-31/IL-31RA interaction, which enhances Ccl 17 and Ccl 22 production and subsequently exacerbates the disease activity of AD.

The mechanism by which IL-31 stimulation enhances IL-4-induced Ccl 17 and Ccl 22 production remains incompletely understood. Several studies have reported that IL-31/IL-31RA interaction mediates STAT1/3/5 and MAP kinase activation [18,19]. Based on the evidence (1) that STAT1 activation induces CCL 17 and CCL 22 in HaCaT cells (human keratinocytes) [20], and (2) that the inhibition of MAP kinase activation reduces CCL 17 and CCL 22 production in HaCaT cells [21], multiple pathway signal transduction such as STAT1/3 and MAP kinase induced by the IL-31/IL-31RA interaction may be involved in the enhancement of Ccl 17 and Ccl 22 production by IL-31 stimulation. However, further studies are required to confirm this.

Since Glyteer inhibits IL-4-induced upregulation of IL-31 RA expression and IL-4-induced Ccl 17 and Ccl 22 production in BMDCs, the dual effects of Glyteer on IL-31RA expression and Ccl 17 and Ccl 22 production contribute to its inhibition of Ccl 17 and Ccl 22 production in AD. These findings suggest that Glyteer treatment potentiates the efficiency of nemolizumab, an IL-31 receptor α-antagonist, and dupilumab, an IL-4 receptor α-antagonist, in the treatment of AD. Nemolizumab has recently been used for the treatment of AD patients and shown to significantly improve clinical outcomes [7]. Although IL-31 is considered to be an important cytokine in the pruritus of AD, the present study revealed a new role of IL-31 in Th2-deviated immune conditions such as the production of CCL 17 and CCL 22 in AD.

In conclusion, we have demonstrated (i) that IL-31/IL-31RA interaction in dendritic cells under Th2-skewed conditions may increase the production of CCL17 and CCL22, contributing to the disease activity of AD, and (ii) that Glyteer treatment could have potential to prevent the production of CCL17 and CCL22 in AD (Figure 5). These findings should also promote our understanding of the roles of dendritic cell functions in AD.

Figure 5. IL-4 augments IL-31/IL-31 RA interaction leading to enhanced Ccl 17 and Ccl 22 production in BMDCs. IL-4 induces upregulation of IL-31RA expression at the mRNA levels ① and the protein levels ②. IL-31RA expression initially upregulated by IL-4 stimulation can lead upregulation of Ccl 17 and Ccl 22 production at the mRNA levels ③ and the protein levels ④, whereas IL-31 stimulation alone without IL-31RA upregulation did not upregulate Ccl 17 and Ccl 22 production ⑤. Impairment of STAT6 signaling pathway activation by Glyteer ⑥ inhibits upregulation of IL-31RA expression and Ccl 17 and Ccl 22 production induced by IL-4 in BMDCs.

4. Materials and Methods

4.1. Reagents

DMSO was purchased from Sigma-Aldrich (St. Louis, MO, USA). Recombinant murine IL-31 and IL-4 were purchased from PeproTech (Rocky Hill, NJ, USA). Glyteer was provided by Fujinaga Pharm Co. Ltd. (Tokyo, Japan) as original sticky-liquid stock. Glyteer is generated from soybean as dry distillated tar after delipidation, which contains wide-ranged organic compounds such as polycyclic aromatic hydrocarbons. Since Glyteer is known to act as a potent AHR ligand, no farther investigations have been conducted to clarify the detailed bioactive components.

4.2. Generation of Bone Marrow-Derived DCs (BMDCs) and Cell Culture

C57BL/6J mice were housed and bred in a clean breeding facility, and the trial was approved by the animal facility of Kyushu University (A30-258-0, 20 Aug 2018–31 Mar 2020). Bone marrow cells were collected freshly from femoral and tibial bones of mice and cultured in RPMI 1640 medium (Sigma-Aldrich) containing 1 mmol/L sodium pyruvate (10 mL; Invitrogen, Waltham, MA, USA), 10 mmol/L 4-(2-hydroxyethyl)-1-piperazineethanesulfonic acid (HEPES) (10 mL; Invitrogen, Waltham, MA, USA), 1% Minimum Essential Medium Non-Essential Amino Acids (MEM NEAA) (10 mL; Invitrogen), 10% FBS (Japan Bio Serum, Fukuyama, Japan), β-mercaptoethanol (50 nmol/L; Invitrogen), 100 U/mL penicillin, and antibiotic-antimycotic 100× (5 mL; 100 mg/mL streptomycin, and 0.25 µg/mL amphotericin B; Invitrogen) with GM-CSF (10 ng/mL) (Miltenyi Biotec, Bergisch Gladbach, Germany). Medium was refreshed twice in 7 days. Non-adherent cells were collected on day 7, and cells were purified immunomagnetically by positive selection with CD11c (N418) MicroBeads (Miltenyi Biotec). Our previous study has reported that the purity of BMDCs was 95–97%, that was confirmed by flow cytometric analysis [15]. Purified BMDCs were cultured with/without stimulants such as IL-4 and IL-31, and/or Glyteer for 24 h or 48 h. Culture supernatants were collected for ELISA analysis. Cell pellets were utilized for qRT-PCR or FACS analysis. This method of generating BMDCs and cell culture matches that in our previous study [15].

4.3. Quantitative Reverse-Transcription (qRT)-PCR Analysis

Total RNA was extracted by using RNeasy® Mini Kit (Qiagen, Hilden, Germany), then reverse transcription for making cDNA was conducted by using PrimeScript™ RT reagent kit (Takara Bio, Kusatsu, Japan). qRT-PCR was performed on CFX Connect Real-time PCR Detection System (Bio-Rad, Hercules, CA, USA) using TB Green® Premix Ex Taq (Takara Bio, Kusatsu, Japan). Amplification was launched as the first step at 95 °C for 30 s, then followed by 40 cycles of qRT-PCR at 95 °C for 5 s and at 61 °C for 20 s as the second step. mRNA expression was measured with normalization by housekeeping gene using β-actin in triplicate, and the mRNA expressions were presented as the fold induction relative to the control group. Each primer sequences are shown in Table 1.

Table 1. The sequences of primers.

Gene		Sequence (5′ to 3′)
β-actin	forward	GGCTGTATTCCCCTCCATCG
	reverse	CCAGTTGGTAACAATGCCATGT
Ccl17	forward	AGGTCACTTCAGATGCTGCTC
	reverse	ACTCTCGGCCTACATTGGTG
Ccl22	forward	GACACCTGACGAGGACACA
	reverse	GCAGAGGGTGACGGATGTAG
IL-31RA	forward	CGATTGTTGTGGAAGAAGGCAA
	reverse	TACTGCTGGGTGGTGATGTTG
OSMRβ	forward	CAGGCGGGTAATCAGACCAATG
	reverse	CATGAGTAAGGGCTGGGACA

Murine Ccl 17 and Ccl 22 ELISA Kit (R&D Systems, Minneapolis, MN, USA) was utilized to measure production of Ccl 17 and Ccl 22 following the manufacturer's protocol. Absorbance of the wells of the ELISA plate was measured using DTX 800 Multimode Detector (Beckman Coulter).

4.5. Fluorescence-Activated Cell Sorting (FACS) Analysis

LIVE/DEAD fixable dead cell staining kit (violet and near IR; Life Technologies) was used to detect dead cells. Then, BMDCs were incubated with anti-CD16/32 antibody (Becton Dickinson, Franklin Lakes, NJ, USA) for 30 min on ice. Anti-murine IL-31 RA antibody (Bioss Antibodies, Boston, MA, USA) was labeled with Zenon R-Phycoerythrin (PE) Rabbit IgG Labeling Kit (Thermo Fisher Scientific, Waltham, MA, USA), in accordance with the manufacturer's protocol. IL-31RA was stained with PE-conjugated anti-murine IL-31RA antibody. Isotype-matched antibodies were used as controls. Stained cells were analyzed on a BD Canto flow cytometer (Becton Dickinson). Stained cells were also observed using a D-Eclipse confocal laser scanning microscope (Nikon, Tokyo, Japan).

4.6. Statistical Analysis

Two-sample Student's t test was used for statistical evaluation of the results. A p-value of <0.05 was considered to show a statistically significant difference. All data are presented as mean ± standard error of the mean (S.E.M.) from three independent experiments.

Author Contributions: S.M., G.T., M.T., A.H.-H., and Y.H.V. performed the experiments. S.M., G.T., M.F. and T.N. designed the experimental protocol and wrote this manuscript.

References

1.   Dillon, S.R.; Sprecher, C.; Hammond, A.; Bilsborough, J.; Rosenfeld-Franklin, M.; Presnell, S.R.; Haugen, H.S.; Maurer, M.; Harder, B.; Johnston, J.; et al. Interleukin 31, a Cytokine Produced by Activated T Cells, Induces Dermatitis in Mice. *Nat. Immunol.* **2004**, *5*, 752–760. [CrossRef] [PubMed]

2.   Zhang, Q.; Putheti, P.; Zhou, Q.; Liu, Q.; Gao, W. Structures and Biological Functions of IL-31 and IL-31 Receptors. *Cytokine Growth Factor Rev.* **2008**, *19*, 347–356. [CrossRef] [PubMed]

3.   Stott, B.; Lavender, P.; Lehmann, S.; Pennino, D.; Durham, S.; Schmidt-Weber, C.B. Human IL-31 is Induced by IL-4 and Promotes TH2-driven Inflammation. *J. Allergy Clin. Immunol.* **2013**, *132*, 446–454.e5. [CrossRef] [PubMed]

4.   Edukulla, R.; Singh, B.; Jegga, A.G.; Sontake, V.; Dillon, S.R.; Madala, S.K. Th2 Cytokines Augment IL-31/IL-31RA Interactions via STAT6-dependent IL-31RA Expression. *J. Biol. Chem.* **2015**, *290*, 13510–13520. [CrossRef] [PubMed]

5.   Furue, M.; Chiba, T.; Tsuji, G.; Ulzii, D.; Kido-Nakahara, M.; Nakahara, T.; Kadono, T. Atopic Dermatitis: Immune Deviation, Barrier Dysfunction, IgE Autoreactivity and New Therapies. *Allergol. Int.* **2017**, *66*, 398–403. [CrossRef] [PubMed]

6.   Simpson, E.L.; Bieber, T.; Guttman-Yassky, E.; Beck, L.A.; Blauvelt, A.; Cork, M.J.; Silverberg, J.I.; Deleuran, M.; Kataoka, Y.; Lacour, J.P.; et al. Two Phase 3 Trials of Dupilumab Versus Placebo in Atopic Dermatitis. *N. Engl. J. Med.* **2016**, *375*, 2335–2348. [CrossRef] [PubMed]

7.   Ruzicka, T.; Hanifin, J.M.; Furue, M.; Pulka, G.; Mlynarczyk, I.; Wollenberg, A.; Galus, R.; Etoh, T.; Mihara, R.; Yoshida, H.; et al. Anti-Interleukin-31 Receptor A Antibody for Atopic Dermatitis. *N. Engl. J. Med.* **2017**, *376*, 826–835. [CrossRef] [PubMed]

8.   Cevikbas, F.; Wang, X.; Akiyama, T.; Kempkes, C.; Savinko, T.; Antal, A.; Kukova, G.; Buhl, T.; Ikoma, A.; Buddenkotte, J.; et al. A Sensory Neuron-expressed IL-31 Receptor Mediates T Helper Cell-dependent Itch: Involvement of TRPV1 and TRPA1. *J. Allergy Clin. Immunol.* **2014**, *133*, 448–460. [CrossRef]

9.   Kato, A.; Fujii, E.; Watanabe, T.; Takashima, Y.; Matsushita, H.; Furuhashi, T.; Morita, A. Distribution of IL-31 and its Receptor Expressing Cells in Skin of Atopic Dermatitis. *J. Dermatol. Sci.* **2014**, *74*, 229–235. [CrossRef]

10. Feld, M.; Garcia, R.; Buddenkotte, J.; Katayama, S.; Lewis, K.; Muirhead, G.; Hevezi, P.; Plesser, K.; Schrumpf, H.; Krjutskov, K.; et al. The Pruritus- and TH2-associated Cytokine IL-31 Promotes Growth of Sensory Nerves. *J. Allergy Clin. Immunol.* **2016**, *138*, 500–508.e24. [CrossRef]

11. Yamamura, K.; Uruno, T.; Shiraishi, A.; Tanaka, Y.; Ushijima, M.; Nakahara, T.; Watanabe, M.; Kido-Nakahara, M.; Tsuge, I.; Furue, M.; et al. The Transcription Factor EPAS1 Links DOCK8 Deficiency to Atopic Skin Inflammation via IL-31 Induction. *Nat. Commun.* **2017**, *8*, 13946. [CrossRef] [PubMed]

12. Stutte, S.; Quast, T.; Gerbitzki, N.; Savinko, T.; Novak, N.; Reifenberger, J.; Homey, B.; Kolanus, W.; Alenius, H.; Förster, I. Requirement of CCL17 for CCR7- and CXCR4-dependent Migration of Cutaneous Dendritic Cells. *Proc. Natl. Acad. Sci. USA* **2010**, *107*, 8736–8741. [CrossRef] [PubMed]

13. Kataoka, Y. Thymus and Activation-regulated Chemokine as a Clinical Biomarker in Atopic Dermatitis. *J. Dermatol.* **2014**, *41*, 221–229. [CrossRef] [PubMed]

14. Hashimoto, S.; Nakamura, K.; Oyama, N.; Kaneko, F.; Tsunemi, Y.; Saeki, H.; Tamaki, K. Macrophage-derived Chemokine (MDC)/CCL22 Produced by Monocyte Derived Dendritic Cells Reflects the Disease Activity in Patients with Atopic Dermatitis. *J. Dermatol. Sci.* **2006**, *44*, 93–99, Epub Sep 27, 2006. [CrossRef] [PubMed]

15. Takemura, M.; Nakahara, T.; Hashimoto-Hachiya, A.; Furue, M.; Tsuji, G. Glyteer, Soybean Tar, Impairs IL-4/Stat6 Signaling in Murine Bone Marrow-Derived Dendritic Cells: The Basis of Its Therapeutic Effect on Atopic Dermatitis. *Int. J. Mol. Sci.* **2018**, *19*, 1169. [CrossRef] [PubMed]

16. Horejs-Hoeck, J.; Schwarz, H.; Lamprecht, S.; Maier, E.; Hainzl, S.; Schmittner, M.; Posselt, G.; Stoecklinger, A.; Hawranek, T.; Duschl, A. Dendritic Cells Activated by IFN-γ/STAT1 Express IL-31 Receptor and Release Proinflammatory Mediators upon IL-31 Treatment. *J. Immunol.* **2012**, *188*, 5319–5326. [CrossRef] [PubMed]

17. Takei, K.; Mitoma, C.; Hashimoto-Hachiya, A.; Uchi, H.; Takahara, M.; Tsuji, G.; Kido-Nakahara, M.; Nakahara, T.; Furue, M. Antioxidant Soybean Tar Glyteer Rescues T-helper-mediated Downregulation of Filaggrin Expression via Aryl Hydrocarbon Receptor. *J. Dermatol.* **2015**, *42*, 171–180. [CrossRef]

18. Dambacher, J.; Beigel, F.; Seiderer, J.; Haller, D.; Göke, B.; Auernhammer, C.J.; Brand, S. Interleukin 31 Mediates MAP Kinase and STAT1/3 Activation in Intestinal Epithelial Cells and its Expression is Upregulated in Inflammatory Bowel Disease. *Gut* **2007**, *56*, 1257–1265. [CrossRef]

19. Kasraie, S.; Niebuhr, M.; Werfel, T. Interleukin (IL)-31 Activates Signal Transducer and Activator of Transcription (STAT)-1, STAT-5, and Extracellular Signal-regulated Kinase 1/2 and Down-regulates IL-12p40 Production in Activated Human Macrophages. *Allergy* **2013**, *68*, 739–747. [CrossRef]

20. Kwon, D.J.; Bae, Y.S.; Ju, S.M.; Goh, A.R.; Youn, G.S.; Choi, S.Y.; Park, J. Casuarinin Suppresses TARC/CCL17 and MDC/CCL22 Production via Blockade of NF-κB and STAT1 Activation in HaCaT Cells. *Biochem. Biophys. Res. Commun.* **2012**, *417*, 1254–1259. [CrossRef]

21. Yano, C.; Saeki, H.; Komine, M.; Kagami, S.; Tsunemi, Y.; Ohtsuki, M.; Nakagawa, H. Mechanism of Macrophage-Derived Chemokine/CCL22 Production by HaCaT Keratinocytes. *Ann. Dermatol.* **2015**, *27*, 152–156. [CrossRef] [PubMed]

14

Aryl Hydrocarbon Receptor in Atopic Dermatitis and Psoriasis

Masutaka Furue [1,2,3,*], **Akiko Hashimoto-Hachiya** [1,2] **and Gaku Tsuji** [1,2]

[1] Department of Dermatology, Graduate School of Medical Sciences, Kyushu University, Maidashi 3-1-1, Higashiku, Fukuoka 812-8582, Japan; ahachi@dermatol.med.kyushu-u.ac.jp (A.H.-H.); gakku@dermatol.med.kyushu-u.ac.jp (G.T.)

[2] Research and Clinical Center for Yusho and Dioxin, Kyushu University, Maidashi 3-1-1, Higashiku, Fukuoka 812-8582, Japan

[3] Division of Skin Surface Sensing, Graduate School of Medical Sciences, Kyushu University, Maidashi 3-1-1, Higashiku, Fukuoka 812-8582, Japan

* Correspondence: furue@dermatol.med.kyushu-u.ac.jp

Abstract: The aryl hydrocarbon receptor (AHR)/AHR-nuclear translocator (ARNT) system is a sensitive sensor for small molecular, xenobiotic chemicals of exogenous and endogenous origin, including dioxins, phytochemicals, microbial bioproducts, and tryptophan photoproducts. AHR/ARNT are abundantly expressed in the skin. Once activated, the AHR/ARNT axis strengthens skin barrier functions and accelerates epidermal terminal differentiation by upregulating filaggrin expression. In addition, AHR activation induces oxidative stress. However, some AHR ligands simultaneously activate the nuclear factor-erythroid 2-related factor-2 (NRF2) transcription factor, which is a master switch of antioxidative enzymes that neutralizes oxidative stress. The immunoregulatory system governing T-helper 17/22 (Th17/22) and T regulatory cells (Treg) is also regulated by the AHR system. Notably, AHR agonists, such as tapinarof, are currently used as therapeutic agents in psoriasis and atopic dermatitis. In this review, we summarize recent topics on AHR related to atopic dermatitis and psoriasis.

Keywords: aryl hydrocarbon receptor (AHR); aryl hydrocarbon receptor-nuclear translocator (ARNT); nuclear factor-erythroid 2-related factor-2 (NRF2); atopic dermatitis; psoriasis; tapinarof; filaggrin; skin barrier; Th17; Th22; Treg; reactive oxygen species; antioxidants

1. Introduction

The skin is the outermost surface of the body and is vulnerable to a myriad of external chemicals and internal substances. To maintain homeostasis, skin cells, including keratinocytes, sebocytes, fibroblasts, dendritic cells, and other immune cells, express several chemical sensors, such as aryl hydrocarbon receptor (AHR), pregnane X receptor, constitutive androstane receptor, and peroxisome proliferator-activated receptors [1–4]. Among these chemical receptors, AHR has gained special attention because it plays a crucial role in photoaging, epidermal differentiation, and immunomodulation [2,3,5–7].

AHR, also called dioxin receptor, binds to environmental polyaromatic hydrocarbons and dioxins with high affinity and induces oxidative stress by generating abundant reactive oxygen species (ROS) [5–7]. Additionally, AHR is a promiscuous receptor and is activated by a plethora of exogenous and endogenous ligands, such as photo-induced chromophores, phytochemicals, and microbial bioproducts [8–12]. Many AHR ligands exert antioxidative activity by activating antioxidative transcription factor nuclear factor-erythroid 2-related factor-2 (NRF2) [10,13]. Medicinal coal tar and soybean tar Glyteer activate both AHR and NRF2 and have been used to treat inflammatory skin diseases, such as atopic dermatitis (AD) and psoriasis [14,15].

AD and psoriasis are common inflammatory skin diseases. An excellent therapeutic response to biologics indicates a pivotal pathogenic role of interleukin (IL)-4/IL-13 signaling in AD [16,17] and the tumor necrosis factor (TNF)-α/IL-23/IL-17A axis in psoriasis [18,19]. Although distinct signaling pathways operate in developing full-blown AD and psoriasis, 81% of dysregulated genes in AD are shared with those in psoriasis in skin lesions [20]. Notably, recent phase II, randomized dose-finding studies have demonstrated that topical application of the natural AHR agonist tapinarof is efficacious and well tolerated in patients with AD and psoriasis [21,22].

The purpose of this article is to summarize the diverse action of AHR signaling in balancing skin homeostasis and to elucidate the fundamental mechanisms of therapeutic AHR potentials in the treatment of AD and psoriasis.

2. AHR Signaling and Modulation of Oxidative and Antioxidative Balance

AHR is a ligand-activated transcription factor [7]. In the absence of ligands, AHR resides in the cytoplasm where it forms a protein complex with heat shock protein 90 (HSP90), hepatitis B virus X-associated protein 2 (XAP-2), and p23 [23,24]. After ligand binding, AHR dissociates from the cytoplasmic complex and a nuclear translocation site of AHR is exposed. Then, AHR is translocated into the nucleus where AHR dimerizes with AHR-nuclear translocator (ARNT), binds DNA responsive elements called xenobiotic responsive elements (XREs), and upregulates the transcription of target genes, such as phase I metabolizing enzyme cytochrome P450 (CYP) members (i.e., *CYP1A1*, *CYP1A2*, and *CYP1B1*) [7,25–29].

Hazardous dioxins such as 2,3,7,8,-tetrachlorodibenzo-p-dioxin (TCDD) activate AHR and upregulate CYP1A1, CYP1A2, and CYP1B1 expression [5,30,31]. Human keratinocytes abundantly express CYP1A1 and to a lesser extent CYP1B1 but not CYP1A2 [32]. CYP1A1 attempts to metabolize TCDD but the continuous efforts of CYP1A1 are unsuccessful because TCDD is structurally stable [33]. The metabolizing process by CYP1A1 generates excessive amounts of ROS and induces oxidative damage in the cell [5,30,31] (Figure 1). To demonstrate these findings, TCDD-induced ROS production was inhibited in AHR-silenced or CYP1A1-silenced cells [30]. As CYP1B1 silencing did not affect TCDD-induced ROS generation, the AHR-CYP1A1 axis is likely to be crucial for generating cellular oxidative stress by hazardous dioxins [30]. A chemical carcinogen β-naphthoflavone also activates CYP1A1 and CYP1A2 via AHR activation in mice [34]. β-Naphthoflavone induces mitochondrial ROS generation. However, this activation is attenuated by an AHR inhibitor or CYP1A1/1A2 silencing [34]. AHR-CYP1A1-mediated oxidative stress is responsible at least in part for the production of proinflammatory cytokines, such as interleukin (IL)-1, IL-6, and IL-8 [35,36].

To survive during oxidative stress, antioxidative machinery is simultaneously activated after AHR activation in the cells. Ligation of AHR also activates antioxidative transcription factor NRF2 and upregulates the expression of phase II antioxidative enzymes (i.e., glutathione S-transferases, heme oxygenase 1 (HMOX1), NAD(P)H dehydrogenase, quinone 1 (NQO1), glutathione S-transferases, and uridine 5'-diphospho-glucuronosyltransferases [13,14,25,26,37–40]. In contrast to proinflammatory consequences after AHR-CYP1A1-ROS induction, the AHR-NRF2 axis is likely to be anti-inflammatory and reduces the production of proinflammatory cytokines [13,39,41]. Many salubrious antioxidative phytochemical extracts (i.e., artichoke (*Cynara scolymus*) in Mediterranean regions, *Opuntia ficus-indica* in Latin America, and *Houttuynia cordata* in Asia) activate the AHR-NRF2 system and upregulate the expression of antioxidative enzymes [13,37,38]. Dioxins activate the AHR-NRF2 battery [40,42,43], however, their powerful AHR-CYP1A1 activation may induce far more oxidative stress that cannot be extinguished by the AHR-NRF2 antioxidative system. Alternatively, salubrious phytochemical AHR ligands stimulate the AHR-NRF2 axis more strongly than the AHR-CYP1A1-ROS pathway and exert antioxidative action [10].

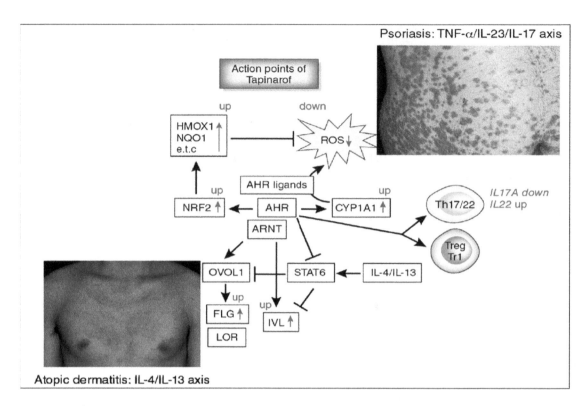

Figure 1. Aryl hydrocarbon receptor (AHR) signal and action points of tapinarof (red words and arrows). AHR is a promiscuous chemical sensor that is activated by various oxidative and antioxidative ligands. Once activated, cytoplasmic AHR translocates into the nucleus where it heterodimerizes with an AHR-nuclear translocator (ARNT) and then induces the transcription of AHR-responsive genes such as cytochrome P450 1A1 (CYP1A1). CYP1A1 degrades AHR ligands. Some ligands such as dioxins are chemically stable and long-lived. Therefore, CYP1A1 generates high amounts of reactive oxygen species (ROS) after sustained efforts to degrade them. Some antioxidative AHR ligands activate nuclear factor-erythroid 2-related factor-2 (NRF2) transcription factor, which upregulates gene expression of various antioxidative enzymes, such as heme oxygenase 1 (HMOX1), NAD(P)H dehydrogenase, and quinone 1 (NQO1), and these antioxidative enzymes neutralize ROS. AHR/ARNT signaling also activates OVO-like 1 (OVOL1) transcription factor and upregulates the expression of filaggrin (FLG) and loricrin (LOR). AHR upregulates the expression of involucrin (IVL) in an OVOL1-independent manner. Therefore, AHR/ARNT signaling accelerates epidermal terminal differentiation and enhances the repair of barrier disruption. Interleukin (IL)-4 and IL-13 activate signal transducer and activator of transcription 6 (STAT6) and inhibit the OVOL1/FLG, OVOL1/LOR, and AHR/IVL axes. However, suitable AHR activation can inhibit the IL-4/IL-13-mediated STAT6 activation and restore the expression of FLG, LOR, and IVL. Regarding immune response, AHR signaling affects T-helper (Th17) differentiation and is essential for IL-22 production. AHR ligation (especially by high concentrations of ligands) induces the differentiation of regulatory cell populations, Treg and Tr1 cells. Tapinarof is an antioxidative AHR ligand and upregulates CYP1A1 expression. Topical tapinarof is efficacious in psoriasis and atopic dermatitis. Current studies demonstrate that tapinarof activates NRF2/antioxidative signaling and reduces oxidative stress. Tapinarof also upregulates FLG and IVL expression. Tapinarof downregulates IL-17A production and increases IL-22 production.

3. AHR and Epidermal Terminal Differentiation

The mammalian epidermis protects the body against injuries from external and environmental factors by providing a barrier-forming cornified layer. Epidermal terminal differentiation or cornified envelope maturation is accomplished by sequential cross-linking of ceramides and various terminal differentiation proteins, such as involucrin (IVL), loricrin (LOR), and filaggrin (FLG) by transglutaminase-1; the majority of these skin barrier-forming proteins map to chromosome 1q21 [44,45].

Notably, activation of the AHR-ARNT axis accelerates epidermal terminal differentiation by coordinately upregulating the production of a series of skin barrier-forming proteins in vivo [46] and in vitro [3,44,47,48]. In parallel, both *Ahr*-deficient and *Ahr*-transgenic mice reveal an abnormality in keratinization [49,50]. Severe abnormalities in keratinization are also observed in *Arnt*-deficient mice [51,52].

Both oxidative and antioxidative ligands for AHR can accelerate epidermal terminal differentiation [3,12,44,47,48]. Slow-metabolizing dioxins induce strong and sustained AHR activation, which results in exaggerated keratinization of keratinocytes and sebocytes and the development of chloracne [2,53]. In contrast, mild and transient AHR activation by antioxidative phytochemical or endogenous AHR ligands are effective in maintaining healthy barrier-intact skin [3,10,54].

Sunlight, especially UVB, generates tryptophan photoderivatives such as formylindolo[3,2-b]carbazole (FICZ), which is a high-affinity ligand for AHR that upregulates CYP1A1 expression [8,55–57]. Compared with slow-metabolizing TCDD, FICZ is rapidly metabolized by CYP1A1 [8,55,56]. Similar to other AHR ligands, FICZ upregulates filaggrin via AHR signaling [57–59]. Although an erythematogenic dose of UVB is harmful through a variety of mechanisms, exposure to a suberythematous dose of UVB prior to tape-stripping results in significantly accelerated barrier recovery rates [60]. Physiological low-dose UVB exposure may be beneficial for skin barrier protection by FICZ-AHR/ARNT-mediated upregulation of filaggrin and other barrier-related proteins [57–59] (Figure 1). In this context, topical application of FICZ significantly attenuated transepidermal water loss and dermatitis score in a murine mite-induced dermatitis model [58].

Mechanisms regarding how AHR signaling accelerates keratinocyte differentiation are not fully understood. Kennedy et al. points to an essential role of ROS production in this regulation [47]. We have demonstrated that AHR signaling upregulates the expression of OVO-like 1 (OVOL1) transcription factor and activates its cytoplasmic to nuclear translocation [3,59,61,62]. Both filaggrin and loricrin are under the control of the AHR-OVOL1 pathway, whereas AHR-mediated involucrin upregulation is independent of OVOL1 [63].

IL-4/IL-13 signaling downregulates the expression of filaggrin, loricrin, and involucrin via signal transducer and activator of transcription 6 (STAT6) activation, impairing the epidermal terminal differentiation and barrier dysfunction [14,15,37,44,61,64,65]. IL-4/IL-13 signaling is likely to impair the cytoplasmic to nuclear translocation of OVOL1, which interferes with the AHR-OVOL1-filaggrin axis [59,61]. Notably, IL-4/IL-13 signaling reciprocally enhances the protein expression of AHR and to a lesser extent ARNT in keratinocytes (Figure 2). Similar results were observed in murine B cells [66]. The implication of IL-4/IL-13-mediated AHR upregulation remains elusive. In addition, IL-4/IL-13-mediated STAT6 activation stimulates keratinocyte to produce periostin, which induces IL-24 production in keratinocytes [67]. IL-24 reduces the filaggrin expression via STAT3 activation [67]. AHR ligands, such as coal tar, Glyteer and FICZ, activate the AHR/ARNT pathway, block the IL-4/IL-13-mediated STAT6 activation, induce the entry of OVOL1 into the nuclei, and restore barrier dysfunction [15,59,61,68].

Figure 2. Human epidermal keratinocytes are stimulated with 10 ng/mL of IL-4 augments the protein expression of aryl hydrocarbon receptor (AHR) and AHR-nuclear translocator (ARNT) compared with untreated control by Western blot analysis.

4. AHR and Immune Modulation

As a crucial chemosensor, AHR activity modulates immune function. AHR and its immunological significance are best characterized in intestinal immunology [28,29,69,70]. *Ahr*-deficient mice have an inherent weak gut barrier [71–73]. In this context, genome-wide association studies have identified AHR as a susceptibility locus in inflammatory bowel diseases [74]. Indeed, the expression of AHR is reduced in the lesioned intestine in inflammatory bowel diseases [75]. This finding may be strongly related to the fact that the intestinal tract is a rich source of AHR ligands derived from dietary materials and microbial bioproducts [69,76].

Early research on AHR-mediated immune modulation was based on toxicological approaches using dioxins [77].   Dioxin-exposed rodents exhibit waste syndrome, dose-dependent thymic involution, depletion of other lymphoid organs, and reduced circulating lymphocyte counts [77].   Antibody production by B cells is also inhibited by toxic doses of dioxins [77]. However, extensive attention by immunologists has recently been focused on the physiological function of AHR in immune regulation [29,69,70,76].

Ligation of AHR by TCDD and endogenous or natural compounds preferentially affects differentiation and propagation of T-helper 17 (Th17) and T regulatory (Treg) cells [29,69,70]. Tryptophan is an essential amino acid and is thought to produce various candidates for endogenous AHR ligands by different metabolic processes.   These metabolic pathways include kynurenine production by indoleamine 2,3-dioxygenase and tryptophan 2,3-dioxygenase, FICZ by UVB exposure, and indole derivatives by bacterial degradation [29,69,70]. Dietary materials such as *Brasicca* contain glucosinolate glucobrassicin, which is metabolized to produce indolo-[3,2-b]-carbazole (ICZ) [29]. The major metabolic pathway of tryptophan is the kynurenine pathway, however, the binding capacity of kynurenine to AHR is very low compared to FICZ and ICZ [29].

In murine CD4$^+$ cells, AHR is highly expressed in Th17 cells, not detectable in Th1 and Th2 cells, and marginally expressed in Treg cells [78]. In addition, Lin-Sca$^+$ and Sca$^-$ progenitor cells in bone marrow, double negative (CD4$^-$ and CD8$^-$) cells in the thymus, innate lymphoid cell type 3 (ILC3) cells, dendritic cells, γδ T cells, and Langerhans cells express high levels of AHR [28,29]. In *Ahr*-deficient mice, *T-bet* and *Ifng* expression in Th1, *Gata3* and *Il4* expression in Th2, and RORγt (*Rorc*) and *Il17a/Il17f* expression in Th17 cells are not significantly affected. However, *Il22* expression in Th17 cells is almost completely abrogated in *Ahr*-deficient mice [78]. FICZ upregulates *Il17a*, *Il17f*, and *Il22* expression in Th17 cells. The expression of AHR is detected in human Th17 cells at higher levels than in Th1 cells and FICZ upregulates the *IL17A*, *IL17F*, and *IL22* expression in Th17 cells [78]. Flowcytometric analysis also revealed that FICZ enhances Th17 differentiation and IL-22 production [69]. In a murine

Th17-mediated experimental autoimmune encephalomyelitis model, injection of FICZ accelerated disease onset whereas it was delayed in *Ahr*-deficient mice. Treg cells were unaffected in this model [78]. In contrast, TCDD treatment increased the number of Treg cells, which exhibited an immunosuppressive function in a murine graft-versus-host disease model [79]. The TCDD-induced increase in Treg number was abrogated in *Ahr*-deficient mice [79]. These studies suggest that prolonged activation of AHR by TCDD may potentiate Treg cell deviation, but transient AHR activation may shift the immune response toward Th17 and more strongly to Th22 cell differentiation (Figure 1).

Th17 and ILC3 cells express high levels of AHR, IL-17, and IL-22 and are crucial for intestinal protective immunity against commensal and pathogenic microbiota [80]. In contrast to the abovementioned experimental autoimmune encephalomyelitis model in which AHR ligation enhances IL-17 and IL-22 production, *Ahr*-deficiency augments Th17 cell differentiation in the intestinal tract where large amounts of dietary- and microbiota-derived AHR ligands are present [80]. In *Ahr*-deficient mice, the amount of microbiota is significantly increased, which is likely to promote Th17 differentiation. Alternatively, *Ahr*-deficient mice exhibit IL-22 reduction, which is consistently found in an experimental autoimmune encephalomyelitis model. Notably, IL-22 supplementation to *Ahr*-deficient mice normalizes the expansion of the microbiota and reduces Th17 deviation, demonstrating that IL-22 is protective against intestinal infection [80]. In addition, ILC3s produce larger amounts of IL-22 than Th17 cells after AHR ligation [80].

In the gut, heterogenous cell populations exist in Foxp3$^+$ Treg cells depending on the expression of neuropilin (Nrp1) and RORγt. Nrp1 is a surface marker to distinguish thymus-derived Tregs (Nrp1$^+$ tTregs) versus peripherally derived Tregs (Nrp1$^-$ pTregs) [70]. In the small and large intestines, all Nrp1$^+$ RORγt$^-$, Nrp1$^-$ RORγt$^+$ and Nrp1$^-$ RORγt$^-$ Treg subpopulations express high levels of AHR [70]. *Ahr* deficiency in these Treg cells induces a significant decrease of Nrp1$^-$ RORγt$^+$ and Nrp1$^-$ RORγt$^-$, but not Nrp1$^+$ RORγt$^-$, Treg subpopulations in the intestine, whereas those in the spleen and mesenteric lymph nodes are not affected [70]. In contrast, AHR activation by FICZ injection preferentially enhances the Nrp1$^-$ RORγt$^-$ Treg subpopulation. High-throughput RNA sequencing revealed that *Ccr6*, *Gpr15*, *Itgae*, *Rgs9*, and *Gzma* genes important for Treg homing and functions in the gut are downregulated in *Ahr*-deficient Tregs while Th1-associated genes *Ifng*, *Ccl5*, and *Tbx21* are upregulated. Moreover, these AHR-expressing Treg cells inhibit T cell-induced wasting disease and colitis [70].

As described above, AHR ligation induces the CYP1A1 production, which efficiently degrades AHR ligands [28,29]. Therefore, constitutive overexpression of CYP1A1 in mice depletes the reservoir of natural AHR ligands, generating a quasi *Ahr*-deficient state [76]. Th17 cells from *Ahr*-deficient mice do not produce IL-22. In parallel, *Cyp1a1*-overexpressed Th17 cells show a reduced IL-22 production [76]. Both *Ahr*-deficient and *Cyp1a1*-overexpressed mice exhibit loss of ILC3 in the small and large intestines. IL-22 derived from ILC3 and Th17 cells is essential in the defense against *Citrobacter rodentium*. Thus, C. *rodentium*-induced colitis becomes life-threatening both in *Ahr*-deficient and *Cyp1a1*-overexpressed mice [76]. Although AHR ligation upregulates CYP1A1, CYP1B1, and CYP1A2 expression, CYP1B1 and CYP1A2 are not crucial for degrading AHR ligands [76]. FICZ-mediated Th17 differentiation and IL-22 production is achieved by extremely low concentrations of FICZ in *Cyp1a1*-deficient CD4$^+$ cells [69]. Furthermore, FICZ promotes IL-17A$^+$ IL-22$^+$, but not IL-17$^+$ IL-22$^-$, cell differentiation [69].

Although AHR ligation tends to affect Th17 and Treg cell differentiation, outcomes are inconsistent in different experimental systems. The dose and the duration of AHR activation by high-affinity AHR ligands are likely the primary factors that explain the fate of T cell differentiation [81]. To this end, Ehrlich et al. examined the effects of low and high doses of four high-affinity AHR ligands (TCDD, FICZ, 2-(1H-Indol-3-ylcarbonyl)-4-thiazolecarboxylic acid (ITE), and 11-Chloro-7H-benzo[de]benzo[4,5]imidazo[2,1-a]isoquinolin-7-one (11-Cl-BBQ)) on CD4$^+$ T cell differentiation using a parent-into-F1 alloresponse mouse model. Intraperitoneal injection of high doses of all agents induced the production of IL-10 producing, Foxp3$^+$ type 1 regulatory T cells (Tr1 cells) on day 2, and increased Foxp3$^+$ Tregs on day 10 in conjunction with suppression of the alloresponse. Alternatively, low doses of the ligands, even when given daily, did not induce Tregs nor alter the alloresponse, but instead increased the percentage of CD4$^+$ cells that produce IL-17 [81]. In summary, accumulating evidence suggests that AHR ligation stimulates Th17 cells to differentiate into Th17/22 cells. AHR ligands may also enhance the regulatory cell population especially in high doses.

5. AHR and Atopic Dermatitis

AD is a common and heterogenous eczematous skin disorder characterized by Th2-deviated skin inflammation, barrier disruption, and chronic pruritus [17,82,83]. Frequent relapse with intense pruritus deteriorates quality of life and decreases treatment satisfaction of the afflicted patients [84–88]. The lifetime incidence of AD is as high as 20% in the general population [89]. Skin barrier dysfunction is associated with the reduced production of terminal differentiation molecules such as filaggrin [15,51]. Abnormal skin barrier integrity also causes an increased colonization of microbes such as *Staphylococcus aureus*, which further exacerbate Th2-deviated skin inflammation [90,91]. In addition, some autoimmune diseases are comorbid with AD [92].

Investigation on *AHR* gene polymorphism reveals that *AHR* rs10249788 and rs2066853 polymorphisms are found in patients with AD, psoriasis, and healthy controls, but no significant differences were detected in genotype or allele frequencies between the three groups [93]. However, the *AHR* rs2066853 (AG + AA) or rs10249788 (CT + TT) genotypes are a risk factor for severe dry skin phenotype and the combined rs10249788 (CT + TT) and rs2066853 (AG + AA) genotypes lead to a higher risk for severe dry skin in Chinese patients with AD [93]. rs10249788 exists in the AHR promoter region where nuclear factor 1C (NF1C) binds and suppresses the transcription and protein expression of AHR [94]. Notably, NF1C prefers to associate with the C allele compared to the T allele at rs10249788. Thus, subjects with the rs10249788 (CC) allele express less AHR than those with the rs10249788 (TT) allele [94]. In fact, AHR mRNA levels for the TT genotype are 1.7-fold higher than those for the CC genotype [95]. No significant differences were obtained in AHR production between the CC and CT genotypes [95]. In parallel with increased levels of AHR, cells with the TT genotype express significantly higher levels of CYP1A1, IL-24, and IL-1β [95]. It is intriguing that IL-24 downregulates the filaggrin expression via STAT3 activation [67].

Immunohistological and real time PCR studies for AHR have been reported in AD [96,97]. Hong et al. showed an increased expression of both AHR and ARNT without CYP1A1 induction in the lesioned skin of AD compared with normal control skin [96]. Alternatively, Kim et al. demonstrated an increased expression of ARNT and CYP1A1 but not AHR in the lesional skin of AD [97]. As the Th2-deviated milieu potently reduces filaggrin and other barrier-related molecules, the upregulation of AHR/ARNT may be compensatory to attenuate the Th2-mediated filaggrin reduction. A recent study by Yu et al. demonstrated the possibility that the Th2-deviated milieu decreases the production of endogenous AHR ligand such as indole-3-aldehyde by commensal skin microbiota [98]. These findings collectively suggest that most AHR likely lack physiological ligands in the Th2-prone milieu in AD. Therefore, rapid-metabolizing AHR ligands, such as FICZ and indole-3-aldehyde, appropriately activate the AHR/ARNT/FLG axis and may be beneficial in treating AD [58,98]. However, vigorous and long-lasting activation of the AHR/ARNT/FLG axis by slow-metabolizing dioxins and environmental pollutants may exacerbate barrier dysfunction and aggravate AD [96,99].

Although the pathogenic implication of AHR and its gene polymorphism in AD remain elusive, recent clinical trials using topical AHR ligand tapinarof have reported its efficacy for AD [100–102]. Tapinarof (5-[(E)-2-phenylethenyl]-2-[propan-2-yl] benzene-1, 3-diol, WBI-1001, GSK2894512 or bentivimod) is a naturally derived (but is now a fully synthetic) hydroxylated stilbene produced by bacterial symbionts of entomopathogenic nematodes [100–103]. Tapinarof is a high affinity AHR ligand with antioxidative activity via NRF2 activation and a ROS-scavenging structure [102] (Figure 1). Tapinarof has gained increased attention because its topical application is efficacious for patients with AD in clinical trials [21,100,104]. Tapinarof activates the AHR/CYP1A1 axis and augments the expression of filaggrin and involucrin [102]. Even in barrier-disrupted AD patients, systemic absorption of topical tapinarof is limited and likely decreases during the treatment course in parallel with treatment success that restores the barrier dysfunction [104]. In general, topical tapinarof is tolerable but frequent adverse events include headaches and folliculitis [104].

In an early clinical trial, patients with AD affecting 3–20% of their body surface area (BSA) and with an Investigator's Global Assessment (IGA; 0: clear, 1: almost clear, 2: mild, 3: moderate, 4: severe, 5: very severe) of 2–4 were randomized (1:1:1) to receive a placebo ($n = 51$), topical tapinarof 0.5% ($n = 50$) or 1% ($n = 47$) in a cream formulation applied twice daily for six weeks [100]. There was a decrease of 1.3 (43%; $p < 0.001$; 95% confidence interval (CI) −1.2 to −0.5) and 1.8 (56.3%; $p < 0.001$; 95% CI −1.6 to −0.9) in IGA at day 42 in the topical tapinarof 0.5% and 1% groups, respectively, compared with a decrease of 0.5 (14.7%) in the placebo group. At day 42, improvement in Eczema Area and Severity Index (EASI) score was 68.9% ($p < 0.001$) and 76.3% ($p < 0.001$) for tapinarof 0.5% and 1%, respectively, compared with 23.3% for placebo. Improvement in pruritus severity score at day 42 was 29.8% ($p < 0.001$) and 66.9% ($p < 0.001$) for tapinarof 0.5% and 1%, respectively, compared with 9.5% for placebo [100]. Adverse events included headaches (placebo: 0%; 0.5% tapinarof: 8%; 1% tapinarof: 14%), migraines (placebo: 0%; 0.5% tapinarof: 4%; 1% tapinarof: 3%), folliculitis (placebo: 0%; 0.5% tapinarof: 6%; 1% tapinarof: 8%), and contact dermatitis (placebo: 0%; 0.5% tapinarof: 3%: 1% tapinarof: 5%) [100].

A phase II, double-blind, vehicle-controlled, randomized, six-arm trial (1:1:1:1:1:1) in patients aged 12 to 65 years, with BSA involvement of at least 5% to 35% and an IGA score of 3 or higher (moderate to severe) at baseline was performed. Primary end points included an IGA score of clear or almost clear (0 or 1) and a minimum two-grade improvement (treatment success) at week 12 [21]. The rates of treatment success with topical tapinarof cream at week 12 were 53% (1% twice daily, $n = 40$), 46% (1% once daily, $n = 41$), 37% (0.5% twice daily, $n = 43$), 34% (0.5% once daily, $n = 41$), 24% (vehicle twice daily, $n = 42$), and 28% (vehicle once daily, $n = 40$). The rate with tapinarof 1% twice daily (53%) was statistically significantly higher than the rate with vehicle twice daily (24%). Notably, treatment success was maintained for four weeks after the end of tapinarof treatment. The proportion of patients achieving EASI75 (75% or greater improvement in EASI) score reduction at week 12 was significantly higher in the groups treated with 1% tapinarof (60% and 51% for twice daily and once daily, respectively) than with vehicle (26% and 25% in the groups receiving vehicle twice daily and once daily, respectively) [21]. Headaches (e.g., 10% (1% twice daily), 2% (0.5% twice daily), and 0% (0.5% twice daily)) and folliculitis (e.g., 10% (1% twice daily), 7% (0.5% twice daily), and 0% (0.5% twice daily)) were again frequent adverse events [21].

In a murine dermatitis model, topically applied FICZ activated AHR and significantly reduced the dermatitis score and histological inflammation with a decrease of *Il22* gene expression in chronic mite antigen-induced dermatitis [58]. In addition, topical FICZ restored the dermatitis-induced filaggrin downregulation [58]. CCL17 and CCL22 are crucial chemokines to recruit Th2 cells [68]. IL-4/IL-13 stimulates dendritic cells to produce CCL17 and CCL22 via STAT6 activation and contributes to the recruitment of Th2 cells in the lesional skin of AD [68]. Soybean tar Glyteer inhibits the IL-4/IL-13-mediated STAT6 activation and subsequent production of CCL17 and CCL22 in dendritic cells [68]. In addition, pruritogenic Th2 cytokine IL-31 synergistically upregulates the IL-4/IL-13-mediated CCL17 and CCL22 production in dendritic cells because IL-4/IL-13 increase IL-31 receptor A (IL31RA) expression [105]. Glyteer again attenuates the IL-4/IL-13-mediated IL31RA upregulation and subsequent CCL17 and CCL22 production by inhibiting STAT6 activation [105]. It is known that coal tar inhibits STAT6 activation via the NRF2-antioxidative pathway [15]. Ligation of AHR by FICZ also reduces the expression of type 1 IgE Fc receptor in Langerhans cells [106].

Although antioxidative AHR ligands are therapeutic for dermatitis, exaggerated activation of AHR by genetic manipulation in transgenic mice or by dioxin treatment induces itchy dermatitis most likely due to an abnormally accelerated keratinization process, epidermal acanthosis, elongation of nerve fibers, and production of pruritogenic artemin [47,99,107]. Therefore, extreme activation of AHR is deleterious for skin. In parallel, ovalbumin-induced delayed hypersensitivity is enhanced by topical benzopyrene with upregulation of IL-5, IL-13, and IL-17 expression in lymph node cells [96].

Since FICZ is an endogenous UVB photoproduct [8], the barrier-protecting effects of FICZ may explain, at least in part, why UVB phototherapy is efficacious for the treatment of AD and psoriasis [108,109].

6. AHR and Psoriasis

Psoriasis is an (auto)immune-mediated disease that manifests as widespread desquamative erythema [110,111]. Males are twice as likely to be affected than females [112,113]. The cosmetic disfigurement associated with psoriasis profoundly impairs the patients' quality of life, treatment satisfaction and adherence, and socioeconomic stability [114,115]. The autoimmune nature of psoriasis is exemplified by its high comorbidity with psoriatic arthritis [110,116–118] and other autoimmune diseases including autoimmune bullous diseases [119–124]. Psoriasis is also comorbid with cardiovascular diseases, metabolic diseases, and renal disorders, which represent a condition called inflammatory skin march [111,125–129]. The excellent therapeutic efficacy of anti-TNF-α/IL-23/IL-17A biologics for psoriasis point to the central role of the TNF-α/IL-23/IL-17A axis in its pathogenesis [18,19,130–134] Additionally, genetic and environmental factors are known to be involved in its pathogenesis [135,136].

As AHR predominantly regulates the immune balance of Th17/22 and Treg cells [28,29,69,70], AHR is expected to play a significant role in psoriasis [102]. In an imiquimod-induced psoriasis model, AhR deficiency exacerbates skin inflammation with upregulated gene expression of Il22, Il17a, and Il23 [137]. The intensity of delayed type-hypersensitivity is also enhanced in Ahr-deficient mice [137]. However, further experiments demonstrated that Ahr-deficiency in nonhematopoietic cells, including keratinocytes, but not in hematopoietic cells, was likely responsible for the exacerbation of inflammation [137]. Notably, intraperitoneal injection of FICZ ameliorated the imiquimod-induced psoriasis-like inflammation. Tapinarof and FICZ also reduced the imiquimod-induced psoriasiform skin inflammation by inhibiting Il17a, Il17f, Il19, Il22, Il23a, and Il1b gene expression [102]. The therapeutic action of tapinarof and FICZ was AHR-dependent because it was not observed in Ahr-deficient mice [102]. In an ex vivo activation assay of skin-resident immunocompetent cells using normal human skin, tapinarof inhibited the expression of IL17A message approximately 50% but increased the IL22 expression [102,138] (Figure 1). In mice, IL-22 is produced from Th17, γδT, ILC3, and CD4$^-$CD8$^-$TCRβ$^+$ cells [139]. AHR was required for IL-22 production by Th17, but not by the three other cell types, in the imiquimod-treated ears [139]. Although imiquimod-induced skin inflammation is popular as a psoriasis model, attention should be paid because imiquimod is degraded by CYP1A1 so the efficacy of AHR agonists may partly rely on this effect in the imiquimod model [140].

Immunohistological and real time PCR studies have demonstrated that the expression of AHR and ARNT is upregulated in the lesional skin of psoriasis, whereas CYP1A1 expression was significantly decreased compared to normal controls [97]. In contrast, serum levels of both AHR and CYP1A1 are elevated in patients with psoriasis compared to normal controls [141]. Further studies are warranted to investigate these controversial data.

In parallel with its preclinical studies, topical tapinarof is efficacious in the treatment of psoriasis. In a randomized, double-blind, placebo-controlled phase II trial, 61 patients with 1–10% BSA covered with plaque psoriasis and a PGA of 2–4 were randomized (2:1) to receive either 1% tapinarof cream or placebo, applied twice daily for 12 weeks [142]. At week 12, the improvement in PGA was 62.8% for patients treated with tapinarof compared with 13.0% for patients randomized to placebo ($p < 0.0001$). The proportion of patients who achieved a PGA of clear or almost clear was significantly higher with tapinarof treatment (67.5%) compared with placebo (4.8%, $p < 0.0001$) [142]. In another double-blind, vehicle-controlled, randomized six-arm trial (1:1:1:1:1:1) in adults with psoriasis with body surface involvement ≥ 1% and ≤ 15% and PGA score ≥ 2 at baseline, treatment success defined by PGA 0 or 1 and a two-grade improvement at week 12 was significantly higher in the tapinarof groups (65% (1% twice daily), 56% (1% once daily), 46% (0.5% twice daily), and 36% (0.5% once daily)) than vehicle groups (11% (twice daily) and 5% (once daily)); this was maintained for four weeks post-treatment [22]. The most commonly (≥5%) reported adverse events that emerged after treatment were folliculitis (19/152, 13% tapinarof groups and 1/75, 1% vehicle groups) and contact dermatitis (12/152, 8% only in the tapinarof groups) [22]. These preclinical and clinical studies reinforce that AHR ligand tapinarof is efficacious in the treatment of psoriasis and atopic dermatitis. In 2019, tapinarof (1% benvitimod cream) was officially approved by the Chinese government for medical use for psoriasis after successful Chinese clinical trials [103]. Overall, why topical and systemic AHR ligands reduce psoriatic inflammation by inhibiting IL-17 and IL-22 in vivo while the same ligands upregulate the expression of IL-17 and IL-22 in vitro is still unknown.

7. Conclusions

Humans empirically utilize natural antioxidative resources to keep their skin healthy, including coal tar, *Galactomyces* fermentation filtrate, *Opuntia ficus-indica* in Latin America, Artichoke in Mediterranean regions, and *Houttuynia cordata* and *Artemisia princeps* in Asia [12,13,15,37,38,62]. These agents are potent AHR ligands which activate the AHR-ARNT system and enhance the terminal differentiation of epidermal keratinocytes [12,13,15,37,38,62]. They also exert antioxidative action via AHR-NRF2 activation [12,13,15,37,38]. The study of the signal transduction mechanisms of the AHR/ARNT system has demonstrated that this system is also deeply involved in immune regulation especially in Th17/22 and Treg maturation [28,29]. A selective AHR agonist, tapinarof is currently being studied because this medicinal agent improves both psoriasis and AD in which different pathomechanisms operate (the TNF-α/IL-23/IL-17 axis in psoriasis and IL-4/IL-13 signaling in AD). Further mechanistic approaches are warranted to develop new drugs targeting the AHR system.

Author Contributions: M.F. wrote the first draft. A.H.-H. and G.T. reviewed the draft. M.F. finalized the article, and all authors approved the submission of the article.

References

1. Furue, K.; Mitoma, C.; Tsuji, G.; Furue, M. Protective role of peroxisome proliferator-activated receptor α agonists in skin barrier and inflammation. *Immunobiology* **2018**, *223*, 327–330. [CrossRef] [PubMed]

2. Furue, M.; Fuyuno, Y.; Mitoma, C.; Uchi, H.; Tsuji, G. Therapeutic agents with AHR inhibiting and NRF2 activating activity for managing chloracne. *Antioxidants (Basel)* **2018**, *7*, 90. [CrossRef]

3. Furue, M.; Hashimoto-Hachiya, A.; Tsuji, G. Antioxidative phytochemicals accelerate epidermal terminal differentiation via the AHR-OVOL1 pathway: Implications for atopic dermatitis. *Acta Derm. Venereol.* **2018**, *98*, 918–923. [CrossRef] [PubMed]

4. Omiecinski, C.J.; Vanden Heuvel, J.P.; Perdew, G.H.; Peters, J.M. Xenobiotic metabolism, disposition, and regulation by receptors: From biochemical phenomenon to predictors of major toxicities. *Toxicol. Sci.* **2011**, *120*, S49–S75. [CrossRef] [PubMed]

5. Esser, C.; Bargen, I.; Weighardt, H.; Haarmann-Stemmann, T.; Krutmann, J. Functions of the aryl 1002 hydrocarbon receptor in the skin. *Semin. Immunopathol.* **2013**, *35*, 677–691. [CrossRef]

6. Furue, M.; Takahara, M.; Nakahara, T.; Uchi, H. Role of AhR/ARNT system in skin homeostasis. *Arch. Dermatol. Res.* **2014**, *306*, 769–779. [CrossRef]

7. Mimura, J.; Fujii-Kuriyama, Y. Functional role of AhR in the expression of toxic effects by TCDD. *Biochim. Biophys. Acta* **2003**, *1619*, 263–268. [CrossRef]

8. Fritsche, E.; Schäfer, C.; Calles, C.; Bernsmann, T.; Bernshausen, T.; Wurm, M.; Hübenthal, U.; Cline, J.E.; Hajimiragha, H.; Schroeder, P.; et al. Lightening up the UV response by identification of the aryl hydrocarbon receptor as a cytoplasmatic target for ultraviolet B radiation. *Proc. Natl. Acad. Sci. USA* **2007**, *104*, 8851–8856. [CrossRef]

9. Rannug, A.; Rannug, U.; Rosenkranz, H.S.; Winqvist, L.; Westerholm, R.; Agurell, E.; Grafström, A.K. Certain photooxidized derivatives of tryptophan bind with very high affinity to the Ah receptor and are likely to be endogenous signal substances. *J. Biol. Chem.* **1987**, *262*, 15422–15427.

10. Furue, M.; Uchi, H.; Mitoma, C.; Hashimoto-Hachiya, A.; Chiba, T.; Ito, T.; Nakahara, T.; Tsuji, G. Antioxidants for healthy skin: The emerging role of aryl hydrocarbon receptors and nuclear factor-erythroid 2-related factor-2. *Nutrients* **2017**, *9*, 223. [CrossRef]

11. Magiatis, P.; Pappas, P.; Gaitanis, G.; Mexia, N.; Melliou, E.; Galanou, M.; Vlachos, C.; Stathopoulou, K.; Skaltsounis, A.L.; Marselos, M.; et al. Malassezia yeasts produce a collection of exceptionally potent activators of the Ah (dioxin) receptor detected in diseased human skin. *J. Investig. Dermatol.* **2013**, *133*, 2023–2030. [CrossRef] [PubMed]

12. Takei, K.; Mitoma, C.; Hashimoto-Hachiya, A.; Takahara, M.; Tsuji, G.; Nakahara, T.; Furue, M. Galactomyces fermentation filtrate prevents T helper 2-mediated reduction of filaggrin in an aryl hydrocarbon receptor-dependent manner. *Clin. Exp. Dermatol.* **2015**, *40*, 786–793. [CrossRef] [PubMed]

13. Takei, K.; Hashimoto-Hachiya, A.; Takahara, M.; Tsuji, G.; Nakahara, T.; Furue, M. Cynaropicrin attenuates UVB-induced oxidative stress via the AhR-Nrf2-Nqo1 pathway. *Toxicol. Lett.* **2015**, *234*, 74–80. [CrossRef] [PubMed]

14. Takei, K.; Mitoma, C.; Hashimoto-Hachiya, A.; Uchi, H.; Takahara, M.; Tsuji, G.; Kido-Nakahara, M.; Nakahara, T.; Furue, M. Antioxidant soybean tar Glyteer rescues T-helper-mediated downregulation of filaggrin expression via aryl hydrocarbon receptor. *J. Dermatol.* **2015**, *42*, 171–180. [CrossRef]

15. Van den Bogaard, E.H.; Bergboer, J.G.; Vonk-Bergers, M.; van Vlijmen-Willems, I.M.; Hato, S.V.; van der Valk, P.G.; Schröder, J.M.; Joosten, I.; Zeeuwen, P.L.; Schalkwijk, J. Coal tar induces AHR-dependent skin barrier repair in atopic dermatitis. *J. Clin. Investig.* **2013**, *123*, 917–927. [CrossRef]

16. Simpson, E.L.; Bieber, T.; Guttman-Yassky, E.; Beck, L.A.; Blauvelt, A.; Cork, M.J.; Silverberg, J.I.; Deleuran, M.; Kataoka, Y.; Lacour, J.P.; et al. Two Phase 3 Trials of dupilumab versus placebo in atopic dermatitis. *N. Engl. J. Med.* **2016**, *375*, 2335–2348. [CrossRef]

17. Furue, M.; Ulzii, D.; Vu, Y.H.; Tsuji, G.; Kido-Nakahara, M.; Nakahara, T. Pathogenesis of atopic dermatitis: Current paradigm. *Iran. J. Immunol.* **2019**, *16*, 97–107.

18. Furue, K.; Ito, T.; Furue, M. Differential efficacy of biologic treatments targeting the TNF-α/IL-23/IL-17 axis in psoriasis and psoriatic arthritis. *Cytokine* **2018**, *111*, 182–188. [CrossRef]

19. Furue, K.; Ito, T.; Tsuji, G.; Kadono, T.; Furue, M. Psoriasis and the TNF/IL23/IL17 axis. *G. Ital. Dermatol. Venereol.* **2019**, *154*, 418–424. [CrossRef]

20. Tsoi, L.C.; Rodriguez, E.; Degenhardt, F.; Baurecht, H.; Wehkamp, U.; Volks, N.; Szymczak, S.; Swindell, W.R.; Sarkar, M.K.; Raja, K.; et al. Atopic dermatitis is an IL-13-dominant disease with greater molecular heterogeneity compared to psoriasis. *J. Investig. Dermatol.* **2019**, *139*, 1480–1489. [CrossRef]

21. Peppers, J.; Paller, A.S.; Maeda-Chubachi, T.; Wu, S.; Robbins, K.; Gallagher, K.; Kraus, J.E. A phase 2, randomized dose-finding study of tapinarof (GSK2894512 cream) for the treatment of atopic dermatitis. *J. Am. Acad. Dermatol.* **2019**, *80*, 89–98. [CrossRef] [PubMed]

22. Robbins, K.; Bissonnette, R.; Maeda-Chubachi, T.; Ye, L.; Peppers, J.; Gallagher, K.; Kraus, J.E. Phase 2, randomized dose-finding study of tapinarof (GSK2894512 cream) for the treatment of plaque psoriasis. *J. Am. Acad. Dermatol.* **2019**, *80*, 714–721. [CrossRef] [PubMed]

23. Kazlauskas, A.; Sundström, S.; Poellinger, L.; Pongratz, I. The hsp90 chaperone complex regulates intracellular localization of the dioxin receptor. *Mol. Cell. Biol.* **2001**, *21*, 2594–2607. [CrossRef] [PubMed]

24. Lees, M.J.; Peet, D.J.; Whitelaw, M.L. Defining the role for XAP2 in stabilization of the dioxin receptor. *J. Biol. Chem.* **2003**, *278*, 35878–35888. [CrossRef]

25. Hayes, J.D.; McMahon, M. Molecular basis for the contribution of the antioxidant responsive element to cancer chemoprevention. *Cancer Lett.* **2001**, *174*, 103–113. [CrossRef]

26. Miao, W.; Hu, L.; Scrivens, P.J.; Batist, G. Transcriptional regulation of NF-E2 p45-related factor (NRF2) expression by the aryl hydrocarbon receptor-xenobiotic response element signaling pathway: Direct cross-talk between phase I and II drug-metabolizing enzymes. *J. Biol. Chem.* **2005**, *280*, 20340–20348. [CrossRef]

27. Esser, C.; Rannug, A. The aryl hydrocarbon receptor in barrier organ physiology, immunology, and toxicology. *Pharmacol. Rev.* **2015**, *67*, 259–279. [CrossRef]

28. Esser, C. The aryl hydrocarbon receptor in immunity: Tools and potential. *Methods Mol. Biol.* **2016**, *1371*, 239–257.

29. Stockinger, B.; Di Meglio, P.; Gialitakis, M.; Duarte, J.H. The aryl hydrocarbon receptor: Multitasking in the immune system. *Annu. Rev. Immunol.* **2014**, *32*, 403–432. [CrossRef]

30. Kopf, P.G.; Walker, M.K. 2,3,7,8-tetrachlorodibenzo-p-dioxin increases reactive oxygen species production in human endothelial cells via induction of cytochrome P4501A. *Toxicol. Appl. Pharmacol.* **2010**, *245*, 91–99. [CrossRef]

31. Denison, M.S.; Soshilov, A.A.; He, G.; DeGroot, D.E.; Zhao, B. Exactly the same but different: Promiscuity and diversity in the molecular mechanisms of action of the aryl hydrocarbon (dioxin) receptor. *Toxicol. Sci.* **2011**, *124*, 1–22. [CrossRef] [PubMed]

32. Baron, J.M.; Höller, D.; Schiffer, R.; Frankenberg, S.; Neis, M.; Merk, H.F.; Jugert, F.K. Expression of multiple cytochrome p450 enzymes and multidrug resistance-associated transport proteins in human skin keratinocytes. *J. Investig. Dermatol.* **2001**, *116*, 541–548. [CrossRef] [PubMed]

33. Inui, H.; Itoh, T.; Yamamoto, K.; Ikushiro, S.; Sakaki, T. Mammalian cytochrome P450-dependent metabolism of polychlorinated dibenzo-p-dioxins and coplanar polychlorinated biphenyls. *Int. J. Mol. Sci.* **2014**, *15*, 14044–14057. [CrossRef] [PubMed]

34. Anandasadagopan, S.K.; Singh, N.M.; Raza, H.; Bansal, S.; Selvaraj, V.; Singh, S.; Chowdhury, A.R.; Leu, N.A.; Avadhani, N.G. β-Naphthoflavone-induced mitochondrial respiratory damage in Cyp1 knockout mouse and in cell culture systems: Attenuation by resveratrol treatment. *Oxid. Med. Cell Longev.* **2017**, *2017*, 5213186. [CrossRef]

35. Tanaka, Y.; Uchi, H.; Hashimoto-Hachiya, A.; Furue, M. Tryptophan photoproduct FICZ upregulates IL1A, IL1B, and IL6 expression via oxidative stress in keratinocytes. *Oxid. Med. Cell. Longev.* **2018**, *2018*, 9298052. [CrossRef]

36. Tsuji, G.; Takahara, M.; Uchi, H.; Takeuchi, S.; Mitoma, C.; Moroi, Y.; Furue, M. An environmental contaminant, benzo(a)pyrene, induces oxidative stress-mediated interleukin-8 production in human keratinocytes via the aryl hydrocarbon receptor signaling pathway. *J. Dermatol. Sci.* **2011**, *62*, 42–49. [CrossRef]

37. Nakahara, T.; Mitoma, C.; Hashimoto-Hachiya, A.; Takahara, M.; Tsuji, G.; Uchi, H.; Yan, X.; Hachisuka, J.; Chiba, T.; Esaki, H.; et al. Antioxidant *Opuntia ficus-indica* extract activates AHR-NRF2 signaling and upregulates filaggrin and loricrin expression in human keratinocytes. *J. Med. Food* **2015**, *18*, 1143–1149. [CrossRef]

38. Doi, K.; Mitoma, C.; Nakahara, T.; Uchi, H.; Hashimoto-Hachiya, A.; Takahara, M.; Tsuji, G.; Nakahara, M.; Furue, M. Antioxidant Houttuynia cordata extract upregulates filaggrin expression in an aryl hydrocarbon-dependent manner. *Fukuoka Igaku Zasshi* **2014**, *105*, 205–213.

39. Tsuji, G.; Takahara, M.; Uchi, H.; Matsuda, T.; Chiba, T.; Takeuchi, S.; Yasukawa, F.; Moroi, Y.; Furue, M. Identification of ketoconazole as an AhR-Nrf2 activator in cultured human keratinocytes: The basis of its anti-inflammatory effect. *J. Investig. Dermatol.* **2012**, *132*, 59–68. [CrossRef]

40. Yeager, R.L.; Reisman, S.A.; Aleksunes, L.M.; Klaassen, C.D. Introducing the "TCDD-inducible AhR-Nrf2 gene battery". *Toxicol. Sci.* **2009**, *111*, 238–246. [CrossRef]

41. Wang, K.; Lv, Q.; Miao, Y.M.; Qiao, S.M.; Dai, Y.; Wei, Z.F. Cardamonin, a natural flavone, alleviates inflammatory bowel disease by the inhibition of NLRP3 inflammasome activation via an AhR/Nrf2/NQO1 pathway. *Biochem. Pharmacol.* **2018**, *155*, 494–509. [CrossRef] [PubMed]

42. Ma, Q.; Kinneer, K.; Bi, Y.; Chan, J.Y.; Kan, Y.W. Induction of murine NAD(P)H:quinone oxidoreductase by 2,3,7,8-tetrachlorodibenzo-p-dioxin requires the CNC (cap 'n' collar) basic leucine zipper transcription factor Nrf2 (nuclear factor erythroid 2-related factor 2): Cross-interaction between AhR (aryl hydrocarbon receptor) and Nrf2 signal transduction. *Biochem. J.* **2004**, *377*, 205–213. [PubMed]

43. Noda, S.; Harada, N.; Hida, A.; Fujii-Kuriyama, Y.; Motohashi, H.; Yamamoto, M. Gene expression of detoxifying enzymes in AhR and Nrf2 compound null mutant mouse. *Biochem. Biophys. Res. Commun.* **2003**, *303*, 105–111. [CrossRef]

44. Furue, M.; Tsuji, G.; Mitoma, C.; Nakahara, T.; Chiba, T.; Morino-Koga, S.; Uchi, H. Gene regulation of filaggrin and other skin barrier proteins via aryl hydrocarbon receptor. *J. Dermatol. Sci.* **2015**, *80*, 83–88. [CrossRef] [PubMed]

45. Kypriotou, M.; Huber, M.; Hohl, D. The human epidermal differentiation complex: Cornified envelope precursors, S100 proteins and the 'fused genes' family. *Exp. Dermatol.* **2012**, *21*, 643–649. [CrossRef] [PubMed]

46. Loertscher, J.A.; Lin, T.M.; Peterson, R.E.; Allen-Hoffmann, B.L. In utero exposure to 2,3,7,8-tetrachlorodibenzo-p-dioxin causes accelerated terminal differentiation in fetal mouse skin. *Toxicol. Sci.* **2002**, *68*, 465–472. [CrossRef]

47. Kennedy, L.H.; Sutter, C.H.; Leon Carrion, S.; Tran, Q.T.; Bodreddigari, S.; Kensicki, E.; Mohney, R.P.; Sutter, T.R. 2,3,7,8-Tetrachlorodibenzo-p-dioxin-mediated production of reactive oxygen species is an essential step in the mechanism of action to accelerate human keratinocyte differentiation. *Toxicol. Sci.* **2013**, *132*, 235–249. [CrossRef]

48. Sutter, C.H.; Bodreddigari, S.; Campion, C.; Wible, R.S.; Sutter, T.R. 2,3,7,8-Tetrachlorodibenzo-p-dioxin increases the expression of genes in the human epidermal differentiation complex and accelerates epidermal barrier formation. *Toxicol. Sci.* **2011**, *124*, 128–137. [CrossRef]

49. Fernandez-Salguero, P.M.; Ward, J.M.; Sundberg, J.P.; Gonzalez, F.J. Lesions of aryl-hydrocarbon receptor-deficient mice. *Vet. Pathol.* **1997**, *34*, 605–614. [CrossRef]

50. Tauchi, M.; Hida, A.; Negishi, T.; Katsuoka, F.; Noda, S.; Mimura, J.; Hosoya, T.; Yanaka, A.; Aburatani, H.; Fujii-Kuriyama, Y.; et al. Constitutive expression of aryl hydrocarbon receptor in keratinocytes causes inflammatory skin lesions. *Mol. Cell. Biol.* **2005**, *25*, 9360–9368. [CrossRef]

51. Geng, S.; Mezentsev, A.; Kalachikov, S.; Raith, K.; Roop, D.R.; Panteleyev, A.A. Targeted ablation of Arnt in mouse epidermis results in profound defects in desquamation and epidermal barrier function. *J. Cell Sci.* **2006**, *119*, 4901–4912. [CrossRef] [PubMed]

52. Takagi, S.; Tojo, H.; Tomita, S.; Sano, S.; Itami, S.; Hara, M.; Inoue, S.; Horie, K.; Kondoh, G.; Hosokawa, K.; et al. Alteration of the 4-sphingenine scaffolds of ceramides in keratinocyte-specific Arnt-deficient mice affects skin barrier function. *J. Clin. Investig.* **2003**, *112*, 1372–1382. [CrossRef]

53. Ju, Q.; Fimmel, S.; Hinz, N.; Stahlmann, R.; Xia, L.; Zouboulis, C.C. 2,3,7,8-Tetrachlorodibenzo-p-dioxin alters sebaceous gland cell differentiation in vitro. *Exp. Dermatol.* **2011**, *20*, 320–325. [CrossRef] [PubMed]

54. Lin, Y.K.; Leu, Y.L.; Yang, S.H.; Chen, H.W.; Wang, C.T.; Pang, J.H. Anti-psoriatic effects of indigo naturalis on the proliferation and differentiation of keratinocytes with indirubin as the active component. *J. Dermatol. Sci.* **2009**, *54*, 168–174. [CrossRef] [PubMed]

55. Rannug, A.; Rannug, U. The tryptophan derivative 6-formylindolo[3,2-b]carbazole, FICZ, a dynamic mediator of endogenous aryl hydrocarbon receptor signaling, balances cell growth and differentiation. *Crit. Rev. Toxicol.* **2018**, *48*, 555–574. [CrossRef]

56. Wincent, E.; Amini, N.; Luecke, S.; Glatt, H.; Bergman, J.; Crescenzi, C.; Rannug, A.; Rannug, U. The suggested physiologic aryl hydrocarbon receptor activator and cytochrome P4501 substrate 6-formylindolo[3,2-b]carbazole is present in humans. *J. Biol. Chem.* **2009**, *284*, 2690–2696. [CrossRef]

57. Furue, M.; Uchi, H.; Mitoma, C.; Hashimoto-Hachiya, A.; Tanaka, Y.; Ito, T.; Tsuji, G. Implications of tryptophan photoproduct FICZ in oxidative stress and terminal differentiation of keratinocytes. *G. Ital. Dermatol. Venereol.* **2019**, *154*, 37–41. [CrossRef]

58. Kiyomatsu-Oda, M.; Uchi, H.; Morino-Koga, S.; Furue, M. Protective role of 6-formylindolo[3,2-b]carbazole (FICZ), an endogenous ligand for arylhydrocarbon receptor, in chronic mite-induced dermatitis. *J. Dermatol. Sci.* **2018**, *90*, 284–294. [CrossRef]

59. Tsuji, G.; Ito, T.; Chiba, T.; Mitoma, C.; Nakahara, T.; Uchi, H.; Furue, M. The role of the OVOL1-OVOL2 axis in normal and diseased human skin. *J. Dermatol. Sci.* **2018**, *90*, 227–231. [CrossRef]

60. Hong, S.P.; Kim, M.J.; Jung, M.Y.; Jeon, H.; Goo, J.; Ahn, S.K.; Lee, S.H.; Elias, P.M.; Choi, E.H. Biopositive effects of low-dose UVB on epidermis: Coordinate upregulation of antimicrobial peptides and permeability barrier reinforcement. *J. Investig. Dermatol.* **2008**, *128*, 2880–2887. [CrossRef]

61. Tsuji, G.; Hashimoto-Hachiya, A.; Kiyomatsu-Oda, M.; Takemura, M.; Ohno, F.; Ito, T.; Morino-Koga, S.; Mitoma, C.; Nakahara, T.; Uchi, H.; et al. Aryl hydrocarbon receptor activation restores filaggrin expression via OVOL1 in atopic dermatitis. *Cell Death Dis.* **2017**, *8*, e2931. [CrossRef]

62. Hirano, A.; Goto, M.; Mitsui, T.; Hashimoto-Hachiya, A.; Tsuji, G.; Furue, M. Antioxidant *Artemisia princeps* extract enhances the expression of filaggrin and loricrin via the AHR/OVOL1 pathway. *Int. J. Mol. Sci.* **2017**, *18*, 1948. [CrossRef]

63. Hashimoto-Hachiya, A.; Tsuji, G.; Murai, M.; Yan, X.; Furue, M. Upregulation of FLG, LOR, and IVL expression by *Rhodiola crenulata* root extract via aryl hydrocarbon receptor: Differential involvement of OVOL. *Int. J. Mol. Sci.* **2018**, *19*, 1654. [CrossRef]

64. Van den Bogaard, E.H.; Podolsky, M.A.; Smits, J.P.; Cui, X.; John, C.; Gowda, K.; Desai, D.; Amin, S.G.; Schalkwijk, J.; Perdew, G.H.; et al. Genetic and pharmacological analysis identifies a physiological role for the AHR in epidermal differentiation. *J. Investig. Dermatol.* **2015**, *135*, 1320–1328. [CrossRef]

65. Zhang, W.; Sakai, T.; Matsuda-Hirose, H.; Goto, M.; Yamate, T.; Hatano, Y. Cutaneous permeability barrier function in signal transducer and activator of transcription 6-deficient mice is superior to that in wild-type mice. *J. Dermatol. Sci.* **2018**, *92*, 54–61. [CrossRef]

66. Tanaka, G.; Kanaji, S.; Hirano, A.; Arima, K.; Shinagawa, A.; Goda, C.; Yasunaga, S.; Ikizawa, K.; Yanagihara, Y.; Kubo, M.; et al. Induction and activation of the aryl hydrocarbon receptor by IL-4 in B cells. *Int. Immunol.* **2005**, *17*, 797–805. [CrossRef]

67. Mitamura, Y.; Nunomura, S.; Nanri, Y.; Ogawa, M.; Yoshihara, T.; Masuoka, M.; Tsuji, G.; Nakahara, T.; Hashimoto-Hachiya, A.; Conway, S.J.; et al. The IL-13/periostin/IL-24 pathway causes epidermal barrier dysfunction in allergic skin inflammation. *Allergy* **2018**, *73*, 1881–1891. [CrossRef] [PubMed]

68. Takemura, M.; Nakahara, T.; Hashimoto-Hachiya, A.; Furue, M.; Tsuji, G. Glyteer, soybean tar, impairs IL-4/Stat6 signaling in murine bone marrow-derived dendritic cells: The basis of its therapeutic effect on atopic dermatitis. *Int. J. Mol. Sci.* **2018**, *19*, 1169. [CrossRef]

69. Schiering, C.; Vonk, A.; Das, S.; Stockinger, B.; Wincent, E. Cytochrome P4501-inhibiting chemicals amplify aryl hydrocarbon receptor activation and IL-22 production in T helper 17 cells. *Biochem. Pharmacol.* **2018**, *151*, 47–58. [CrossRef] [PubMed]

70. Ye, J.; Qiu, J.; Bostick, J.W.; Ueda, A.; Schjerven, H.; Li, S.; Jobin, C.; Chen, Z.E.; Zhou, L. The aryl hydrocarbon receptor preferentially marks and promotes gut regulatory T cells. *Cell Rep.* **2017**, *21*, 2277–2290. [CrossRef] [PubMed]

71. Kiss, E.A.; Vonarbourg, C.; Kopfmann, S.; Hobeika, E.; Finke, D.; Esser, C.; Diefenbach, A. Natural aryl hydrocarbon receptor ligands control organogenesis of intestinal lymphoid follicles. *Science* **2011**, *334*, 1561–1565. [CrossRef] [PubMed]

72. Lee, J.S.; Cella, M.; McDonald, K.G.; Garlanda, C.; Kennedy, G.D.; Nukaya, M.; Mantovani, A.; Kopan, R.; Bradfield, C.A.; Newberry, R.D.; et al. AHR drives the development of gut ILC22 cells and postnatal lymphoid tissues via pathways dependent on and independent of Notch. *Nat. Immunol.* **2011**, *13*, 144–151. [CrossRef] [PubMed]

73. Qiu, J.; Heller, J.J.; Guo, X.; Chen, Z.M.; Fish, K.; Fu, Y.X.; Zhou, L. The aryl hydrocarbon receptor regulates gut immunity through modulation of innate lymphoid cells. *Immunity* **2012**, *36*, 92–104. [CrossRef] [PubMed]

74. Liu, J.Z.; van Sommeren, S.; Huang, H.; Ng, S.C.; Alberts, R.; Takahashi, A.; Ripke, S.; Lee, J.C.; Jostins, L.; Shah, T.; et al. Association analyses identify 38 susceptibility loci for inflammatory bowel disease and highlight shared genetic risk across populations. *Nat. Genet.* **2015**, *47*, 979–986. [CrossRef]

75. Monteleone, I.; Rizzo, A.; Sarra, M.; Sica, G.; Sileri, P.; Biancone, L.; MacDonald, T.T.; Pallone, F.; Monteleone, G. Aryl hydrocarbon receptor-induced signals up-regulate IL-22 production and inhibit inflammation in the gastrointestinal tract. *Gastroenterology* **2011**, *141*, 237–248. [CrossRef]

76. Schiering, C.; Wincent, E.; Metidji, A.; Iseppon, A.; Li, Y.; Potocnik, A.J.; Omenetti, S.; Henderson, C.J.; Wolf, C.R.; Nebert, D.W.; et al. Feedback control of AHR signalling regulates intestinal immunity. *Nature* **2017**, *542*, 242–245. [CrossRef]

77. Holsapple, M.P.; Morris, D.L.; Wood, S.C.; Snyder, N.K. 2,3,7,8-tetrachlorodibenzo-p-dioxin-induced changes in immunocompetence: Possible mechanisms. *Annu. Rev. Pharmacol. Toxicol.* **1991**, *31*, 73–100. [CrossRef]

78. Veldhoen, M.; Hirota, K.; Westendorf, A.M.; Buer, J.; Dumoutier, L.; Renauld, J.C.; Stockinger, B. The aryl hydrocarbon receptor links TH17-cell-mediated autoimmunity to environmental toxins. *Nature* **2008**, *453*, 106–109. [CrossRef]

79. Funatake, C.J.; Marshall, N.B.; Steppan, L.B.; Mourich, D.V.; Kerkvliet, N.I. Cutting edge: Activation of the aryl hydrocarbon receptor by 2,3,7,8-tetrachlorodibenzo-p-dioxin generates a population of CD4+ CD25+ cells with characteristics of regulatory T cells. *J. Immunol.* **2005**, *175*, 4184–4188. [CrossRef]

80. Qiu, J.; Guo, X.; Chen, Z.M.; He, L.; Sonnenberg, G.F.; Artis, D.; Fu, Y.X.; Zhou, L. Group 3 innate lymphoid cells inhibit T-cell-mediated intestinal inflammation through aryl hydrocarbon receptor signaling and regulation of microflora. *Immunity* **2013**, *39*, 386–399. [CrossRef]

81. Ehrlich, A.K.; Pennington, J.M.; Bisson, W.H.; Kolluri, S.K.; Kerkvliet, N.I. TCDD, FICZ, and other high affinity AhR ligands dose-dependently determine the fate of CD4+ T cell differentiation. *Toxicol. Sci.* **2018**, *161*, 310–320. [CrossRef] [PubMed]

82. Furue, M.; Chiba, T.; Tsuji, G.; Ulzii, D.; Kido-Nakahara, M.; Nakahara, T.; Kadono, T. Atopic dermatitis: Immune deviation, barrier dysfunction, IgE autoreactivity and new therapies. *Allergol. Int.* **2017**, *66*, 398–403. [CrossRef] [PubMed]

83. Seo, E.; Yoon, J.; Jung, S.; Lee, J.; Lee, B.H.; Yu, J. Phenotypes of atopic dermatitis identified by cluster analysis in early childhood. *J. Dermatol.* **2019**, *46*, 117–123. [CrossRef]

84. Arima, K.; Gupta, S.; Gadkari, A.; Hiragun, T.; Kono, T.; Katayama, I.; Demiya, S.; Eckert, L. Burden of atopic dermatitis in Japanese adults: Analysis of data from the 2013 National Health and Wellness Survey. *J. Dermatol.* **2018**, *45*, 390–396. [CrossRef]

85. Igarashi, A.; Fujita, H.; Arima, K.; Inoue, T.; Dorey, J.; Fukushima, A.; Taguchi, Y. Health-care resource use and current treatment of adult atopic dermatitis patients in Japan: A retrospective claims database analysis. *J. Dermatol.* **2019**, *46*, 652–661. [CrossRef]

86. Jung, H.J.; Bae, J.Y.; Kim, J.E.; Na, C.H.; Park, G.H.; Bae, Y.I.; Shin, M.K.; Lee, Y.B.; Lee, U.H.; Jang, Y.H.; et al. Survey of disease awareness, treatment behavior and treatment satisfaction in patients with atopic dermatitis in Korea: A multicenter study. *J. Dermatol.* **2018**, *45*, 1172–1180. [CrossRef]

87. Komura, Y.; Kogure, T.; Kawahara, K.; Yokozeki, H. Economic assessment of actual prescription of drugs for treatment of atopic dermatitis: Differences between dermatology and pediatrics in large-scale receipt data. *J. Dermatol.* **2018**, *45*, 165–174. [CrossRef]

88. Takeuchi, S.; Oba, J.; Esaki, H.; Furue, M. Non-corticosteroid adherence and itch severity influence perception of itch in atopic dermatitis. *J. Dermatol.* **2018**, *45*, 158–164. [CrossRef]

89. Williams, H.; Stewart, A.; von Mutius, E.; Cookson, W.; Anderson, H.R. Is eczema really on the increase worldwide? *J. Allergy Clin. Immunol.* **2008**, *121*, 947–954. [CrossRef] [PubMed]

90. Furue, M.; Iida, K.; Imaji, M.; Nakahara, T. Microbiome analysis of forehead skin in patients with atopic dermatitis and healthy subjects: Implication of *Staphylococcus* and *Corynebacterium*. *J. Dermatol.* **2018**, *45*, 876–877. [CrossRef]

91. Iwamoto, K.; Moriwaki, M.; Miyake, R.; Hide, M. Staphylococcus aureus in atopic dermatitis: Strain-specific cell wall proteins and skin immunity. *Allergol. Int.* **2019**, *68*, 309–315. [CrossRef] [PubMed]

92. Furue, M.; Kadono, T. "Inflammatory skin march" in atopic dermatitis and psoriasis. *Inflamm. Res.* **2017**, *66*, 833–842. [CrossRef] [PubMed]

93. Li, Z.Z.; Zhong, W.L.; Hu, H.; Chen, X.F.; Zhang, W.; Huang, H.Y.; Yu, B.; Dou, X. Aryl hydrocarbon receptor polymorphisms are associated with dry skin phenotypes in Chinese patients with atopic dermatitis. *Clin. Exp. Dermatol.* **2019**, *44*, 613–619. [CrossRef] [PubMed]

94. Li, D.; Takao, T.; Tsunematsu, R.; Morokuma, S.; Fukushima, K.; Kobayashi, H.; Saito, T.; Furue, M.; Wake, N.; Asanoma, K. Inhibition of AHR transcription by NF1C is affected by a single-nucleotide polymorphism, and is involved in suppression of human uterine endometrial cancer. *Oncogene* **2013**, *32*, 4950–4959. [CrossRef]

95. Liu, G.; Asanoma, K.; Takao, T.; Tsukimori, K.; Uchi, H.; Furue, M.; Kato, K.; Wake, N. Aryl hydrocarbon receptor SNP -130 C/T associates with dioxins susceptibility through regulating its receptor activity and downstream effectors including interleukin. *Toxicol. Lett.* **2015**, *232*, 384–392. [CrossRef]

96. Hong, C.H.; Lee, C.H.; Yu, H.S.; Huang, S.K. Benzopyrene, a major polyaromatic hydrocarbon in smoke fume, mobilizes Langerhans cells and polarizes Th2/17 responses in epicutaneous protein sensitization through the aryl hydrocarbon receptor. *Int. Immunopharmacol.* **2016**, *36*, 111–117. [CrossRef]

97. Kim, H.O.; Kim, J.H.; Chung, B.Y.; Choi, M.G.; Park, C.W. Increased expression of the aryl hydrocarbon receptor in patients with chronic inflammatory skin diseases. *Exp. Dermatol.* **2014**, *23*, 278–281. [CrossRef] [PubMed]

98. Yu, J.; Luo, Y.; Zhu, Z.; Zhou, Y.; Sun, L.; Gao, J.; Sun, J.; Wang, G.; Yao, X.; Li, W. A tryptophan metabolite of the skin microbiota attenuates inflammation in patients with atopic dermatitis through the aryl hydrocarbon receptor. *J. Allergy Clin. Immunol.* **2019**, *143*, 2108–2119. [CrossRef] [PubMed]

99. Hidaka, T.; Ogawa, E.; Kobayashi, E.H.; Suzuki, T.; Funayama, R.; Nagashima, T.; Fujimura, T.; Aiba, S.; Nakayama, K.; Okuyama, R.; et al. The aryl hydrocarbon receptor AhR links atopic dermatitis and air pollution via induction of the neurotrophic factor artemin. *Nat. Immunol.* **2017**, *18*, 64–73. [CrossRef]

100. Bissonnette, R.; Poulin, Y.; Zhou, Y.; Tan, J.; Hong, H.C.; Webster, J.; Ip, W.; Tang, L.; Lyle, M. Efficacy and safety of topical WBI-1001 in patients with mild to severe atopic dermatitis: Results from a 12-week, multicentre, randomized, placebo-controlled double-blind trial. *Br. J. Dermatol.* **2012**, *166*, 853–860. [CrossRef]

101. Richardson, W.H.; Schmidt, T.M.; Nealson, K.H. Identification of an anthraquinone pigment and a hydroxystilbene antibiotic from Xenorhabdus luminescens. *Appl. Environ. Microbiol.* **1988**, *54*, 1602–16055.

102. Smith, S.H.; Jayawickreme, C.; Rickard, D.J.; Nicodeme, E.; Bui, T.; Simmons, C.; Coquery, C.M.; Neil, J.; Pryor, W.M.; Mayhew, D.; et al. Tapinarof is a natural AhR agonist that resolves skin inflammation in mice and humans. *J. Investig. Dermatol.* **2017**, *137*, 2110–2119. [CrossRef]

103. Zang, Y.N.; Jiang, D.L.; Cai, L.; Chen, X.; Wang, Q.; Xie, Z.W.; Liu, Y.; Zhang, C.Y.; Jing, S.; Chen, G.H.; et al. Use of a dose-response model to guide future clinical trial of Benvitimod cream to treat mild and moderate psoriasis. *Int. J. Clin. Pharmacol. Ther.* **2016**, *54*, 87–95. [CrossRef]

104. Bissonnette, R.; Vasist, L.S.; Bullman, J.N.; Collingwood, T.; Chen, G.; Maeda-Chubachi, T. Systemic pharmacokinetics, safety, and preliminary efficacy of topical AhR agonist Tapinarof: Results of a phase 1 study. *Clin. Pharmacol. Drug Dev.* **2018**, *7*, 524–531. [CrossRef]

105. Miake, S.; Tsuji, G.; Takemura, M.; Hashimoto-Hachiya, A.; Vu, Y.H.; Furue, M.; Nakahara, T. IL-4 augments IL-31/IL-31 receptor alpha interaction leading to enhanced Ccl17 and Ccl22 production in dendritic cells: Implications for atopic dermatitis. *Int. J. Mol. Sci.* **2019**, *20*, 4053. [CrossRef]

106. Koch, S.; Stroisch, T.J.; Vorac, J.; Herrmann, N.; Leib, N.; Schnautz, S.; Kirins, H.; Forster, I.; Weighardt, H.; Bieber, T. AhR mediates an anti-inflammatory feedback mechanism in human Langerhans cells involving FcεRI and IDO. *Allergy* **2017**, *72*, 1686–1693. [CrossRef]

107. Edamitsu, T.; Taguchi, K.; Kobayashi, E.H.; Okuyama, R.; Yamamoto, M. Aryl hydrocarbon receptor directly regulates artemin gene expression. *Mol. Cell Biol.* **2019**, *39*. [CrossRef]

108. Morita, A. Current developments in phototherapy for psoriasis. *J. Dermatol.* **2018**, *45*, 287–292. [CrossRef]

109. Ortiz-Salvador, J.M.; Pérez-Ferriols, A. Phototherapy in Atopic Dermatitis. *Adv. Exp. Med. Biol.* **2017**, *996*, 279–286.

110. Boehncke, W.H.; Schön, M.P. Psoriasis. *Lancet* **2015**, *386*, 983–994. [CrossRef]

111. Furue, M.; Kadono, T. The contribution of IL-17 to the development of autoimmunity in psoriasis. *Innate Immun.* **2019**, *25*, 337–343. [CrossRef]

112. Ogawa, E.; Okuyama, R.; Seki, T.; Kobayashi, A.; Oiso, N.; Muto, M.; Nakagawa, H.; Kawada, A. Epidemiological survey of patients with psoriasis in Matsumoto city, Nagano Prefecture, Japan. *J. Dermatol.* **2018**, *45*, 314–317. [CrossRef]

113. Ito, T.; Takahashi, H.; Kawada, A.; Iizuka, H.; Nakagawa, H. Epidemiological survey from 2009 to 2012 of psoriatic patients in Japanese Society for Psoriasis Research. *J. Dermatol.* **2018**, *45*, 293–301. [CrossRef]

114. Ichiyama, S.; Ito, M.; Funasaka, Y.; Abe, M.; Nishida, E.; Muramatsu, S.; Nishihara, H.; Kato, H.; Morita, A.; Imafuku, S.; et al. Assessment of medication adherence and treatment satisfaction in Japanese patients with psoriasis of various severities. *J. Dermatol.* **2018**, *45*, 727–731. [CrossRef]

115. Takahashi, H.; Satoh, K.; Takagi, A.; Iizuka, H. Cost-efficacy and pharmacoeconomics of psoriatic patients in Japan: Analysis from a single outpatient clinic. *J. Dermatol.* **2019**, *46*, 478–481. [CrossRef]

116. Komatsu-Fujii, T.; Honda, T.; Otsuka, A.; Kabashima, K. Improvement of nail lesions in a patient with psoriatic arthritis by switching the treatment from an anti-interleukin-17A antibody to an anti-tumor necrosis factor-α antibody. *J. Dermatol.* **2019**, *46*, e158–e160. [CrossRef]

117. Tsuruta, N.; Narisawa, Y.; Imafuku, S.; Ito, K.; Yamaguchi, K.; Miyagi, T.; Takahashi, K.; Fukamatsu, H.; Morizane, S.; Koketsu, H.; et al. Cross-sectional multicenter observational study of psoriatic arthritis in Japanese patients: Relationship between skin and joint symptoms and results of treatment with tumor necrosis factor-α inhibitors. *J. Dermatol.* **2019**, *46*, 193–198. [CrossRef]

118. Yamamoto, T.; Ohtsuki, M.; Sano, S.; Morita, A.; Igarashi, A.; Okuyama, R.; Kawada, A. Late-onset psoriatic arthritis in Japanese patients. *J. Dermatol.* **2019**, *46*, 169–170. [CrossRef]

119. Chujo, S.; Asahina, A.; Itoh, Y.; Kobayashi, K.; Sueki, H.; Ishiji, T.; Umezawa, Y.; Nakagawa, H. New onset of psoriasis during nivolumab treatment for lung cancer. *J. Dermatol.* **2018**, *45*, e55–e56. [CrossRef]

120. Furue, K.; Ito, T.; Tsuji, G.; Kadono, T.; Nakahara, T.; Furue, M. Autoimmunity and autoimmune co-morbidities in psoriasis. *Immunology* **2018**, *154*, 21–27. [CrossRef]

121. Ho, Y.H.; Hu, H.Y.; Chang, Y.T.; Li, C.P.; Wu, C.Y. Psoriasis is associated with increased risk of bullous pemphigoid: A nationwide population-based cohort study in Taiwan. *J. Dermatol.* **2019**, *46*, 604–609. [CrossRef]

122. Ichiyama, S.; Hoashi, T.; Kanda, N.; Hashimoto, H.; Matsushita, M.; Nozawa, K.; Ueno, T.; Saeki, H. Psoriasis vulgaris associated with systemic lupus erythematosus successfully treated with apremilast. *J. Dermatol.* **2019**, *46*, e219–e221. [CrossRef]

123. Kamata, M.; Asano, Y.; Shida, R.; Maeda, N.; Yoshizaki, A.; Miyagaki, T.; Kawashima, T.; Tada, Y.; Sato, S. Secukinumab decreased circulating anti-BP180-NC16a autoantibodies in a patient with coexisting psoriasis vulgaris and bullous pemphigoid. *J. Dermatol.* **2019**, *46*, e216–e217. [CrossRef]

124. Masaki, S.; Bayaraa, B.; Imafuku, S. Prevalence of inflammatory bowel disease in Japanese psoriatic patients. *J. Dermatol.* **2019**, *46*, 590–594. [CrossRef]

125. Chiu, H.Y.; Chang, W.L.; Shiu, M.N.; Huang, W.F.; Tsai, T.F. Psoriasis is associated with a greater risk for cardiovascular procedure and surgery in patients with hypertension: A nationwide cohort study. *J. Dermatol.* **2018**, *45*, 1381–1388. [CrossRef]

126. Momose, M.; Asahina, A.; Fukuda, T.; Sakuma, T.; Umezawa, Y.; Nakagawa, H. Evaluation of epicardial adipose tissue volume and coronary artery calcification in Japanese patients with psoriasis vulgaris. *J. Dermatol.* **2018**, *45*, 1349–1352. [CrossRef]

127. Takamura, S.; Takahashi, A.; Inoue, Y.; Teraki, Y. Effects of tumor necrosis factor-α, interleukin-23 and interleukin-17A inhibitors on bodyweight and body mass index in patients with psoriasis. *J. Dermatol.* **2018**, *45*, 1130–1134. [CrossRef]

128. Han, J.H.; Lee, J.H.; Han, K.D.; Kim, H.N.; Bang, C.H.; Park, Y.M.; Lee, J.Y.; Kim, T.Y. Increased risk of psoriasis in subjects with abdominal obesity: A nationwide population-based study. *J. Dermatol.* **2019**, *46*, 695–701. [CrossRef]

129. Yamazaki, F.; Takehana, K.; Tamashima, M.; Okamoto, H. Improvement in abnormal coronary arteries estimated by coronary computed tomography angiography after secukinumab treatment in a Japanese psoriatic patient. *J. Dermatol.* **2019**, *46*, e51–e52. [CrossRef]

130. Bayaraa, B.; Imafuku, S. Sustainability and switching of biologics for psoriasis and psoriatic arthritis at Fukuoka University Psoriasis Registry. *J. Dermatol.* **2019**, *46*, 389–398. [CrossRef]

131. Nakajima, K.; Sano, S. Mouse models of psoriasis and their relevance. *J. Dermatol.* **2018**, *45*, 252–263. [CrossRef]

132. Ogawa, E.; Sato, Y.; Minagawa, A.; Okuyama, R. Pathogenesis of psoriasis and development of treatment. *J. Dermatol.* **2018**, *45*, 264–272. [CrossRef]

133. Kamata, M.; Tada, Y. Safety of biologics in psoriasis. *J. Dermatol.* **2018**, *45*, 279–286. [CrossRef]

134. Tada, Y.; Ishii, K.; Kimura, J.; Hanada, K.; Kawaguchi, I. Patient preference for biologic treatments of psoriasis in Japan. *J. Dermatol.* **2019**, *46*, 466–477. [CrossRef]

135. Bayaraa, B.; Imafuku, S. Relationship between environmental factors, age of onset and familial history in Japanese patients with psoriasis. *J. Dermatol.* **2018**, *45*, 715–718. [CrossRef]

136. Elder, J.T. Expanded genome-wide association study meta-analysis of psoriasis expands the catalog of common psoriasis-associated variants. *J. Investig. Dermatol. Symp. Proc.* **2018**, *19*, S77–S78. [CrossRef]

137. Di Meglio, P.; Duarte, J.H.; Ahlfors, H.; Owens, N.D.; Li, Y.; Villanova, F.; Tosi, I.; Hirota, K.; Nestle, F.O.; Mrowietz, U.; et al. Activation of the aryl hydrocarbon receptor dampens the severity of inflammatory skin conditions. *Immunity* **2014**, *40*, 989–1001. [CrossRef]

138. Smith, S.H.; Peredo, C.E.; Takeda, Y.; Bui, T.; Neil, J.; Rickard, D.; Millerman, E.; Therrien, J.P.; Nicodeme, E.; Brusq, J.M.; et al. Development of a topical treatment for psoriasis targeting RORγ: From bench to skin. *PLoS ONE* **2016**, *11*, e0147979. [CrossRef]

139. Cochez, P.M.; Michiels, C.; Hendrickx, E.; Van Belle, A.B.; Lemaire, M.M.; Dauguet, N.; Warnier, G.; de Heusch, M.; Togbe, D.; Ryffel, B.; et al. AhR modulates the IL-22-producing cell proliferation/recruitment in imiquimod-induced psoriasis mouse model. *Eur. J. Immunol.* **2016**, *46*, 1449–1459. [CrossRef]

140. Mescher, M.; Tigges, J.; Rolfes, K.M.; Shen, A.L.; Yee, J.S.; Vogeley, C.; Krutmann, J.; Bradfield, C.A.; Lang, D.; Haarmann-Stemmann, T. The Toll-like receptor agonist imiquimod is metabolized by aryl hydrocarbon receptor-regulated cytochrome P450 enzymes in human keratinocytes and mouse liver. *Arch. Toxicol.* **2019**, *93*, 1917–1926. [CrossRef]

141. Beranek, M.; Fiala, Z.; Kremlacek, J.; Andrys, C.; Krejsek, J.; Hamakova, K.; Palicka, V.; Borska, L. Serum levels of aryl hydrocarbon receptor, cytochromes P450 1A1 and 1B1 in patients with exacerbated psoriasis vulgaris. *Folia Biol. (Praha)* **2018**, *64*, 97–102. [PubMed]

142. Bissonnette, R.; Bolduc, C.; Maari, C.; Nigen, S.; Webster, J.M.; Tang, L.; Lyle, M. Efficacy and safety of topical WBI-1001 in patients with mild to moderate psoriasis: Results from a randomized double-blind placebo-controlled, phase II trial. *J. Eur. Acad. Dermatol. Venereol.* **2012**, *26*, 1516–1521. [CrossRef] [PubMed]

15

The EGFR-ERK/JNK-CCL20 Pathway in Scratched Keratinocytes May Underpin Koebnerization in Psoriasis Patients

Kazuhisa Furue [1], Takamichi Ito [1], Yuka Tanaka [1], Akiko Hashimoto-Hachiya [2], Masaki Takemura [1], Maho Murata [1], Makiko Kido-Nakahara [1], Gaku Tsuji [2], Takeshi Nakahara [3] and Masutaka Furue [1,2,3,*]

[1]   Department of Dermatology, Faculty of Medical Sciences, Kyushu University, Maidashi 3-1-1, Fukuoka 812-8582, Japan; ffff5113@gmail.com (K.F.); takamiti@dermatol.med.kyushu-u.ac.jp (T.I.); yukat53@med.kyushu-u.ac.jp (Y.T.); take0917@dermatol.med.kyushu-u.ac.jp (M.T.); muratama@dermatol.med.kyushu-u.ac.jp (M.M.); macky@dermatol.med.kyushu-u.ac.jp (M.K.-N.)
[2]   Research and Clinical Center for Yusho and Dioxin, Kyushu University Hospital, Maidashi 3-1-1, Fukuoka 812-8582, Japan; ahachi@dermatol.med.kyushu-u.ac.jp (A.H.-H.); gakku@dermatol.med.kyushu-u.ac.jp (G.T.)
[3]   Division of Skin Surface Sensing, Department of Dermatology, Faculty of Medical Sciences, Kyushu University, Maidashi 3-1-1, Fukuoka 812-8582, Japan; nakahara@dermatol.med.kyushu-u.ac.jp
*   Correspondence: furue@dermatol.med.kyushu-u.ac.jp

Abstract: Epidermal keratinocytes represent a rich source of C-C motif chemokine 20 (CCL20) and recruit CCR6$^+$ interleukin (IL)-17A–producing T cells that are known to be pathogenic for psoriasis. A previous study revealed that scratch injury on keratinocytes upregulates CCL20 production, which is implicated in the Koebner phenomenon characteristically seen in psoriasis patients. However, the molecular mechanisms leading to scratch-induced CCL20 production remain elusive. In this study, we demonstrate that scratch injury upregulates the phosphorylation of epidermal growth factor receptor (EGFR) and that the specific EGFR inhibitor PD153035 attenuates scratch-induced CCL20 upregulation in an extracellular signal-related kinase (ERK)-dependent, and to a lesser extent, a c-Jun N-terminal kinase (JNK)-dependent but p38 mitogen-activated protein kinase (MAPK)–independent manner. Immunoreactive CCL20 was visualized in the keratinocytes that lined the scratched wound. IL-17A also induced the phosphorylation of EGFR and further augmented scratch-induced CCL20 upregulation. The EGFR-ERK/JNK-CCL20 pathway in scratched keratinocytes may explain why Koebnerization is frequently seen in psoriasis patients.

Keywords: CCL20; IL-17A; psoriasis; scratch injury; epidermal growth factor receptor; Koebner phenomenon; ERK; JNK; p38 MAPK; keratinocyte

1. Introduction

Psoriasis is an immune-mediated skin disease characterized by epidermal hyperproliferation and dermal inflammatory cell infiltrates such as dendritic cells and T cells [1]. Psoriasis has shown a diverse prevalence across populations worldwide: 2.5% in Europeans, 0.05–3% in Africans, and 0.1–0.5% in Asians [1,2]. Psoriasis markedly diminishes the quality of life, treatment adherence/satisfaction, and socioeconomic stability of afflicted patients [3,4]. Skin injury triggers or exacerbates psoriatic lesions in a condition named the Koebner phenomenon [5,6]. Although the Koebner phenomenon is observed in other skin diseases such as lichen planus and vitiligo, it is particularly associated with psoriasis [5,6]. However, the pathogenetic mechanism of Koebnerization is not clear [5,6].

A number of biologic therapies are currently approved for the management of moderate to severe psoriasis. These biologics target specific molecules in the immune system, and they have a favorable safety and efficacy profiles than the traditional systemic agents such as methotrexate and cyclosporine [7]. Therapeutic success by specific biologics points to the pathogenic role of the tumor necrosis factor-α (TNF-α) axis and the interleukin (IL)-23/IL-17A axis in psoriasis [8–13]. The gene expression of *TNF*, *IL23*, and *IL17A* is upregulated in the skin lesions of psoriasis patients [13–15]. Infiltration of IL-17A–producing T helper (Th17) cells is detected in the lesional skin of psoriatic patients, and certain Th17 cells are reactive to selective autoantigens [16–18].

The recruitment of Th17 cells into the lesion is governed by CCL20-CCR6 engagement [19,20]. The expression of CCR6 has been confirmed in other IL-17A–producing cytotoxic T cells (Tc17) [21,22], innate lymphoid cell group3 (ILC3) [23,24], and $\gamma\delta$T cells [25,26]. CCL20 is a potent chemoattractant for CCR6$^+$ T cells as well as dendritic cells [20,27–29]. Psoriatic lesions are associated with abundant epidermal CCL20 expression and dermal skin–homing CCR6$^+$ Th17 cells [17,30,31]. Epidermal keratinocytes represent a rich source of CCL20 secretion [32]. In addition, mechanical suctioning or scratching upregulates the mRNA and protein expression of CCL20 [27,32], and keratinocytes release large amounts of CCL20 in a time- and scratch line number-dependent manner [32]. In a murine psoriasis model generated by intradermal IL-23 injection, treatment with an anti–CCL20 antibody significantly reduced the recruitment of CCR6$^+$ cells and attenuated IL-23–induced psoriasiform dermatitis [33]. Getschman et al. designed a CCL20 variant, CCL20S64C, that acts as a partial agonist of CCR6 [34]. After administration, CCL20S64C competes with CCL20 and significantly attenuates IL-23–induced psoriasiform inflammation in mice [34]. These preclinical studies reinforce the crucial role of the CCL20-CCR6 axis in the pathogenesis of psoriasis.

We have previously demonstrated an upregulated production of CCL20 following scratch injury in keratinocytes and proposed a potential link to the Koebner phenomenon in psoriasis [32]. However, the subcellular mechanisms of scratch-induced CCL20 production in keratinocytes remain elusive. One of the prominent biological alterations following scratch wounding is the activation of epidermal growth factor receptor (EGFR) in epithelial cells, including keratinocytes and corneal cells [35,36]. Therefore, we hypothesized that EGFR activation induces upstream signal transduction for CCL20 production. In this study, we demonstrated that scratch-induced CCL20 production was mediated by EGFR-extracellular signal-related kinase (ERK), and to a lesser extent, by the EGFR–c-Jun N-terminal kinase (JNK) pathway in keratinocytes. IL-17A also upregulated CCL20 production via EGFR activation and further potentiated scratch-induced CCL20 production, suggesting that epidermal CCL20 production is an integral part in the pathogenesis of psoriasis and Koebnerization.

2. Results

2.1. Scratch-Induced CCL20 Expression Is Ameliorated by EGFR Inhibition

Consistent with our previous report [32], scratch injury augmented the protein production of CCL20 compared with non-scratched control human keratinocytes (Figure 1). Significant amounts of CCL20 were released from scratched keratinocytes as early as 3 h after scratch injury (Figure 1). Notably, the EGFR inhibitor PD153035 significantly inhibited scratch-induced CCL20 upregulation (Figure 2A). Moreover, PD153035 significantly decreased the baseline production of CCL20 even in non-scratched controls (Figure 2A). We next examined whether or not scratch injury phosphorylates EGFR. In accordance with previous reports [35,36], scratch injury upregulated the phosphorylation of EGFR (P-EGFR) compared with non-scratched controls, and scratch-induced P-EGFR upregulation was attenuated in the presence of PD153035 (Figure 2B). These results suggest a pivotal regulatory role of EGFR signaling in scratch-induced CCL20 production in keratinocytes.

Figure 1. Scratch injury–induced CCL20 production. The production of CCL20 was measured at 3, 6, and 24 h after the initiation of culture in non-scratched control and scratched keratinocyte cultures. Representative data of three independent experiments are shown. ** $p < 0.01$. *** $p < 0.001$.

Figure 2. Scratch injury-induced CCL20 production depends on activation of epidermal growth factor receptor (EGFR). (**A**) Scratch injury-induced CCL20 production was measured in the presence or absence of PD153035 (EGFR inhibitor, 300 or 600 nM) at 24 h after scratching. (**B**) The phosphorylation of EGFR (P-EGFR) was measured by western blot analysis at 1 h after scratching. Representative enzyme-linked immunosorbent assay (ELISA) data and Western blot images of three independent experiments are shown. ** $p < 0.01$. *** $p < 0.001$.

2.2. Spatial Distribution of CCL20 Expression in Keratinocytes

Subsequently, we attempted to visualize the CCL20 expression using an immunofluorescence technique. Compared with IgG staining in negative controls (Figure 3A), the immunoreactive CCL20 was positively but faintly and diffusely stained in the non-scratched control keratinocytes (Figure 3B). Compared with staining in negative controls (Figure 3C), CCL20 expression was clearly enhanced in the keratinocytes residing along the scratch-edge area (Figure 3D, arrows). These findings strongly suggest that the scratch injury triggers CCL20 production in keratinocytes adjacent to the wound.

Figure 3. Immunofluorescent visualization of CCL20 at 6 h after scratching. (**A**) Non-scratched control keratinocytes stained with control IgG. (**B**) Non-scratched control keratinocytes stained with anti–CCL20 antibody. (**C**) Scratched keratinocytes stained with control IgG. (**D**) Scratched keratinocytes stained with anti–CCL20 antibody. Original magnification 100×. Representative data of three independent experiments are shown.

2.3. Scratch-Induced CCL20 Production Depends on ERK and, to a Lesser Extent, JNK, but Not the p38 Mitogen-Activated Protein Kinase (MAPK) Pathway

The variable involvement of MAPKs (ERK, JNK, and p38 MAPK) in CCL20 expression has been reported in stimuli-specific and cell type–specific manners [37–41]. Therefore, we examined whether scratch injury activates MAPKs in our system. As shown in Figure 4, scratch injury phosphorylated ERK, JNK, and p38 MAPK molecules compared with nonscratched controls. We then investigated whether scratch-induced CCL20 expression is affected by the ERK inhibitor U0126, the JNK inhibitor SP600125, and the p38 MAPK inhibitor SB203580 (Figure 5). Of note, the scratch-induced CCL20 expression was strongly and significantly inhibited by U0126 and partially by SP600125 (Figure 5). U0126 and SP600125 also inhibited the baseline production of CCL20 in nonscratched keratinocytes (Figure 5). SB203580 did not inhibit baseline and scratch-induced CCL20 production (Figure 5). These results indicate that scratch-induced CCL20 expression is regulated by ERK and partially by JNK activation in keratinocytes.

Figure 4. Scratch injury induces phosphorylation of ERK1/2, JNK, and p38 MAPK at 1 h after scratching. Phosphorylation of ERK1/2, JNK, and p38 MAPK was examined by western blotting in non-scratched control and scratched keratinocytes. Representative blot images of three independent experiments (**A**) and the relative expressions of phosphorylated proteins (**B**) are shown. * $p < 0.05$. ** $p < 0.01$. *** $p < 0.001$.

Figure 5. Scratch-induced CCL20 (24 h after scratching) upregulation depends on ERK1/2 and JNK activation. The CCL20 production was measured in nonscratched control and scratched keratinocytes in the presence or absence of U0126 (ERK1/2 inhibitor, 10 μM), SB203580 (p38 MAPK inhibitor, 10 μM), and SP600125 (JNK inhibitor, 10 μM). Representative data of three independent experiments are shown. * $p < 0.05$. ** $p < 0.01$. *** $p < 0.001$.

2.4. IL-17A Synergistically Enhances Scratch-Induced CCL20 Production

Because IL-17A feasibly upregulates CCL20 production in keratinocytes [42], we next checked whether IL-17A augments scratch-induced CCL20 expression. IL-17A alone upregulated CCL20 production in non-scratched control keratinocytes in a dose-dependent fashion (Figure 6A).

When combined with scratch injury, IL-17A additively or synergistically enhanced scratch-induced CCL20 production (Figure 6A). Interestingly, the IL-17A–induced CCL20 production was also attenuated by the EGFR inhibitor PD153035 (Figure 6B). In accordance with this result, IL-17A alone induced the phosphorylation of EGFR and was attenuated by PD153035 in non-scratched control keratinocytes (Figure 7). IL-17A induced similar levels of EGFR activation as did scratch injury. Significant enhancement of phosphorylated EGFR (P-EGFR) was not observed in combined treatment with scratch and IL-17A compared with IL-17A monotreatment (Figure 7). These results stress the crucial role of EGFR activation in IL-17A–induced, as well as in scratch-induced CCL20 production.

Figure 6. IL-17A augments scratch-induced CCL20 upregulation at 3 h after scratching. (**A**) CCL20 production was measured in non-scratched control and scratched keratinocytes in the presence or absence of IL-17A (0.1 or 1 ng/mL). (**B**) Non-scratched keratinocytes were stimulated with IL-17A (0.1 or 1 ng/mL) with or without PD153035 (EGFR inhibitor, 300 nM). Representative data of three independent experiments are shown. * $p < 0.05$. ** $p < 0.01$. *** $p < 0.001$.

Figure 7.   IL-17A upregulates the phosphorylation of EGFR at 3 h after scratching. The phosphorylation of EGFR was measured by western blot in non-scratched control keratinocytes and scratched-keratinocytes in the presence or absence of IL-17A (1 ng/mL) or PD153035 (EGFR inhibitor, 300 nM). Representative blot images of three independent experiments and the relative expressions of phosphorylated proteins are shown. * $p < 0.05$. ** $p < 0.01$. *** $p < 0.001$.

3. Discussion

CCR6 is a representative surface marker for IL-17A–producing immune cells [19–21,23,28,43]. CCL20 and CCR6 engagement is critical for the recruitment of CCR6$^+$ Th17 cells [27,29,44]. Although immune cells can feasibly produce CCL20 [45–48], the expression of CCL20 seems to be confined to peripheral tissues, including skin [32,42,44]. Epidermal keratinocytes constitutively produce CCL20 in culture conditions [32,42]. The lesional epidermal keratinocytes express abundant CCL20 in patients with psoriasis [30,31]. Following stimulation with IL-17A, keratinocyte production of CCL20 is markedly enhanced [42].

We have previously shown that mechanical scratching also upregulates CCL20 production in keratinocytes [32]. However, the underlying mechanisms remain elusive. In this study, we demonstrated that scratch-induced CCL20 expression is mediated by the EGFR-ERK (and, to a lesser extent, by the EGFR-JNK) pathway. The scratch injury induced the phosphorylation of EGFR in keratinocytes. The scratch-induced activation of EGFR is consistent with previous reports [35,36]. The production of CCL20 was detected as early as 3 h after scratch injury, and the blockade of EGFR activation by its specific inhibitor, PD153035, significantly reduced scratch-induced CCL20 upregulation. PD153035 also significantly decreased the baseline production of CCL20 in non-scratched control keratinocytes. These results indicate that CCL20 production is highly dependent on EGFR signaling. Notably, the immunofluorescence study revealed that CCL20 expression was markedly augmented in keratinocytes lining the scratched edge, suggesting a clear relationship between scratch injury and CCL20 upregulation.

Scratch injury activated and induced the phosphorylation of ERK1/2, JNK, and p38 MAPK in keratinocytes. However, in the present study, scratch-induced CCL20 protein upregulation was strongly blocked by an ERK inhibitor and partially by a JNK inhibitor but not by a p38 MAPK inhibitor. In hepatocellular carcinoma cells and murine colonic epithelial cells, CCL20 expression is known to depend on the ERK pathway [37,38]. TNF-α–induced CCL20 upregulation depends on ERK and p38 MAPK in bronchial epithelial cells [39]. Prolactin upregulated CCL20 expression in keratinocytes and was dependent on ERK and JNK [40]. Evidence from our own and previous studies suggests that the ERK (partially JNK) pathway plays a pivotal role in scratch/EGFR-mediated CCL20 production. Although p38 MAPK is not directly involved in scratch-induced CCL20 production, a recent study suggests that p38 MAPK may regulate the recycling of EGFR by accelerating the latter's endocytosis [49].

Positive therapeutic responses to biologics and lesional transcriptomic analysis have highlighted the critical pathogenic role of IL-17A in psoriasis [15,32,50]. Scratch injury triggers the development of psoriatic lesions (Koebner phenomenon) in patients with psoriasis [6]. Therefore, we next examined the effects of IL-17A on scratch-induced CCL20 production. IL-17A dose-dependently increased CCL20 production in non-scratched control keratinocytes, as reported previously [42]. When they were combined with the scratch injury, we observed an additive or synergistic augmentation of CCL20 production by scratch and IL-17A. In line with a previous study that elucidated EGFR activation by IL-17A [51,52], we also demonstrated that IL-17A upregulated the phosphorylation of EGFR and that the EGFR inhibitor PD153035 attenuated IL-17A–mediated CCL20 production. These results suggest that, in patients with psoriasis, the scratch injury stimulates keratinocytes to produce CCL20, which attracts circulating Th17 cells into the scratched skin. IL-17A produced from recruited Th17 cells may further accelerate CCL20 production from the scratched epidermis and further recruit circulating Th17 cells to the injured skin, leading to a feed-forward positive loop that develops into the Koebnerized psoriatic eruption. Both scratch-induced and IL-17A–induced CCL20 expression depend on EGFR activation. Consistent with the present results, it has been demonstrated that the inhibition of EGFR by erlotinib or cetuximab successfully improves severe psoriasis [53–56].

A first-in-human study using a humanized anti–CCL20 antibody, GSK3050002, has already been reported for the treatment of psoriasis [27]. Intravenous GSK305002 inhibits the infiltration of Th17 cells, but not Th1 or Th2 cells, into the suction blisters (rich in CCL20) in treated individuals, suggesting the active and selective involvement of the CCL20/CCR6 axis in Th17 cell homing into the skin [27]. In addition, preclinical studies reveal that a humanized anti–CCR6 antibody or a small-molecule CCR6 antagonist efficiently inhibits the infiltration of immune cells and inflammatory symptoms in a murine psoriatic model [29,43]. These studies stress the significance of CCL20 as a potential therapeutic target for psoriasis. In parallel, the increased expression of CCL20 and CCR6 has been demonstrated in lichen planus which also manifests Koebnerization [57]. There are several limitations in this study. We only examined the effects of scratch injury on the monolayer keratinocyte culture system. Further studies are warranted using three-dimensional skin equivalent, ex vivo human skin, or in vivo mouse models. Fibroblasts may affect the scratch-induced, keratinocyte-derived CCL20 expression in coculture models. More extensive studies may be necessary to draw a concrete conclusion.

In conclusion, scratch-induced CCL20 production depends on the EGFR-ERK (and partially on the JNK) pathway. As has been proposed previously [58], EGFR signaling may be a significant and integral component in the pathogenesis of Koebnerization and psoriasis. Our study underscores the potential role of new therapies such as anti-CCL20 antibody and EGFR/ERK inhibitors in the management of psoriasis.

4. Materials and Methods

4.1. Reagents and Antibodies

Dimethyl sulfoxide (DMSO) was purchased from Sigma-Aldrich (St. Louis, MO, USA). $CaCl_2$ (Fujifilm Wako Pure Chemical Corporation, Osaka, Japan) was dissolved in UltraPure distilled water (Invitrogen, Carlsbad, CA, USA) and added to culture medium at a final concentration of 1.6 mM. In the same way, recombinant human IL-17A (PeproTech, Rocky Hill, NJ, USA) was used at final concentrations of 0.1 and 1.0 ng/mL. An EGFR–tyrosine kinase inhibitor, PD153035 (ChemScene LLC, Monmouth Junction, NJ, USA), was dissolved in DMSO and added to culture medium at final concentrations of 300 and 600 nM. Control cultures contained comparable amounts of DMSO (0.01%) and UltraPure distilled water (1.6%). Signal-transduction inhibitors U0126 (ERK1/2 inhibitor) and SB203580 (p38 inhibitor) were purchased from Tocris Bioscience (Bristol, UK), and SP600125 (JNK inhibitor) was obtained from Abcam (Cambridge, UK). The antibodies used for immunofluorescence staining were as follows: rabbit anti–human macrophage inflammatory protein 3 alpha (MIP-3α, CCL20) polyclonal antibody, and normal rabbit polyclonal IgG (all from Abcam); and goat anti–rabbit IgG (H + L) cross-adsorbed secondary antibody with Alexa Fluor 488 dye (Thermo Fisher Scientific, Waltham, MA, USA). The antibodies (catalog numbers) used for western blotting were as follows: rabbit anti–human ERK1/2 (9102S), JNK (9252S), p38 MAPK (8690S), phospho-ERK1/2 (4370S, Thr202/Tyr204), phospho-JNK (4668S, Thr183/Tyr185), phospho-p38 MAPK (4511S, Thr180/Tyr182), EGFR (4267S), phosphor-EGFR (3777S, Tyr1068), and β-actin (4970S) monoclonal antibodies (all from Cell Signaling Technology, Danvers, MA, USA) as primary antibodies, and goat anti-rabbit IgG HRP-linked antibody (7074S) (Cell Signaling Technology) as a secondary antibody.

4.2. Cell Culture

Normal human epidermal keratinocytes (NHEKs) from neonatal foreskin were cultured in KBM-GOLD Keratinocyte Basal Medium supplemented with KGM-GOLD SingleQuots (all from Lonza, Basel, Switzerland) containing bovine pituitary extract, recombinant epidermal growth factor, insulin, hydrocortisone, transferrin, gentamicin sulfate–amphotericin (GA-1000) (Lonza), and epinephrine and were maintained at 37 °C in 5% CO_2. The culture medium was replaced every day, and the cells were serially passaged at 70–80% confluence. In all experiments, cells were used at the third passage. Cells (3.5×10^5 cells/well) were seeded in 6-well culture plates (Corning Inc., Corning, NY, USA), and the culture medium was replaced every day. At 100% confluence, cells were treated with a high level of $CaCl_2$ (1.6 mM, high-Ca^{2+} conditions), which converted the cells from the proliferative state to the differentiating state.

4.3. CCL20 Secretion in an In Vitro Scratched Keratinocyte Model

The in vitro scratched keratinocyte model was performed as previously described [32]. Briefly, NHEKs at 100% confluence were incubated for 24 h under high-Ca^{2+} conditions at 37 °C in 5% CO_2. Then, the cell sheets were scratched (10 lines) with a 250-µL Long Tip (Watson Bio Lab, Tokyo, Japan). In several assays, the scratched cell sheets were also treated with IL-17A (0.1 or 1.0 ng/mL) [42,59], PD153035 (300 or 600 nM) [60], U0126 (10 µM), SB203580 (10 µM), or SP600125 (10 µM).

4.4. Enzyme-Linked Immunosorbent Assay (ELISA)

Culture supernatants were collected, and the concentrations of CCL20 were measured using Quantikine Human CCL20 ELISA Kits (R&D Systems, Minneapolis, MN, USA) in accordance with the manufacturer's instructions. Absorbance at 450 nM was measured with an iMark microplate reader (Bio-Rad Laboratories Inc., Hercules, CA, USA), and the concentrations of CCL20 were determined in each sample by comparison with a standard curve.

4.5. Western Blotting

Protein lysates of NHEKs were isolated from cells with 100 µL/well of lysis buffer (25 mM HEPES, 10 mM $Na_4P_2O_7$/10 H_2O, 100 mM NaF, 5 mM EDTA, 2 mM Na_3VO_4, and 1% Triton X-100), supplemented with 10 µL/well of proteinase inhibitor cocktail (Sigma-Aldrich). The lysates were then centrifuged at 14,000 rpm for 20 min, and the supernatants were used for analysis. The protein concentration of each lysate was measured with a BCA protein assay kit (Thermo Fisher Scientific). Equal amounts of protein (30 µg for EGFR, phosphor-EGFR; 20 µg for the other proteins) were mixed with 2× sample buffer (Nacalai Tesque, Inc., Kyoto, Japan), boiled at 95 °C for 5 min, loaded onto Bolt 4–12% Bis-Tris Plus Gels (Invitrogen), and electrophoresed at 200 V and 160 mA for 22 min. The proteins were then transferred to a polyvinylidene fluoride (PVDF) membrane (Invitrogen) using the Power Blotter XL System (Invitrogen). Membranes were blocked with 2% bovine serum albumin (BSA; Sigma-Aldrich) in 0.1% tris buffered saline with tween (TBS-T). Membranes were probed with primary antibodies overnight at 4 °C. After incubation with anti–rabbit IgG HRP-linked secondary antibody at room temperature for 1 h, protein bands were visualized with SuperSignal West Pico Chemiluminescent Substrate (Thermo Fisher Scientific) using the ChemiDoc Touch Imaging System (Bio-Rad Laboratories Inc.).

4.6. Immunofluorescence Analysis

Immunofluorescence analysis was performed as reported previously [61]. The cells were cultured in 4-well slide chambers (1.5×10^5 cells/well) (Lab-Tek, Rochester, NY, USA) in accordance with the culture methods described herein. Then, the cell sheets were scratched and incubated for 6 h at 37 °C in 5% CO_2. The cell sheets were washed with PBS 3 times for 5 min each and fixed in cold acetone for 10 min at room temperature. The cell sheets were blocked with 10% BSA (Roche Diagnostics, Basel, Switzerland) and incubated with rabbit anti-human CCL20 polyclonal antibody or control normal rabbit polyclonal IgG. Goat anti-rabbit IgG (H + L) cross-adsorbed secondary antibody with Alexa Fluor 488 dye was used as the secondary antibody. The nucleus was stained with 4′,6-diamino-2-phenylindole (DAPI). Slides were then mounted with Ultra Cruz mounting medium (Santa Cruz Biotechnology, Dallas, TX, USA) and were observed using a D-Eclipse confocal laser scanning microscope (Nikon, Tokyo, Japan).

4.7. Statistical Analysis

All data are presented as mean ± standard deviation (SD). The significance of differences between groups was assessed using unpaired 2-tailed student's t-test (2 groups) or 1-way analysis of variance (ANOVA), followed by Tukey's multiple comparison test (multiple groups) using GraphPad

PRISM 7.0 software (GraphPad Software, La Jolla, CA, USA). A p-value of < 0.05 was considered statistically significant.

Author Contributions: K.F. performed all the experiments with the help and advice of T.I., Y.T., A.H.-H., M.T., M.M., M.K.-N., G.T. and T.N. K.F. wrote the first draft of the article. M.F. designed the experimental protocol finalized the article. All authors approved the finalized article. All authors have read and agreed to the published version of the manuscript.

References

1. Boehncke, W.H.; Schön, M.P. Psoriasis. *Lancet* **2015**, *386*, 983–994. [CrossRef]
2. Furue, K.; Yamamura, K.; Tsuji, G.; Mitoma, C.; Uchi, H.; Nakahara, T.; Kido-Nakahara, M.; Kadono, T.; Furue, M. Highlighting interleukin-36 signalling in plaque psoriasis and pustular psoriasis. *Acta Derm. Venereol.* **2018**, *98*, 5–13. [CrossRef]
3. Ichiyama, S.; Ito, M.; Funasaka, Y.; Abe, M.; Nishida, E.; Muramatsu, S.; Nishihara, H.; Kato, H.; Morita, A.; Imafuku, S.; et al. Assessment of medication adherence and treatment satisfaction in Japanese patients with psoriasis of various severities. *J. Dermatol.* **2018**, *45*, 727–731. [CrossRef]
4. Takahashi, H.; Satoh, K.; Takagi, A.; Iizuka, H. Cost-efficacy and pharmacoeconomics of psoriatic patients in Japan: Analysis from a single outpatient clinic. *J. Dermatol.* **2019**, *46*, 478–481. [CrossRef]
5. Miller, R.A. The Koebner phenomenon. *Int. J. Dermatol.* **1982**, *21*, 192–197. [CrossRef]
6. Weiss, G.; Shemer, A.; Trau, H. The Koebner phenomenon: Review of the literature. *J. Eur. Acad. Dermatol. Venereol.* **2002**, *16*, 241–248. [CrossRef]
7. Kaushik, S.B.; Lebwohl, M.G. Review of safety and efficacy of approved systemic psoriasis therapies. *Int. J. Dermatol.* **2019**, *58*, 649–658. [CrossRef]
8. Nakajima, K.; Sano, S. Mouse models of psoriasis and their relevance. *J. Dermatol.* **2018**, *45*, 252–263. [CrossRef]
9. Ogawa, E.; Sato, Y.; Minagawa, A.; Okuyama, R. Pathogenesis of psoriasis and development of treatment. *J. Dermatol.* **2018**, *45*, 264–272. [CrossRef]
10. Furue, K.; Ito, T.; Furue, M. Differential efficacy of biologic treatments targeting the TNF-α/IL-23/IL-17 axis in psoriasis and psoriatic arthritis. *Cytokine* **2018**, *111*, 182–188. [CrossRef]
11. Furue, K.; Ito, T.; Tsuji, G.; Kadono, T.; Furue, M. Psoriasis and the TNF/IL23/IL17 axis. *G. Ital. Dermatol. Venereol.* **2019**, *154*, 418–424. [CrossRef]
12. Sano, S.; Kubo, H.; Morishima, H.; Goto, R.; Zheng, R.; Nakagawa, H. Guselkumab, a human interleukin-23 monoclonal antibody in Japanese patients with generalized pustular psoriasis and erythrodermic psoriasis: Efficacy and safety analyses of a 52-week, phase 3, multicenter, open-label study. *J. Dermatol.* **2018**, *45*, 529–539. [CrossRef]
13. Krueger, J.G.; Brunner, P.M. Interleukin-17 alters the biology of many cell types involved in the genesis of psoriasis, systemic inflammation and associated comorbidities. *Exp. Dermatol.* **2018**, *27*, 115–123. [CrossRef]
14. Lowes, M.A.; Russell, C.B.; Martin, D.A.; Towne, J.E.; Krueger, J.G. The IL-23/T17 pathogenic axis in psoriasis is amplified by keratinocyte responses. *Trends Immunol.* **2013**, *34*, 174–181. [CrossRef]
15. Tsoi, L.C.; Rodriguez, E.; Degenhardt, F.; Baurecht, H.; Wehkamp, U.; Volks, N.; Szymczak, S.; Swindell, W.R.; Sarkar, M.K.; Raja, K.; et al. Atopic dermatitis is an IL-13-dominant disease with greater molecular heterogeneity compared to psoriasis. *J. Investig. Dermatol.* **2019**, *139*, 1480–1489. [CrossRef]
16. Furue, M.; Kadono, T. The contribution of IL-17 to the development of autoimmunity in psoriasis. *Innate Immun.* **2019**, *25*, 337–343. [CrossRef]
17. Pène, J.; Chevalier, S.; Preisser, L.; Vénéreau, E.; Guilleux, M.H.; Ghannam, S.; Molès, J.P.; Danger, Y.; Ravon, E.; Lesaux, S.; et al. Chronically inflamed human tissues are infiltrated by highly differentiated Th17 lymphocytes. *J. Immunol.* **2008**, *180*, 7423–7430. [CrossRef]
18. Villanova, F.; Flutter, B.; Tosi, I.; Grys, K.; Sreeneebus, H.; Perera, G.K.; Chapman, A.; Smith, C.H.; Di Meglio, P.; Nestle, F.O. Characterization of innate lymphoid cells in human skin and blood demonstrates increase of NKp44+ ILC3 in psoriasis. *J. Investig. Dermatol.* **2014**, *134*, 984–991. [CrossRef]
19. Singh, S.P.; Zhang, H.H.; Foley, J.F.; Hedrick, M.N.; Farber, J.M. Human T cells that are able to produce IL-17 express the chemokine receptor CCR6. *J. Immunol.* **2008**, *180*, 214–221. [CrossRef]
20. Sallusto, F.; Impellizzieri, D.; Basso, C.; Laroni, A.; Uccelli, A.; Lanzavecchia, A.; Engelhardt, B. T-cell trafficking in the central nervous system. *Immunol. Rev.* **2012**, *248*, 216–227. [CrossRef]

21. Diani, M.; Casciano, F.; Marongiu, L.; Longhi, M.; Altomare, A.; Pigatto, P.D.; Secchiero, P.; Gambari, R.; Banfi, G.; Manfredi, A.A.; et al. Increased frequency of activated CD8$^+$ T cell effectors in patients with psoriatic arthritis. *Sci. Rep.* **2019**, *9*, 10870. [CrossRef]

22. Steel, K.J.A.; Srenathan, U.; Ridley, M.; Durham, L.E.; Wu, S.Y.; Ryan, S.E.; Hughes, C.D.; Chan, E.; Kirkham, B.W.; Taams, L.S. Synovial IL-17A+ CD8+ T cells display a polyfunctional, pro-inflammatory and tissue-resident memory phenotype and function in psoriatic arthritis. *Arthritis Rheumatol.* **2019**. [CrossRef]

23. Bando, J.K.; Gilfillan, S.; Song, C.; McDonald, K.G.; Huang, S.C.; Newberry, R.D.; Kobayashi, Y.; Allan, D.S.J.; Carlyle, J.R.; Cella, M.; et al. The tumor necrosis f actor superfamily member RANKL suppresses effector cytokine production in group 3 innate lymphoid cells. *Immunity* **2018**, *48*, 1208–1219. [CrossRef]

24. Talayero, P.; Mancebo, E.; Calvo-Pulido, J.; Rodríguez-Muñoz, S.; Bernardo, I.; Laguna-Goya, R.; Cano-Romero, F.L.; García-Sesma, A.; Loinaz, C.; Jiménez, C.; et al. Innate lymphoid cells groups 1 and 3 in the epithelial compartment of functional human intestinal allografts. *Am. J. Transplant.* **2016**, *16*, 72–82. [CrossRef]

25. Campbell, J.J.; Ebsworth, K.; Ertl, L.S.; McMahon, J.P.; Newland, D.; Wang, Y.; Liu, S.; Miao, Z.; Dang, T.; Zhang, P.; et al. IL-17-secreting γδ T cells are completely dependent upon CCR6 for homing to inflamed skin. *J. Immunol.* **2017**, *199*, 3129–3136. [CrossRef]

26. Mabuchi, T.; Takekoshi, T.; Hwang, S.T. Epidermal CCR6+ γδ T cells are major producers of IL-22 and IL-17 in a murine model of psoriasiform dermatitis. *J. Immunol.* **2011**, *187*, 5026–5031. [CrossRef]

27. Bouma, G.; Zamuner, S.; Hicks, K.; Want, A.; Oliveira, J.; Choudhury, A.; Brett, S.; Robertson, D.; Felton, L.; Norris, V.; et al. CCL20 neutralization by a monoclonal antibody in healthy subjects selectively inhibits recruitment of CCR6$^+$ cells in an experimental suction blister. *Br. J. Clin. Pharmacol.* **2017**, *83*, 1976–1990. [CrossRef]

28. Maecker, H.T.; McCoy, J.P.; Nussenblatt, R. Standardizing immunophenotyping for the Human Immunology Project. *Nat. Rev. Immunol.* **2012**, *12*, 191–200. [CrossRef]

29. Robert, R.; Ang, C.; Sun, G.; Juglair, L.; Lim, E.X.; Mason, L.J.; Payne, N.L.; Bernard, C.C.; Mackay, C.R. Essential role for CCR6 in certain inflammatory diseases demonstrated using specific antagonist and knockin mice. *JCI Insight* **2017**, *2*, e94821. [CrossRef]

30. Homey, B.; Dieu-Nosjean, M.C.; Wiesenborn, A.; Massacrier, C.; Pin, J.J.; Oldham, E.; Catron, D.; Buchanan, M.E.; Müller, A.; de Waal Malefyt, R.; et al. Up-regulation of macrophage inflammatory protein-3 alpha/CCL20 and CC chemokine receptor 6 in psoriasis. *J. Immunol.* **2000**, *164*, 6621–6632. [CrossRef]

31. Kim, T.G.; Jee, H.; Fuentes-Duculan, J.; Wu, W.H.; Byamba, D.; Kim, D.S.; Kim, D.Y.; Lew, D.H.; Yang, W.I.; Krueger, J.G.; et al. Dermal clusters of mature dendritic cells and T cells are associated with the CCL20/CCR6 chemokine system in chronic psoriasis. *J. Investig. Dermatol.* **2014**, *134*, 1462–1465. [CrossRef]

32. Furue, K.; Ito, T.; Tanaka, Y.; Yumine, A.; Hashimoto-Hachiya, A.; Takemura, M.; Murata, M.; Yamamura, K.; Tsuji, G.; Furue, M. Cyto/chemokine profile of in vitro scratched keratinocyte model: Implications of significant upregulation of CCL20, CXCL8 and IL36G in Koebner phenomenon. *J. Dermatol. Sci.* **2019**, *94*, 244–251. [CrossRef]

33. Mabuchi, T.; Singh, T.P.; Takekoshi, T.; Jia, G.F.; Wu, X.; Kao, M.C.; Weiss, I.; Farber, J.M.; Hwang, S.T. CCR6 is required for epidermal trafficking of γδ-T cells in an IL-23-induced model of psoriasiform dermatitis. *J. Investig. Dermatol.* **2013**, *133*, 164–171. [CrossRef]

34. Getschman, A.E.; Imai, Y.; Larsen, O.; Peterson, F.C.; Wu, X.; Rosenkilde, M.M.; Hwang, S.T.; Volkman, B.F. Protein engineering of the chemokine CCL20 prevents psoriasiform dermatitis in an IL-23-dependent murine model. *Proc. Natl. Acad. Sci. USA* **2017**, *114*, 12460–12465. [CrossRef]

35. Tokumaru, S.; Higashiyama, S.; Endo, T.; Nakagawa, T.; Miyagawa, J.I.; Yamamori, K.; Hanakawa, Y.; Ohmoto, H.; Yoshino, K.; Shirakata, Y.; et al. Ectodomain shedding of epidermal growth factor receptor ligands is required for keratinocyte migration in cutaneous wound healing. *J. Cell Biol.* **2000**, *151*, 209–220. [CrossRef]

36. Xu, K.P.; Ding, Y.; Ling, J.; Dong, Z.; Yu, F.S. Wound-induced HB-EGF ectodomain shedding and EGFR activation in corneal epithelial cells. *Invest. Ophthalmol. Vis. Sci.* **2004**, *45*, 813–820. [CrossRef]

37. Benkheil, M.; Paeshuyse, J.; Neyts, J.; van Haele, M.; Roskams, T.; Liekens, S. HCV-induced EGFR-ERK signaling promotes a pro-inflammatory and pro-angiogenic signature contributing to liver cancer pathogenesis. *Biochem. Pharmacol.* **2018**, *155*, 305–315. [CrossRef]

38. Dutta, P.; Ta, A.; Thakur, B.K.; Dasgupta, N.; Das, S. Biphasic Ccl20 regulation by toll-like receptor 9 through the activation of ERK-AP-1 and non-canonical NF-κB signaling pathways. *Biochim. Biophys. Acta Gen. Subj.* **2017**, *1861*, 3365–3377. [CrossRef]

39. Zijlstra, G.J.; Fattahi, F.; Rozeveld, D.; Jonker, M.R.; Kliphuis, N.M.; van den Berge, M.; Hylkema, M.N.; ten Hacken, N.H.; van Oosterhout, A.J.; Heijink, I.H. Glucocorticoids induce the production of the chemoattractant CCL20 in airway epithelium. *Eur. Respir. J.* **2014**, *44*, 361–370. [CrossRef]

40. Kanda, N.; Shibata, S.; Tada, Y.; Nashiro, K.; Tamaki, K.; Watanabe, S. Prolactin enhances basal and IL-17-induced CCL20 production by human keratinocytes. *Eur. J. Immunol.* **2009**, *39*, 996–1006. [CrossRef]

41. Liu, Y.; Lagowski, J.P.; Gao, S.; Raymond, J.H.; White, C.R.; Kulesz-Martin, M.F. Regulation of the psoriatic chemokine CCL20 by E3 ligases Trim32 and Piasy in keratinocytes. *J. Investig. Dermatol.* **2010**, *130*, 1384–1390. [CrossRef]

42. Harper, E.G.; Guo, C.; Rizzo, H.; Lillis, J.V.; Kurtz, S.E.; Skorcheva, I.; Purdy, D.; Fitch, E.; Iordanov, M.; Blauvelt, A. Th17 cytokines stimulate CCL20 expression in keratinocytes in vitro and in vivo: Implications for psoriasis pathogenesis. *J. Investig. Dermatol.* **2009**, *129*, 2175–2183. [CrossRef]

43. Campbell, J.J.; Ebsworth, K.; Ertl, L.S.; McMahon, J.P.; Wang, Y.; Yau, S.; Mali, V.R.; Chhina, V.; Kumamoto, A.; Liu, S.; et al. Efficacy of Chemokine Receptor Inhibition in Treating IL-36α-Induced Psoriasiform Inflammation. *J. Immunol.* **2019**, *202*, 1687–1692. [CrossRef]

44. Schutyser, E.; Struyf, S.; Van Damme, J. The CC chemokine CCL20 and its receptor CCR6. *Cytokine Growth Factor Rev.* **2003**, *14*, 409–426. [CrossRef]

45. Bridgewood, C.; Watad, A.; Russell, T.; Palmer, T.M.; Marzo-Ortega, H.; Khan, A.; Millner, P.A.; Dunsmuir, R.; Rao, A.; Loughenbury, P.; et al. Identification of myeloid cells in the human enthesis as the main source of local IL-23 production. *Ann. Rheum. Dis.* **2019**, *78*, 929–933. [CrossRef]

46. Hedrick, M.N.; Lonsdorf, A.S.; Shirakawa, A.K.; Lee, C.C.R.; Liao, F.; Singh, S.P.; Zhang, H.H.; Grinberg, A.; Love, P.E.; Hwang, S.T.; et al. CCR6 is required for IL-23-induced psoriasis-like inflammation in mice. *J. Clin. Investig.* **2009**, *119*, 2317–2329. [CrossRef]

47. Komatsu, N.; Okamoto, K.; Sawa, S.; Nakashima, T.; Oh-hora, M.; Kodama, T.; Tanaka, S.; Bluestone, J.A.; Takayanagi, H. Pathogenic conversion of Foxp3+ T cells into TH17 cells in autoimmune arthritis. *Nat. Med.* **2014**, *20*, 62–68. [CrossRef]

48. Yamazaki, T.; Yang, X.O.; Chung, Y.; Fukunaga, A.; Nurieva, R.; Pappu, B.; Martin-Orozco, N.; Kang, H.S.; Ma, L.; Panopoulos, A.D.; et al. CCR6 regulates the migration of inflammatory and regulatory T cells. *J. Immunol.* **2008**, *181*, 8391–8401. [CrossRef]

49. Tanaka, T.; Zhou, Y.; Ozawa, T.; Okizono, R.; Banba, A.; Yamamura, T.; Oga, E.; Muraguchi, A.; Sakurai, H. Ligand-activated epidermal growth factor receptor (EGFR) signaling governs endocytic trafficking of unliganded receptor monomers by non-canonical phosphorylation. *J. Biol. Chem.* **2018**, *293*, 2288–2301. [CrossRef]

50. Momose, M.; Asahina, A.; Umezawa, Y.; Nakagawa, H. Long-term clinical efficacy and safety of secukinumab for Japanese patients with psoriasis: A single-center experience. *J. Dermatol.* **2018**, *45*, 318–321. [CrossRef]

51. Acciani, T.H.; Suzuki, T.; Trapnell, B.C.; Le Cras, T.D. Epidermal growth factor receptor signalling regulates granulocyte-macrophage colony-stimulating factor production by airway epithelial cells and established allergic airway disease. *Clin. Exp. Allergy* **2016**, *46*, 317–328. [CrossRef]

52. Chen, X.; Cai, G.; Liu, C.; Zhao, J.; Gu, C.; Wu, L.; Hamilton, T.A.; Zhang, C.J.; Ko, J.; Zhu, L.; et al. IL-17R-EGFR axis links wound healing to tumorigenesis in Lrig1+ stem cells. *J. Exp. Med.* **2019**, *216*, 195–214. [CrossRef]

53. Goepel, L.; Jacobi, A.; Augustin, M.; Radtke, M.A. Rapid improvement of psoriasis in a patient with lung cancer after treatment with erlotinib. *J. Eur. Acad. Dermatol. Venereol.* **2018**, *32*, e311–e313. [CrossRef]

54. Overbeck, T.R.; Griesinger, F. Two cases of psoriasis responding to erlotinib: Time to revisiting inhibition of epidermal growth factor receptor in psoriasis therapy? *Dermatology* **2012**, *225*, 179–182. [CrossRef]

55. Trivin, F.; Boucher, E.; Raoul, J.L. Complete sustained regression of extensive psoriasis with cetuximab combination chemotherapy. *Acta Oncol.* **2004**, *43*, 592–593. [CrossRef]

56. Neyns, B.; Meert, V.; Vandenbroucke, F. Cetuximab treatment in a patient with metastatic colorectal cancer and psoriasis. *Curr. Oncol.* **2008**, *15*, 196–197. [CrossRef]

57. Ichimura, M.; Hiratsuka, K.; Ogura, N.; Utsunomiya, T.; Sakamaki, H.; Kondoh, T.; Abiko, Y.; Otake, S.; Yamamoto, M. Expression profile of chemokines and chemokine receptors in epithelial cell layers of oral lichen planus. *J. Oral Pathol. Med.* **2006**, *35*, 167–174. [CrossRef]

58. Johnston, A.; Gudjonsson, J.E.; Aphale, A.; Guzman, A.M.; Stoll, S.W.; Elder, J.T. EGFR and IL-1 signaling synergistically promote keratinocyte antimicrobial defenses in a differentiation-dependent manner. *J. Investig. Dermatol.* **2011**, *131*, 329–337. [CrossRef]

59. Tohyama, M.; Hanakawa, Y.; Shirakata, Y.; Dai, X.; Yang, L.; Hirakawa, S.; Tokumaru, S.; Okazaki, H.; Sayama, K.; Hashimoto, K. IL-17 and IL-22 mediate IL-20 subfamily cytokine production in cultured keratinocytes via increased IL-22 receptor expression. *Eur. J. Immunol.* **2009**, *39*, 2779–2788. [CrossRef]

60. Sutter, C.H.; Yin, H.; Li, Y.; Mammen, J.S.; Bodreddigari, S.; Stevens, G.; Cole, J.A.; Sutter, T.R. EGF receptor signaling blocks aryl hydrocarbon receptor-mediated transcription and cell differentiation in human epidermal keratinocytes. *Proc. Natl. Acad. Sci. USA* **2009**, *106*, 4266–4271. [CrossRef]

61. Ulzii, D.; Kido-Nakahara, M.; Nakahara, T.; Tsuji, G.; Furue, K.; Hashimoto-Hachiya, A.; Furue, M. Scratching counteracts IL-13 signaling by upregulating the decoy receptor IL-13Rα2 in deratinocytes. *Int. J. Mol. Sci.* **2019**, *20*, 3324. [CrossRef] [PubMed]

16

Recent Advances in Psoriasis Research: The Clue to Mysterious Relation to Gut Microbiome

Mayumi Komine [1,2]

[1] Department of Dermatology, Jichi Medical University, 3311-1 Yakushiji, Shimotsuke, Tochigi 329-0498, Japan; mkomine12@jichi.ac.jp

[2] Department of Biochemistry, Jichi Medical University, 3311-1 Yakushiji, Shimotsuke, Tochigi 329-0498, Japan

Abstract: Psoriasis is a chronic inflammatory cutaneous disease, characterized by activated plasmacytoid dendritic cells, myeloid dendritic cells, Th17 cells, and hyperproliferating keratinocytes. Recent studies revealed skin-resident cells have pivotal roles in developing psoriatic skin lesions. The balance in effector T cells and regulatory T cells is disturbed, leading Foxp3-positive regulatory T cells to produce proinflammatory IL-17. Not only acquired but also innate immunity is important in psoriasis pathogenesis, especially in triggering the disease. Group 3 innate lymphoid cell are considered one of IL-17-producing cells in psoriasis. Short chain fatty acids produced by gut microbiota stabilize expression of Foxp3 in regulatory T cells, thereby stabilizing their function. The composition of gut microbiota influences the systemic inflammatory status, and associations been shown with diabetes mellitus, cardiovascular diseases, psychomotor diseases, and other systemic inflammatory disorders. Psoriasis has been shown to frequently comorbid with diabetes mellitus, cardiovascular diseases, psychomotor disease and obesity, and recent report suggested the similar abnormality in gut microbiota as the above comorbid diseases. However, the precise mechanism and relation between psoriasis pathogenesis and gut microbiota needs further investigation. This review introduces the recent advances in psoriasis research and tries to provide clues to solve the mysterious relation of psoriasis and gut microbiota.

Keywords: psoriasis; tissue resident cells; innate lymphoid cells; regulatory T cells; Foxp3; gut microbiome; systemic inflammation

1. Introduction

Psoriasis is a chronic inflammatory skin disease, with diverse disease severity and clinical phenotypes. Currently, no curative treatment exists, however, recent advances in therapeutics have made it possible to suppress the disease almost to disappearance. Progress in immunology and molecular biology has dramatically changed understanding of psoriasis pathogenesis, enabling development of novel treatment modalities.

In this review, several recent findings in psoriasis research are reviewed, to support further investigation.

2. Present Understanding of Psoriasis Pathogenesis

Plaque psoriasis is clinically defined as a cutaneous disease with multiple plaques of scaly erythematous lesions. The diagnosis is usually simple with macroscopic findings, but sometimes difficult to differentiate from eczematous, lichenoid, or other conditions. Microscopic investigation is sometimes helpful, but macroscopically difficult cases are also usually difficult to diagnose microscopically. The reason may be that there are heterogeneous clinical groups of psoriasis patients, suggesting that there are heterogenous pathogenetic groups in psoriasis patients. This is supported by the fact certain biologic drugs are efficient in some psoriasis patients but not in others. It has also been postulated that there is mixed pathogenesis of autoimmune and autoinflammatory conditions in psoriasis [1], and the balance of these conditions may differ among patients.

Krueger and Guttman [2] proposed a novel concept which positioned psoriasis and atopic dermatitis at the both ends of the same inflammatory disease spectrum: Psoriasis is located at pure Th17 inflammation, and atopic dermatitis is a combination of Th17, Th2, and Th1 inflammation.

Recent development of biologics for psoriasis treatment produced a novel skin condition, named "paradoxical psoriasis-like eruption" [3]. Paradoxical reactions have been noted for the first time in rheumatoid arthritis patients treated with anti-tumor necrosis factor (TNF) antibodies who developed psoriasis-like skin eruptions. Recently other immunological conditions provoked by targeted biological agents are included in paradoxical reactions, considered "class-effect of targeted biological agents". The interaction between genetically predisposed conditions and targeted biological agents may result in the development of paradoxical reaction development. This itself is of scientific interest, in the context of understanding mechanisms of inflammatory diseases.

The present understanding of psoriasis pathogenesis is summarized in Figure 1. Dendritic cells, T lymphocytes, and keratinocytes are the three major cellular players. Genetic background predisposes patients susceptible to psoriasis: epithelial cells exposed to various stimuli such as bacteria, virus, ultraviolet light, or mechanical stress, leads to apoptosis or necrosis of these cells resulting in exposure of self nucleic acids to tissues [4]. Self DNA bound to LL-37, a part of antimicrobial peptide cathelicidine produced by keratinocytes (KC), stimulating plasmacytoid dendritic cells (pDC) to produce large amount of type I interferons. Simultaneously, self RNA bound to LL-37 stimulate myeloid dendritic cells (mDC) produce tumor necrosis factor alpha (TNFα) and inducible nitric oxide synthase (iNOS). These cytokines produced by DCs stimulate immature T cells to develop into inflammatory T cells, especially Th17 cells, producing interleukin (IL)-17 and IL-22, which develop psoriatic phenotype in KC. KCs produce antimicrobial peptides such as cathelicidine, beta defensine (BD), psoriasin and S100 proteins, chemokines e.g., CXCL1, 2, 8, 10, 11, and CCL20 which attract neutrophils and Th17 cells; and proinflammatory cytokines, such as TNFα, IL-1, and IL-17. These inflammatory reactions cause an inflammatory loop sustaining chronic psoriasis [4].

Recent findings also imply psoriasis inflammation's systemic nature. Obesity's genetic background is distinct from that of psoriasis, however, psoriasis is highly associated with obesity. One explanation is adipose tissue in obese persons produce inflammatory adipocytokines, such as leptin, resistin, and TNFα, leading genetically predisposed patients to develop psoriasis. Increased amount of inflammatory adipocytokines and decreased regulatory adipocytokines have been reported in psoriasis patients, which also correlate with disease severity. This adipocytokine imbalance accelerates insulin resistance and endothelial dysfunction, leading to atherosclerosis and cardiovascular events [5].

3. Tissue Resident Cells

Tissue resident cells have been identified and have focused attention on the possibility of disclosing one of the unsolved mysteries: why systemic inflammation of psoriasis chooses skin and articular as the most involved inflammatory sites.

Clark R. et al. [6] proposed resident memory T cells as pathogenic cells of fixed and recurrent skin lesions of psoriasis. Resident memory T cells are a recently identified T cell subset residing in epithelial barrier tissues such as skin, gut, lung, and reproductive tracts. They are highly protective against pathogens frequently encountered in each tissue. Boyman O et al. [7] in 2004 disclosed that normal appearing, uninvolved skin of psoriasis patients transplanted on immune deficient mice developed psoriatic lesions, indicating that there existed pathogenic skin resident immune cells in non-lesional skin of psoriasis patients. Subsequent studies revealed almost 20 billion T cells reside in healthy human skin, twice as many T cells in the entire blood volume. These skin resident T cells express CD45RO, CLA, and CCR4, and strong effector functions with various T cell receptor (TCR) repertoires.

Large numbers of antigenically active tissue resident T cells have subsequently been disclosed in the gastrointestinal tract, lung, reproductive tract, peritoneum, and bone marrow [8–13].

Clinical trials of anti-E-selectin which completely block the migration of circulating T cells from blood to skin on psoriasis patients revealed its ineffectiveness, suggesting the clue to Tissue resident cell involvement in psoriasis [14]. Another study demonstrating transplanted normal-appearing uninvolved skin of psoriasis patients on immunodeficient mice developed psoriasis lesions suggested psoriasis patients' normal-appearing skin contains pathogenic cells which can develop psoriasis lesions without the circulating blood cells [7]. Subsequent studies revealed CD4-positive T cells with IL-22 and CD8-positive T cells producing IL-17 remained resident in previously involved psoriasis lesions after complete clinical resolution from a variety of treatments [15,16].

Gallais serezal I et al. [17] proposed a skewed pool of resident T cells in psoriasis patients trigger non-lesional skin of psoriasis patients to develop psoriasis lesion. They collected never lesional psoriasis (NLP) skin from mild psoriasis patients instead of from severe psoriasis, because in severe psoriasis, patients' uninvolved skin shows psoriatic gene expression profiles. These NLP with normal gene expression profiles exhibited IL-17- and IFN-γ-producing T cell accumulation after stimulation, which triggers keratinocytes to produce IFNα introducing an alternative source of Type I interferons in initiation of psoriasis. Their analysis revealed skewed T cell population in NLP with CD8-positive CD49a-negative T cells, and CCR6-positive T cells producing IL-22, IL-17, and IFNγ. NLP keratinocytes produce increased amounts of CCL20 upon stimulation with *Candida albicans* or mannan suggesting the role of KC, weakly stimulated by resident fungi, in accumulation of IL-17 and IL-22 producing CCR6-positive resident T cells in NLP skin of psoriasis patients. Resident T cells are insufficient to develop psoriasis lesions, but upon stimulation with various stimuli, such as mechanical stress, viral infection, and bacterial infection, these skewed population of resident memory T cells produce inflammatory cytokines, such as IL-17, IL-22, and IFNγ, which initiate psoriasis inflammation (Figure 2). Their study also demonstrated for the first time the role of KC in production of IFNα in psoriasis pathogenesis.

4. Innate Lymphoid Cells

Innate lymphoid cells (ILCs) are recently identified innate immune cells. They were found among lineage-negative cell populations not expressing any mature cell markers, such as Mac-1 for myeloid cells, CD4 and CD8 for T cells, CD19 for B cells, or Ter-119 for erythrocytes. They have a high potency for cytokine production without specific antigen stimulation [18]. Psoriasis has been considered an "autoimmune" disease; however, no specific antigens have been identified so far. The innate immune system is a relatively primitive immune system, directly activated by components of virus, bacteria, fungi, or self-DNAs and RNAs, without specific antigens. Many cell types were included in innate immune cells, such as neutrophils, mast cells, and natural killer cells as well as innate lymphoid cells. It is not surprising that these innate immune cells take part in psoriasis pathogenesis.

ILCs have been subdivided into three groups: ILC1, ILC2, and ILC3. ILC1 (group 1 ILC) characteristically produces IFN gamma, perforin, and granzyme, while ILC2 (group 2 ILC) produces IL-5, IL-13, and IL-4, with nuclear expression of GATA3. ILC3 (group 3 ILC) expresses IL-7Rα, matures with IL-7 and IL-23, and produces IL-17, IL-22, and lymphotoxin with nuclear expression of RORγt [18,19]. ILC3 in humans is further divided into three subsets on the basis of expression of natural cytotoxicity receptors: NKp44, NKp46, and NKp30. NKp44-positive ILC3 produces IL-22 and is dependent on aryl hydrocarbon receptor (AhR). NKp44-negative ILC3 produces IL-17A following stimulation, but NKp44-negative ILC3s have plasticity, and they are able to develop into NKp44-positive ILC3s or into ILC1s with IFNγ production [20]. In inflammatory bowel diseases, ILC3s have been shown to produce IL-17 in the gut [21]. Therefore, the world of ILCs looks as if it were the parallel world of helper T cells (Figure 3).

Soare A et al. [22] reported increased numbers of ILC3 exist in the circulating blood of psoriatic arthritis patients, and ILC3/ILC2 ratios correlated well with disease severity. ILC3 also increased in the lesional and non-lesional skin of psoriasis patients. Keren A et al. [23] revealed that injection of NKp44-positive ILC3 without T cells was able to develop psoriatic skin eruption in SCID mice with implantation of healthy human skin.

These results indicate that ILC3 may have a pathogenic role in psoriasis, which compensates the absence of specific self-antigen.

5. Regulatory T Cells

Regulatory T cells (Treg) have immune suppressive function to suppress excess immunity against a diverse range of antigens, such as self-antigens, commensal bacteria-derived antigens, and environmental allergens. Many autoimmune and inflammatory diseases, such as systemic erythematosus, inflammatory bowel diseases, and rheumatoid arthritis, show decreased Treg numbers and function. Foxp3 (Forkhead box P3) is a transcription factor playing a crucial role in development, maintenance and function of Tregs. Deficiency of Foxp3 results in lack of Tregs, and causes severe systemic inflammatory diseases characterized by autoimmunity, colitis, and allergies.

Tregs usually develop in the thymus from CD4−, CD8−, double negative thymocytes, called thymus-derived regulatory T cells (tTregs) or natural occurring Tregs (nTregs). Expression of Foxp3 are strongly induced through T cell receptor (TCR) signals after the recognition of self-antigen-MHC complex present on antigen presenting cells (APCs). tTregs are believed to comprise most of the systemic Treg population. A second subset of Tregs is induced in the peripheral tissues from CD4-positive naïve T cells by stimulation with cytokine combination, such as TGFβ and IL-2. This type of Tregs is called induced Tregs (iTregs) or peripherally induced Tregs (pTregs). iTregs usually represent Tregs induced in vitro, while pTregs indicates Tregs developed from naïve T cells in vivo.

tTregs matured in thymus have constitutive and stable expression of Foxp3, supported by the binding of several transcription factors to its corresponding promoter and enhancer regions. Several enhancer regions are identified, designated as conserved non-coding sequences (CNS) 1, 2, and 3, and CNS0 has recently been identified upstream of CNS1 [24].

Promoter region and each CNS binds specific transcription factors, which regulate the expression of Foxp3.

The most fundamental transcription factor for Foxp3 expression may be the recently identified Satb1, which binds to CNS0 inducing both transcriptional and epigenetic regulation. Satb1 binds to CNS0 at the beginning of Treg commitment and serves as a pioneering element involved in the transcriptional regulation sequence in Treg development. Nr4a is a transcription factor which binds to CNS2 and the promoter region of Foxp3, necessary for both pTerg and tTreg development. TCR activation induces Nr4a expression, which is essential for pTreg and tTreg development and maintenance after TCR activation. IL-2 and TGFβ are well-known inducers of Tregs, and IL-2 is essential in inducing both tTregs and pTregs, while TGFβ is needed in pTreg development. STAT5 is activated downstream of IL-2R, and STAT5 response elements exist in CNS2 and Foxp3 promoter region. CNS1 contains binding sites for Smads, NFAT, AP-1, and retinoic acid receptor (RAR). Smad2 and Smad3 are redundantly essential for development of iTregs/pTregs in the downstream of TGFβ. CNS2 region contains biding sites for multiple transcription factors, such as STAT5, NFAT, Runx1/Cbfβ, CREB, and Foxp3. This enhancer is very important in maintaining its own expression under inflammatory circumstances where Tregs are subjected to inflammatory cytokines and stronger TCR stimulation. CNS2 locus has multiple CpG sites making this region susceptible for methylation/demethylation status. In tTregs, CNS2 is fully demethylated: full sets of transcription factors bind to this locus enabling stable expression of Foxp3, and stable phenotype of tTregs. In pTregs, CNS2 locus is also demethylated, but with a slightly lower stability compared to tTregs. In iTregs, CNS2 locus is rarely demethylated, which makes this subset very unstable. This CNS2 locus is the major Treg-specific demethylated resion (TSDR) whose demethylated status confers the stability of Foxp3 expression, and the function of Tregs [25] (Figure 4).

The inducers and stabilizers of Foxp3 expression are summarized in Table 1.

Table 1. Factors which induce or stabilize Foxp3 expression.

Factors	Mechanism
Retinoic acids	Binding to *Foxp3* enhancer CNS1 through RAR
Progesterone	Suppression of mTOR
Vitamine D3	Binding to *Foxp3* enhancer CNS1 through VDR
Short chain fatty acids	Activation of GPR43
Butyrates	Inhibition of HDAC
Vitamine C	Activation of TET enzymes
Hydrogen sulfide	Induction of TET1 and TET2
Rapamycin	Inhibition of mTOR
JAK1 inhibitor	Suppression of Th17
AhR ligands	Suppression of Th17

Modified from Kanamori M. et al. Trends in Immunol 2016 [24].

Retinoic acids and vitamin D3 are ligands for their specific nuclear receptors, retinoic acid receptor (RAR), retinoid X receptor (RXR), and vitamin D receptor (VDR). Retinoids binds to RARs and/or RXRs, which make homo or heterodimers to bind to their binding sequences in regulatory region in the target genes. Butyrate induces retinoic acid production in gut dendritic cells, resulting in induction and stabilization of Foxp3 expression in regulatory T cells.

Active form of vitamin D3, generated through the enzymes produced in skin or in liver and kidney, binds to VDR, which makes heterodimers with RXR and binds to response element usually resides in distal area of target genes and exert its functions. Ultraviolet (UV) B and antimicrobial peptides, such as cathelicidin and S100 proteins, are inducers of active vitamin D3 production in epidermis. Active vitamin D3 systemically distribute through blood flow binding to vitamin D binding protein (DBP), enter target cells through binding to heat shock protein (HSP) 70 in cytoplasm, and finally transported to the nucleus binding to VDR [26]. VDR binds to its binding site in enhancer regions of Foxp3 gene, resulting in induction and stabilization of Foxp3 expression. Alternative receptors other than VDR have been reported, such as retinoid orphan receptor (ROR)α, RORγ [27], and aryl hydrocarbon receptor (AhR) [28]. By binding to these alternative receptors, vitamin D3 derivatives have been reported to suppress inflammatory reactions, such as Th17-type inflammation, through suppressing the transactivation function of these nuclear receptors [27].

pTregs are induced by CD103-positive dendritic cells (DCs) in mesenteric lymph nodes dependent on TGFβ and retinoic acid. Cutaneous CD103-positive DCs have also been reported to induce pTregs [29]. Recent report indicated that DCs in cervical lymph nodes induce Tregs, but are not CD103-positive DCs [30,31].

Recently, Gagliani et al. [32] reported intestinal Th17 can lose the ability to produce IL-17 and behave like regulatory T cells resembling CD4+Foxp3- Type 1 Tregs (Tr1). This functional reprogramming is irreversible, and these transdifferentiated Tr1 cells show anti-inflammatory properties and suppress Th17-mediated colitis.

Psoriasis patients have a decreased number of regulatory T cells with disturbed function. Several reports indicated that successful treatment of psoriasis restored the function and number of Tregs in peripheral blood [33,34]. Bovenschen [35] reported that Foxp3-positive regulatory T cells are easily converted into Foxp3-low, IL-17 producing, and RORγt-expressing cells. The plasticity of Treg/Th17 cells makes pathophysiology of the disease more complex (Figure 5).

6. Microbiome

Advancement in computer science and next generation sequencing (NGS) technique has enabled analysis of huge amounts of genetic data at once, revealing composition of microorganisms without culture. High throughput 16S rRNA sequencing of gut microbial populations or total genome sequencing and mass-spectrometry-based metabolomic analysis can characterize gut microbiome and metabolites. Gut microbiota is a dense and diverse microbial community composed of more than 100 trillion cells and 5 million genes over 3-fold and 100-fold more than host cells and genes. Gut microbiota is composed of thousands of species. However, the majority belong to six bacterial phyla: *Actinobacteria*, *Bacteroides*, *Firmicutes*, *Fusobacteria*, *Proteobacteria*, and *Verrucomicrobia*. Fungi, Archaea, protozoa, and viruses are also included in gut microbiota. The composition of microbiota is highly influenced by environmental factors such as food, drug, and hygiene conditions, and also dependent on age and genetic background. Microbiota functions as natural digestive organs, as they digest plant polysaccharides indigestible by the host, can biosynthesize essential amino acids and vitamins, and also detoxicate hazardous materials. Recent studies revealed they also have important roles in immune system development and resistance to pathogens. Biotransformation of drugs can occur through gut microbiota altering the effects of drugs expected in vitro studies or catalyzing them to cause undesirable effects. Human genome analysis has revealed genetic susceptibility to certain diseases, and analysis of microbiota as a "second genome" would reveal more important information for disease susceptibility and drug metabolism. Further studies on gut microbiota are needed to understand the precise mechanisms in disease susceptibility variance and drug effects and side effects profiles between individuals. Such research could enhance development of precision medicine [36].

Recent studies linked cardiac disease, insulin resistance, and metabolic syndrome to gut microbiota [37,38]. Several reports supported the contribution of gut microbiota in the production of TMA (trimethylamine), the precursor of TMAO (trimethylamine N-oxide), which is a known proatherogenic molecule independent of traditional cardiovascular disease (CVD) risk factors. TMAO is involved in host cholesterol metabolism and activates macrophages leading to increased risk of CVD, myocardial infarction, and stroke. Higher TMAO producers had more *Firmicutes* than *Bacteroides* within the stool. TMAO has also been suggested to be a candidate molecule of developing type 2 diabetes mellitus (DM). Dietary supplementation with TMAO in mice resulted in impaired glucose tolerance and adipose tissue inflammation promotion. Crasiun and Balskus reported that *cutC* gene expression by bacteria such as *Disulfovibrio* can cause increased conversion of choline to TMA. Compared to healthy controls, phyla *Bacteroides* and *Proteobacteria* were reduced and phyla *Firmicutes* and *Fusobacteria* were increased in coronary artery diseases (CAD) patients [39]. Similar results were reported revealing decrease in phylum *Bacteroides* and increase in phylum *Firmicutes* in CAD patients [40]. Sanchez-Alcoholado et al. [36] compared CAD patients with type 2 DM to CAD patients without type 2 DM and revealed these two groups had different composition of gut microbiota. CAD patients with type 2 DM had decreased phylum *Bacteroides* and increased phyla *Firmicutes* and *Proteobacteria*. They also revealed plasma TMAO levels were significantly higher in CAD with DM patients compared to CAD without DM patients, which correlated with the increase in phyla *Enterobacteriaceae* and *Desulfovibrio* and a decrease in phylum *Faecalibacterium*.

Obesity is related to gut dysbiosis and increased gut permeability, resulting in abnormal translocation of bacteria and bacterial component in blood circulation. The increase in gut barrier permeability caused increase in blood lipopolysaccharide (LPS) levels, resulting in systemic low-grade inflammation and metabolic disease including type 2 diabetes [41]. Glucagon-like protein (GLP) 2 is produced by L cells in the gut, which is regulated by the host nutritional status, and increases nutrient absorption. It induces gut epithelial cell proliferation and expression of tight junction proteins. It also regulates production of antimicrobial peptides by Paneth cells. Gut microbiota in lean individuals have been reported to induce endogenous GLP2 production, resulting in improvement in gut barrier function, while that of obese patients suppresses GLP2 production leading to gut barrier impairment and bacterial translocation in blood [42].

Zonulin is a protein modulating permeability of tight junctions in the digestive tract. It was originally discovered in patients with Celiac disease and type 1 diabetes. Zonulin binds to its receptor and activates the pathway of tight junction openings resulting in increased gut permeability. Increased permeability in gut epithelial tissues leads to increased passage of antigens, and triggers autoimmunity in susceptible individuals. Recent study reported gliadin binds to CXCR3 triggering the release of zonulin. Zonulin activates PKC and PLC resulting in actin poymelization and rearrangement of cytoskeleton inducing loosening of tight junctions in a reversible manner. Increased serum level and increased excretion in the feces of zonulin have been reported in patients with gut barrier disruption, such as patients with Celiac disease, as well as type-1 diabetes, obesity, and non-alcoholic fatty liver disease [43].

Activated effector cells are anabolic, consuming glucose as their carbon source, and utilizing glycolysis to obtain ATP. Memory and regulatory cells are catabolic, utilizing fatty acids, amino acids, as well as glucose for their energy source, and utilize oxidative phosphorylation to obtain ATP. Key molecules promoting the glycolytic and lipogenic pathway are mammalian target of Rapamycin (mTOR) and adenosine monophosphate-activated kinase (AMPK). AMPK and mTOR are energy sensors regulated by nutrients availability. Th17 cells depend on glycolytic-lipogenic pathway and fatty acid synthesis for their development, while Tregs depend on oxidative phosphorylation and consume exogenous fatty acids. HIF1α is the transcription factor which upregulates glycolytic pathway in Th17 cells binding to RORγt promoter and enhancing its expression, while also suppressing Foxp3 expression. It promotes differentiation of naïve T cells towards Th17 cells and inhibits differentiation into Treg cells under normoxic and hypoxic conditions. Inflammation sites are usually in hypoxic condition and show increased extracellular ATP concentration, which induces HIF1αactivation required for Th17 cell development, and AhR inactivation needed in Tr1 metabolism. Thus, metabolic factors have immune-modifying ability by skewing Th17/Treg balance resulting in skewed balance in inflammation or immune tolerance [44].

Gut microbiota profoundly affect T cell differentiation and response to immune stimuli. Segmented filamentous bacteria (SFB), a *Clostridia*-related species found mainly in rodents, specifically induces Th17 cells in the small intestine and other sites in autoimmune condition. SFB colonization is usually beneficial because it attenuates bacteria-induced colitis, while it also induces colitis in genetically susceptible mice strains. The abundance of SFB and the gut barrier function is regulated by IL-23R/IL-22 pathway. The disruption of gut barrier resulting in systemic distribution of bacteria or their components induces IL-23 pathway, initiating barrier repair, and Th17 responses in order to neutralize invading microbes. IL-23 induced by SFB stimulates production of IL-22 from ILC3 causing serum amyloid A production by epithelial cells [45] (Figure 6).

Psoriasis is considered a systemic and chronic inflammatory disease, involving skin, as well as the cardiovascular system, insulin homeostasis, psychomotor systems, and lipid metabolism. A recent study has detected bacterial DNA in blood in active psoriasis patients (bacterial translocation; BT), and those with bacterial DNA-positive psoriasis patients showed higher serum inflammatory cytokine levels, longer duration of disease and younger onset of disease. They suggested that psoriasis eruption may be related to bacterial DNA in blood originating in the gut [46]. Codoner et al. revealed phylum *Bacteroides* decreased and phylum *Faecalibacterium* increased in psoriasis patients. They compared the microbiome between BT-positive patients and BT-negative patients and did not find specific phyla of microbiome. They speculated that dysbiosis in psoriasis patient guts caused insufficient gut barrier permeability resulting in bacterial translocation into the blood stream [47]. Hidalgo-Cantabrana et al. reported recently the increase in *Bacteroides* and decrease in *Firmicutes* in psoriasis patients compared to healthy controls [48].

Bacteroides can produce short chain fatty acids (SCFA) such as propionates and butyrates. These SCFA bind to the G-protein-coupled receptor, GPR41 and GPR43, and induce GLP-1 and GLP-2 production in L cells, which influence the energy metabolism and improve gut barrier function [49]. *Akkermansia muciniphila* has also been suggested to produce SCFA to improve energy metabolism, which are decreased in obese patients compared to healthy controls. SCFA are also involved in the stabilization of Foxp3 expression as discussed above, resulting in improvement of regulatory T cell function. GPR41 and GPR43, the receptors for SCFA, are expressed on the surface of regulatory T cells distributed in the gut. The number of Tregs increased in mice supplemented with SCFA. Experimentally induced autoimmune encephalomyelitis was suppressed in mice supplemented with SCFA [49].

Scher et al. [50] reported gut microbiota composition was different in psoriatic arthritis patients and psoriasis without arthritis patients. They found that phylum *Actinobacteria* was significantly decreased in psoriatic arthritis patients. *Actinobacteria* phylum includes *Bifidobacterium* species, of which supplementation lowered the serum levels of CRP and TNFαa in psoriasis patients.

Another approach altering the gut microbial effect is to influence the pathway the microbiome uses. Farnesoid X receptor (FXR) is the essential nuclear receptor whose antagonist can inhibit high-fat diet-induced obesity in mice. FXR is involved in the metabolism of bile acid, lipid, and glucose. Intestine-specific FXR knockout mice were resistant to high-fat diet-induced obesity. However, contradictory results have been reported: FXR-null mice showed increased glucose intolerance on a chow diet, and FXR-agonist was effective in improving insulin sensitivity in genetically obese mice. Other studies presented that FXR-null mice showed increased glucose tolerance and FXR-agonist exacerbated insulin resistance and lipid metabolism in obese mice models. Li et al. speculated this discrepancy is due to differences in gut microbiota composition and the distinct roles of liver FXR and intestine FXR. Their study provided evidence that FXR inhibition in the intestine by antioxidant "tempol" or by genetic ablation of FXR is effective in suppressing diet-induced obesity and insulin resistance [51,52]. Other molecules in the context of microbiome signaling are peroxisome proliferator activated receptor (PPAR)s. Gut microbiota influence the expression of PPARs, and PPARs transduce signals to induce or suppress many molecules involved in inflammation, obesity, and insulin resistance [53].

7. Discussion and Conclusions

Many novel findings revealed the importance of innate immunity in psoriasis pathogenesis. The roles of skin resident cells and Tregs have been drawing attention in psoriasis pathogenesis. Epidemiological study revealed the relation between psoriasis and comorbid diseases such as cardiovascular diseases, diabetes mellitus and obesity, and the gut dysbiosis in psoriasis patients has recently been demonstrated. However, the underling mechanism and pathogenic roles of gut microbiome has to be clarified further. This review tried to hunt the findings in basic science and in metabolic diseases, and to combine them to be applied to future psoriasis research.

It is not clear whether dysbiosis in gut microbiota in psoriasis patients has the pathogenic roles or just the result of systemic inflammation in psoriasis. However, the recent study on gut microbiota and the immune regulatory mechanism suggests that dysbiosis in gut microbiota by inducing disfunction of Tregs and activation of Th17 and ILC3 could lead genetically susceptible individuals to develop psoriasis. It may also cause obesity, diabetes mellitus, and cardiovascular diseases, among individuals with distinct genetic backgrounds. The increase in number of psoriasis patients in Japan with westernization of life could be explained by the change of diet, resulting in a change in microbiota. Decrease of dietary fibers may reduce SCFA-producing phyla in gut microbiota, resulting in activation of gut dendritic cells to produce IL-23, which in turn may stimulate unstable Foxp3-positive Tregs to differentiate into IL-17-producing cells. Psoriasis has been recognized as a multifactorial genetic disease, not only depending on genetic background, but also on environmental factors including lifestyle habits, which could also be well-explained.

Skewed balance of skin resident cells may be generated by activation of epidermal keratinocytes producing slightly higher amount of CCL20 by commensal microbe stimulation in genetically susceptible individuals, which could be enhanced under the environment of disturbed Treg function and increased Th17 cytokines in individuals with dysbiosis.

In this review, the gut–skin axis is the main target of discussion, thus skin-specific cells, such as epidermal keratinocytes and dermal fibroblasts, are not discussed. The nuclear receptors such as RARs, VDR, and RORs are expressed not only in immune cells, but also in epidermal keratinocytes [26], making the epidermal keratinocytes another target of immune regulation. Skin has its own microbiome, through influencing the homeostasis of epidermis, it regulates the immune status of the whole body. The discussion on these issues have been left at another opportunity.

Systemic inflammation in psoriasis patients has led researchers to investigate the relation of psoriasis to metabolic diseases and has significantly deepened recent psoriasis investigation. A systemic approach to treat psoriasis has long been attempted with etretinate and cyclosporine, and recent biologics have shown remarkable therapeutic effects. Knowledge in skin resident cells are preferential to topical treatment, however, accumulating evidence in the gut–skin axis [54] would favor a nutritional approach or signal inhibition to change microbiome composition. Therefore, increasing therapeutic options may be available for future psoriasis treatment.

8. Figures, Tables, and Schemes

Figure 1. Pathogenesis of psoriasis. Modified from Lowes M.A. et al. Trends in Immunol 2016 [4].

External immune triggers, LL37 bound to self-DNA or RNA activate plasmacytoid and myeloid dendritic cells (pDC and mDC). Activated plasmacytoid cells produce type 1 interferons, and myeloid dendritic cells produce TNFα, iNOS, and IL-23, which activate Th17 cells to produce IL-17 and IL-22. IL-17 and IL-22 induce proliferation, production of cytokines, chemokines and antimicrobial peptides from epidermal keratinocytes, thus resulting in psoriatic phenotype.

Figure 2. Skewed balance of tissue resident immune cells induces psoriasis in never-lesional skin of psoriasis patients. Modified from Gallais Sérézal I et al. J Allergy Clin Immunol 2018 [17].

Weak stimulation by commensal bacteria and fungi causes sparse production of CCL20 from the epidermal keratinocytes, resulting in skewed distribution of CCR6-positive, IL-17-producing cells in the never-lesional skin of psoriasis patients (NLP) over IFNγ-producing cells, which prepare conditions for psoriasis eruption when appropriate insults, such as bacterial or viral infection, or trauma occurs.

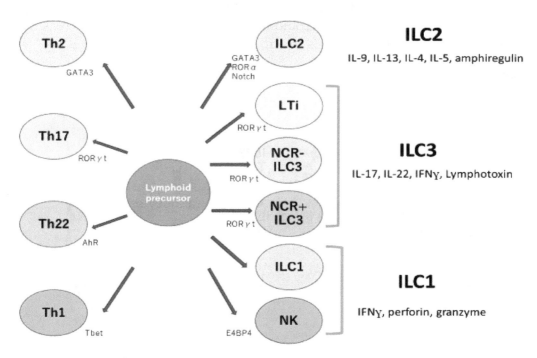

Figure 3. Three groups of innate lymphoid cells parallel three types of T helper cells. Modified from Walker JA et al. Nat Rev Immunol 2013 [18].

Innate lymphoid cells are divided into three groups; group 1, 2, and 3. Function and essential nuclear factors seem similar to those of corresponding T helper cells.

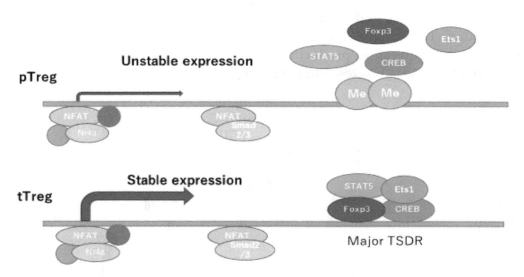

Figure 4. Expression of FOXP3 in pTreg is unstable. Modified from Kanamori M et al. Trends in Immunol 2016, and Iizuka-Koga et al. J Autoimmun 2017 [24,25].

Promoter lesion of FOXP3 gene contains major Treg-specific demethylated resion (TSDR), which binds transcription factors, such as FOXP3, CREB, Ets1, and STAT5 constitutively in tTregs, but just transiently in pTregs. TSDR in pTregs are partially methylated, which makes it difficult to bind transcription factors needed for the stable expression of FOXP3.

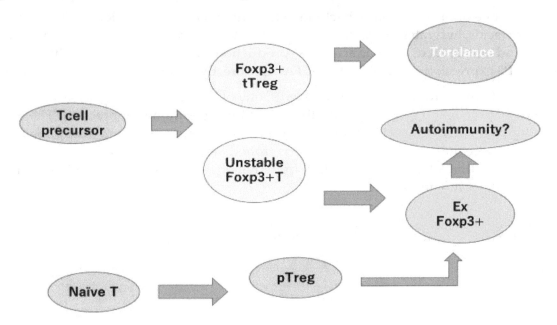

Figure 5. Foxp3-positive Tregs, but with unstable expression, would easily lose FOXP3 expression and become inflammatory. Modified from Iizuka-Koga M et al. J Autoimmun 2017 [25].

tTregs differentiated in thymus stably express FOXP3 and are involved in immune tolerance. Peripherally induced Tregs and Tregs with unstable FOXP3 expression can lose FOXP3 expression and become inflammatory cells, which may contribute to autoimmunity.

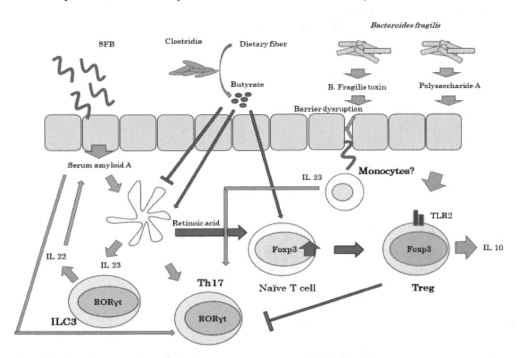

Figure 6. Gut microbiota regulates the balance of Th17 vs. Tregs. Modified from Omenetti S and Pizzaro TT. Frontiers Immuno 2015 [43].

Segmented filamentous bacteria (SFB) colonization allow them to closely contact to intestinal epithelium, which induce cytokines, such as serum amyloid A (SAA), and activate Th17. SAA also induces IL-23 production from dendritic cells, which indirectly activate Th17 and ILC3 to produce pro-inflammatory IL-17, and IL-22. IL-22 stimulate intestinal epithelial cells to produce SAA.

Clostridia is one of the commensal bacteria in the gut, which ferment dietary fibers and produce short chain fatty acids; butyrates. SCFA suppresses dendritic cell production of inflammatory cytokines, such as IL-6, and also induces retinoic acid (RA) production from dendritic cells, which induces and stabilizes FOXP3 expression in naïve Tcells. SCFA also directly act on naïve T cells to express FOXP3.

There are different strains of *Bacteroides fragilis*, one of which produces polysaccharide A (PSA) and induce IL-10 production from Treg cells, thereby inducing immune suppression. The other strain produces B. fragilis toxin (BFA), which causes impairment of tight junctions and disruption of intestinal barrier function. Recognition of microbial products from disseminated bacteria by microbe associated molecular patterns stimulates IL-23 production from monocytes and stimulates Th17 cells to produce IL-17 and exacerbates inflammation.

Author Contributions: M.K. contributed to reading and writing the whole manuscript and drawing the figures. All authors have read and agreed to the published version of the manuscript.

Abbreviations

IL	Interleukin
Th	T helper
DNA	Deoxy ribonucleic acid
RNA	Ribonucleic acid
CCL	CC chemokine ligand
CXCL	CXC chemokine ligand
CCR	CC chemokine receptor
CXCR	CXC chemokine receptor
TGFβ	Transforming growth factor beta
STAT	Signal transducers and activators of transcription
NFAT	Nuclear factor for activated T cells
AP-1	Activator protein 1
CREB	cAMP response element bunding protein
PKC	Protein kinase C
PLC	Phospholipase C
ATP	Adenosine triphosphate
HIF1	Hypoxia inducible factor
ROR	RAR-related orphan receptor
GATA	GATA binding protein
GPR	G-protein coupled receptor
CRP	C reactive protein
TCR	T cell receptor
CLA	Cutaneous lymphocyte associated antigen
IFN	Interferon
NK	Natural killer

References

1.   Liang, Y.; Sarkar, M.K.; Tsoi, L.C.; Gudjonsson, J.E. Psoriasis: A mixed autoimmune and autoinflammatory disease. *Curr. Opin. Immunol.* **2017**, *49*, 1–8. [CrossRef] [PubMed]

2.   Guttman-Yassky, E.; Krueger, J.G. Atopic dermatitis and psoriasis: Two different immune diseases or one spectrum? *Curr. Opin. Immunol.* **2017**, *48*, 68–73. [CrossRef] [PubMed]

3. Moy, A.P.; Murali, M.; Kroshinsky, D.; Horn, T.D.; Nazarian, R.M. T-helper immune phenotype may underlie 'paradoxical' tumour necrosis factor-α inhibitor therapy-related psoriasiform dermatitis. *Clin. Exp. Derm.* **2018**, *43*, 19–26. [CrossRef] [PubMed]

4. Lowes, M.A.; Russell, C.B.; Martin, D.A.; Towne, J.E.; Krueger, J.G. The IL-23/T17 pathogenic axis in psoriasis is amplified by keratinocyte responses. *Trends Immunol.* **2013**, *34*, 174–181. [CrossRef]

5. Jensen, P.; Skov, L. Psoriasis and Obesity. *Dermatology* **2016**, *232*, 633–639. [CrossRef]

6. Clark, R.A. Resident memory T cells in human health and disease. *Sci. Transl. Med.* **2015**, *7*, 269rv1. [CrossRef]

7. Boyman, O.; Hefti, H.P.; Conrad, C.; Nickoloff, B.J.; Suter, M.; Nestle, F.O. Spontaneous development of psoriasis in a new animal model shows an essential role for resident T cells and tumor necrosis factor-alpha. *J. Exp. Med.* **2004**, *199*, 731–736. [CrossRef]

8. Clark, R.A.; Chong, B.; Mirchandani, N.; Brinster, N.K.; Yamanaka, K.; Dowgiert, R.K.; Kupper, T.S. The vast majority of CLA+ T cells are resident in normal skin. *J. Immunol.* **2006**, *176*, 4431. [CrossRef]

9. Booth, J.S.; Toapanta, F.R.; Salerno-Goncalves, R.; Patil, S.; Kader, H.A.; Safta, A.M.; Czinn, S.J.; Greenwald, B.D.; Sztein, M.B. Characterization and functional properties of gastric tissue-resident memory T cells from children, adults, and the elderly. *Front. Immunol.* **2014**, *5*, 294. [CrossRef]

10. Okhrimenko, A.; Grün, J.R.; Westendorf, K.; Fang, Z.; Reinke, S.; von Roth, P.; Wassilew, G.; Kühl, A.A.; Kudernatsch, R.; Demski, S.; et al. Human memory T cells from the bone marrow are resting and maintain long-lasting systemic memory. *Proc. Nat. Acad. Sci.* **2014**, *111*, 9229–9234. [CrossRef]

11. Turner, D.L.; Bickham, K.L.; Thome, J.J.; Kim, C.Y.; D'Ovidio, F.; Wherry, E.J.; Farber, D.L. Lung niches for the generation and maintenance of tissue-resident memory T cells. *Mucosal Immunol.* **2014**, *7*, 501–510. [CrossRef] [PubMed]

12. Roberts, G.W.; Baird, D.; Gallagher, K.; Jones, R.E.; Pepper, C.J.; Williams, J.D.; Topley, N. Functional effector memory T cells enrich the peritoneal cavity of patients treated with peritoneal dialysis. *J. Am. Soc. Nephrol.* **2009**, *20*, 1895–1900. [CrossRef] [PubMed]

13. Purwar, R.; Campbell, J.; Murphy, G.; Richards, W.G.; Clark, R.A.; Kupper, T.S. Resident Memory T Cells (T(RM)) Are Abundant in Human Lung: Diversity, Function, and Antigen Specificity. *PLoS ONE* **2011**, *6*, e16245. [CrossRef] [PubMed]

14. Bhushan, M.; Bleiker, T.O.; Ballsdon, A.E.; Allen, M.H.; Sopwith, M.; Robinson, M.K.; Clarke, C.; Weller, R.P.; Graham-Brown, R.A.; Keefe, M.; et al. Anti-E-selectin is ineffective in the treatment of psoriasis: A randomized trial. *Br. J. Dermatol.* **2002**, *146*, 824–831. [CrossRef] [PubMed]

15. Cheuk, S.; Wikén, M.; Blomqvist, L.; Nylén, S.; Talme, T.; Ståhle, M.; Eidsmo, L. Epidermal Th22 and Tc17 cells form a localized disease memory in clinically healed psoriasis. *J. Immunol.* **2014**, *192*, 3111–3120. [CrossRef] [PubMed]

16. Matos, T.R.; O'Malley, J.T.; Lowry, E.L.; Hamm, D.; Kirsch, I.R.; Robins, H.S.; Kupper, T.S.; Krueger, J.G.; Clark, R.A. Clinically resolved psoriatic lesions contain psoriasis-specific IL-17-producing αβ T cell clones. *J. Clin. Invest.* **2017**, *127*, 4031–4041. [CrossRef] [PubMed]

17. Gallais Sérézal, I.; Hoffer, E.; Ignatov, B.; Martini, E.; Zitti, B.; Ehrström, M.; Eidsmo, L. A skewed pool of resident T cells triggers psoriasis-associated tissue responses in never-lesional skin from patients with psoriasis. *J. Allergy Clin. Immunol.* **2019**, *143*, 1444–1454. [CrossRef]

18. Walker, J.A.; Barlow, J.L.; McKenzie, A.N. Innate lymphoid cells–how did we miss them? *Nat. Rev. Immunol.* **2013**, *13*, 75–87. [CrossRef]

19. Bernink, J.H.; Peters, C.P.; Munneke, M.; te Velde, A.A.; Meijer, S.L.; Weijer, K.; Hreggvidsdottir, H.S.; Heinsbroek, S.E.; Legrand, N.; Buskens, C.J.; et al. Human type 1 lymphoid cells accumulate in inflamed mucosal tissues. *Nat. Immunol.* **2013**, *14*, 221–229. [CrossRef]

20. Villanova, F.; Flutter, B.; Tosi, I.; Grys, K.; Sreeneebus, H.; Perera, G.K.; Chapman, A.; Smith, C.H.; Di Meglio, P.; Nestle, F.O. Characterization of innate lymphoid cells in human skin and blood demonstrates increase of NKp44+ ILC3 in psoriasis. *J. Investig. Derm.* **2014**, *134*, 984–991. [CrossRef]

21. Zeng, B.; Shi, S.; Ashworth, G.; Dong, C.; Liu, J.; Xing, F. ILC3 function as a double-edged sword in inflammatory bowel diseases. *Cell Death Dis.* **2019**, *10*, 315. [CrossRef] [PubMed]

22. Soare, A.; Weber, S.; Maul, L.; Rauber, S.; Gheorghiu, A.M.; Luber, M.; Houssni, I.; Kleyer, A.; von Pickardt, G.; Gado, M.; et al. Cutting Edge: Homeostasis of Innate Lymphoid Cells Is Imbalanced in Psoriatic Arthritis. *J. Immunol.* **2018**, *200*, 1249–1254. [CrossRef] [PubMed]

23. Keren, A.; Shemer, A.; Ginzburg, A.; Ullmann, Y.; Schrum, A.G.; Paus, R.; Gilhar, A. Innate lymphoid cells 3 induce psoriasis in xenotransplanted healthy human skin. *J. Allergy Clin. Immunol.* **2018**, *142*, 305–308.e6. [CrossRef] [PubMed]

24. Kanamori, M.; Nakatsukasa, H.; Okada, M.; Lu, Q.; Yoshimura, A. Induced Regulatory T Cells: Their Development, Stability, and Applications. *Trends Immunol.* **2016**, *37*, 803–811. [CrossRef]

25. Iizuka-Koga, M.; Nakatsukasa, H.; Ito, M.; Akanuma, T.; Lu, Q.; Yoshimura, A. Induction and maintenance of regulatory T cells by transcription factors and epigenetic modifications. *J. Autoimmun.* **2017**, *83*, 113–121. [CrossRef]

26. Bikle, D.; Christakos, S. New aspects of vitamin D metabolism and action - addressing the skin as source and target. *Nat. Rev. Endocrinol.* **2020**, *16*, 234–252. [CrossRef]

27. Slominski, A.T.; Kim, T.K.; Takeda, Y.; Janjetovic, Z.; Brozyna, A.A.; Skobowiat, C.; Wang, J.; Postlethwaite, A.; Li, W.; Tuckey, R.C.; et al. RORα and ROR γ are expressed in human skin and serve as receptors for endogenously produced noncalcemic 20-hydroxy- and 20,23-dihydroxyvitamin D. *FASEB J.* **2014**, *28*, 2775–2789. [CrossRef]

28. Slominski, A.T.; Kim, T.K.; Janjetovic, Z.; Brożyna, A.A.; Żmijewski, M.A.; Xu, H.; Sutter, T.R.; Tuckey, R.C.; Jetten, A.M.; Crossman, D.K. Differential and Overlapping Effects of $20,23(OH)_2D3$ and $1,25(OH)_2D3$ on Gene Expression in Human Epidermal Keratinocytes: Identification of AhR as an Alternative Receptor for $20,23(OH)_2D3$. *Int. J. Mol. Sci.* **2018**, *19*, 3072. [CrossRef]

29. Shiokawa, A.; Kotaki, R.; Takano, T.; Nakajima-Adachi, H.; Hachimura, S. Mesenteric lymph node CD11b- $CD103_+$ PD-L1$_{High}$ dendritic cells highly induce regulatory T cells. *Immunology* **2017**, *152*, 52–64. [CrossRef]

30. Yamazaki, S.; Maruyama, A.; Okada, K.; Matsumoto, M.; Morita, A.; Seya, T. Dendritic cells from oral cavity induce Foxp3(+) regulatory T cells upon antigen stimulation. *PLoS ONE* **2012**, *7*, e51665. [CrossRef]

31. Yamazaki, S.; Odanaka, M.; Nishioka, A.; Kasuya, S.; Shime, H.; Hemmi, H.; Imai, M.; Riethmacher, D.; Kaisho, T.; Ohkura, N.; et al. Ultraviolet B-Induced Maturation of CD11b-Type Langerin_ Dendritic Cells Controls the Expansion of Foxp3$_+$ Regulatory T Cells in the Skin. *J. Immunol.* **2018**, *200*, 119–129. [CrossRef] [PubMed]

32. Gagliani, N.; Vesely, M.C.A.; Iseppon, A.; Brockmann, L.; Xu, H.; Palm, N.W.; de Zoete, M.R.; Licona-Limón, P.; Paiva, R.S.; Ching, T.; et al. TH17 cells transdifferentiate into regulatory T cells during resolution of inflammation. *Nature* **2015**, *523*, 221–225. [CrossRef] [PubMed]

33. Quaglino, P.; Ortoncelli, M.; Comessatti, A.; Ponti, R.; Novelli, M.; Bergallo, M.; Costa, C.; Cicchelli, S.; Savoia, P.; Bernengo, M.G. Circulating CD4+CD25brightFOXP3+ T cells are up-regulated by biological therapies and correlate with the clinical response in psoriasis patients. *Dermatology* **2009**, *219*, 250–258. [CrossRef] [PubMed]

34. Saito, C.; Maeda, A.; Morita, A. Bath-PUVA therapy induces circulating regulatory T cells in patients with psoriasis. *J. Derm. Sci.* **2009**, *53*, 231–233. [CrossRef] [PubMed]

35. Bovenschen, H.J.; van de Kerkhof, P.C.; van Erp, P.E.; Woestenenk, R.; Joosten, I.; Koenen, H.J. Foxp3+ regulatory T cells of psoriasis patients easily differentiate into IL-17A-producing cells and are found in lesional skin. *J. Invest. Derm.* **2011**, *131*, 1853–1860. [CrossRef] [PubMed]

36. Spanogiannopoulos, P.; Bess, E.N.; Carmody, R.N.; Turnbaugh, P.J. The microbial pharmacists within us: A metagenomic view of xenobiotic metabolism. *Nat. Rev. Microbiol.* **2016**, *14*, 273–287. [CrossRef]

37. Sanchez-Alcoholado, L.; Castellano-Castillo, D.; Jordán-Martínez, L.; Moreno-Indias, I.; Cardila-Cruz, P.; Elena, D.; Muñoz-Garcia, A.J.; Queipo-Ortuño, M.I.; Jimenez-Navarro, M. Role of Gut Microbiota on Cardio-Metabolic Parameters and Immunity in Coronary Artery Disease Patients with and without Type-2 Diabetes Mellitus. *Front. Microbiol.* **2017**, *8*, 1936. [CrossRef]

38. Larsen, N.; Vogensen, F.K.; van den Berg, F.W.; Nielsen, D.S.; Andreasen, A.S.; Pedersen, B.K.; Al-Soud, W.A.; Sørensen, S.J.; Hansen, L.H.; Jakobsen, M. Gut microbiota in human adults with type 2 diabetes differs from non-diabetic adults. *PLoS ONE* **2010**, *5*, e9085. [CrossRef]

39. Cui, L.; Zhao, T.; Hu, H.; Zhang, W.; Hua, X. Association Study of Gut Flora in Coronary Heart Disease through High-Throughput Sequencing. *Biomed. Res. Int.* **2017**, *2017*, 3796359. [CrossRef]

40. Emoto, T.; Yamashita, T.; Kobayashi, T.; Sasaki, N.; Hirota, Y.; Hayashi, T.; So, A.; Kasahara, K.; Yodoi, K.; Matsumoto, T.; et al. Characterization of gut microbiota profiles in coronary artery disease patients using data mining analysis of terminal restriction fragment length polymorphism: Gut microbiota could be a diagnostic marker of coronary artery disease. *Heart Vessel.* **2017**, *32*, 39–46. [CrossRef]

41. Cani, P.D.; Everard, A.; Duparc, T. Gut microbiota, enteroendocrine functions and metabolism. *Curr. Opin. Pharm.* **2013**, *13*, 935–940. [CrossRef] [PubMed]

42. Cani, P.D.; Possemiers, S.; Van de Wiele, T.; Guiot, Y.; Everard, A.; Rottier, O.; Geurts, L.; Naslain, D.; Neyrinck, A.; Lambert, D.M.; et al. Changes in gut microbiota control inflammation in obese mice through a mechanism involving GLP-2-driven improvement of gut permeability. *Gut* **2009**, *58*, 1091–1103. [CrossRef] [PubMed]

43. Omenetti, S.; Pizarro, T.T. The Treg/Th17 Axis: A Dynamic Balance Regulated by the Gut Microbiome. *Front. Immunol.* **2015**, *6*, 639. [CrossRef] [PubMed]

44. Rahman, M.T.; Ghosh, C.; Hossain, M.; Linfield, D.; Rezaee, F.; Janigro, D.; Marchi, N.; van Boxel-Dezaire, A.H.H. IFN-γ, IL-17A, or zonulin rapidly increase the permeability of the blood-brain and small intestinal epithelial barriers: Relevance for neuro-inflammatory diseases. *Biochem. Biophys. Res. Commun.* **2018**, *507*, 274–279. [CrossRef] [PubMed]

45. Martin, A.M.; Sun, E.W.; Rogers, G.B.; Keating, D.J. The Influence of the Gut Microbiome on Host Metabolism Through the Regulation of Gut Hormone Release. *Front. Physiol.* **2019**, *10*, 428. [CrossRef]

46. Ramírez-Boscá, A.; Navarro-López, V.; Martínez-Andrés, A.; Such, J.; Francés, R.; Horga de la Parte, J.; Asín-Llorca, M. Identification of Bacterial DNA in the Peripheral Blood of Patients With Active Psoriasis. *Jama Derm.* **2015**, *151*, 670–671. [CrossRef]

47. Codoñer, F.M.; Ramírez-Bosca, A.; Climent, E.; Carrión-Gutierrez, M.; Guerrero, M.; Pérez-Orquín, J.M.; Horga de la Parte, J.; Genovés, S.; Ramón, D.; Navarro-López, V.; et al. Gut microbial composition in patients with psoriasis. *Sci. Rep.* **2018**, *8*, 3812. [CrossRef]

48. Hidalgo-Cantabrana, C.; Gómez, J.; Delgado, S.; Requena-López, S.; Queiro-Silva, R.; Margolles, A.; Coto, E.; Sánchez, B.; Coto-Segura, P. Gut microbiota dysbiosis in a cohort of patients with psoriasis. *Br. J. Dermatol.* **2019**, *181*, 1287–1295. [CrossRef]

49. Smith, P.M.; Howitt, M.R.; Panikov, N.; Michaud, M.; Gallini, C.A.; Bohlooly-Y., M.; Glickman, J.N.; Garrett, W.S. The microbial metabolites, short-chain fatty acids, regulate colonic Treg cell homeostasis. *Science* **2013**, *341*, 569–573. [CrossRef]

50. Scher, J.U.; Ubeda, C.; Artacho, A.; Attur, M.; Isaac, S.; Reddy, S.M.; Marmon, S.; Neimann, A.; Brusca, S.; Patel, T.; et al. Decreased bacterial diversity characterizes the altered gut microbiota in patients with psoriatic arthritis, resembling dysbiosis in inflammatory bowel disease. *Arthritis Rheumatol.* **2015**, *67*, 128–139. [CrossRef]

51. Jiang, C.; Xie, C.; Lv, Y.; Li, J.; Krausz, K.W.; Shi, J.; Brocker, C.N.; Desai, D.; Amin, S.G.; Bisson, W.H.; et al. Intestine-selective farnesoid X receptor inhibition improves obesity-related metabolic dysfunction. *Nat. Commun.* **2015**, *6*, 10166. [CrossRef] [PubMed]

52. Li, F.; Jiang, C.; Krausz, K.W.; Li, Y.; Albert, I.; Hao, H.; Fabre, K.M.; Mitchell, J.B.; Patterson, A.D.; Gonzalez, F.J. Microbiome remodelling leads to inhibition of intestinal farnesoid X receptor signalling and decreased obesity. *Nat Commun.* **2013**, *4*, 2384. [CrossRef] [PubMed]

53. den Besten, G.; Bleeker, A.; Gerding, A.; van Eunen, K.; Havinga, R.; van Dijk, T.H.; Oosterveer, M.H.; Jonker, J.W.; Groen, A.K.; Reijngoud, D.J.; et al. Short-Chain Fatty Acids Protect Against High-Fat Diet-Induced Obesity via a PPARγ-Dependent Switch From Lipogenesis to Fat Oxidation. *Diabetes* **2015**, *64*, 2398–2408. [CrossRef] [PubMed]

54. Salem, I.; Ramser, A.; Isham, N.; Ghannoum, M.A. The Gut Microbiome as a Major Regulator of the Gut-Skin Axis. *Front. Microbiol.* **2018**, *9*, 1459. [CrossRef]

Permissions

List of Contributors

Markus Blaess
Institute of Precision Medicine, Medical and Life Sciences Faculty, Furtwangen University, Jakob-Kienzle-Strasse 17, 78054 Villingen-Schwenningen, Germany

Hans-Peter Deigner
Institute of Precision Medicine, Medical and Life Sciences Faculty, Furtwangen University, Jakob-Kienzle-Strasse 17, 78054 Villingen-Schwenningen, Germany
EXIM Department, Fraunhofer Institute IZI Leipzig, Schillingallee 68, 18057 Rostock, Germany

Raj Chovatiya
Department of Dermatology, Northwestern University Feinberg School of Medicine, Chicago, IL 60611, USA

Jonathan I. Silverberg
Department of Dermatology, George Washington University School of Medicine, Washington, DC 20037, USA

Piotr Wójcik, Michał Biernacki, Wojciech Łuczaj and Elżbieta Skrzydlewska
Department of Analytical Chemistry, Medical University of Bialystok, 15-089 Białystok, Poland

Adam Wroński
Dermatological Specialized Center "DERMAL" NZOZ in Bialystok, 15-453 Białystok, Poland

Georg Waeg
Institute of Molecular Biosciences, University of Graz, 8010 Graz, Austria

Neven Žarković
LabOS, Rudjer Boskovic Institute, Laboratory for Oxidative Stress, 10000 Zagreb, Croatia

Agnieszka Owczarczyk-Saczonek, Marta Kasprowicz-Furmańczyk and Waldemar Placek
Department of Dermatology, Sexually Transmitted Diseases and Clinical Immunology, The University of Warmia and Mazury, Al. Wojska Polskiego 30, 10-229 Olsztyn, Poland

Magdalena Krajewska-Włodarczyk
Department of Rheumatology, Municipal Hospital in Olsztyn, 10-229 Olsztyn, Poland
Department of Internal Medicine, School of Medicine, Collegium Medicum, University of Warmia and Mazury, 10-900 Olsztyn, Poland

Chun-Ming Shih and Chun-Yao Huang
Department of Internal Medicine, School of Medicine, College of Medicine, Taipei Medical University, Taipei 11031, Taiwan
Cardiovascular Research Center, Taipei Medical University Hospital, Taipei 11031, Taiwan
Taipei Heart Institute, Taipei Medical University, Taipei 11031, Taiwan

Chang-Cyuan Chen
Department of Anatomy and Cell Biology, School of Medicine, College of Medicine, Taipei Medical University, Taipei 11031, Taiwan

Ai-Wei Lee
Cardiovascular Research Center, Taipei Medical University Hospital, Taipei 11031, Taiwan
Taipei Heart Institute, Taipei Medical University, Taipei 11031, Taiwan
Department of Anatomy and Cell Biology, School of Medicine, College of Medicine, Taipei Medical University, Taipei 11031, Taiwan

Chen-Kuo Chu
Department of Emergency Medicine, Taichung Veterans General Hospital, Taichung 40705, Taiwan

Kuo-Hsien Wang
Department of Dermatology, Taipei Medical University Hospital, Taipei 11031, Taiwan

Kazuhisa Furue
Department of Dermatology, Graduate School of Medical Sciences, Kyushu University, Maidashi 3-1-1, Higashiku, Fukuoka 812-8582, Japan

Gaku Tsuji
Department of Dermatology, Graduate School of Medical Sciences, Kyushu University, Maidashi 3-1-1, Higashiku, Fukuoka 812-8582, Japan
Research and Clinical Center for Yusho and Dioxin, Kyushu University, Maidashi 3-1-1, Higashiku, Fukuoka 812-8582, Japan

Takeshi Nakahara
Department of Dermatology, Graduate School of Medical Sciences, Kyushu University, Maidashi 3-1-1, Higashiku, Fukuoka 812-8582, Japan
Division of Skin Surface Sensing, Graduate School of Medical Sciences, Kyushu University, Maidashi 3-1-1, Higashiku, Fukuoka 812-8582, Japan

Kento Mizutani, Yoshiaki Matsushima, Ai Umaoka, Karin Okada and Keiichi Yamanaka
Department of Dermatology, Graduate School of Medicine, Mie University, Mie, Tsu 514-8507, Japan

Eri Shirakami
Department of Dermatology, Graduate School of Medicine, Mie University, Mie, Tsu 514-8507, Japan
Department of Dermatology, Faculty of Medicine, Shimane University, Shimane, Izumo 693-8501, Japan

Eishin Morita
Department of Dermatology, Faculty of Medicine, Shimane University, Shimane, Izumo 693-8501, Japan

Masako Ichishi and Masatoshi Watanabe
Department of Oncologic Pathology, Graduate School of Medicine, Mie University, Mie, Tsu 514-8507, Japan

Yukie Yamaguchi
Department of Environmental Immuno-Dermatology, School of Medicine, Yokohama City University Graduate, Yokohama 236-0027, Japan

Marco Diani and Gianfranco Altomare
Department of Dermatology and Venereology, IRCCS Istituto Ortopedico Galeazzi, 20161 Milan, Italy

Silvia Perego, Veronica Sansoni, Marta Gomarasca and Martina Faraldi
Laboratory of Experimental Biochemistry and Molecular Biology, IRCCS Istituto Ortopedico Galeazzi, 20161 Milan, Italy

Lucrezia Bertino
Department of Clinical and Experimental Medicine, section of Dermatology, University of Messina, 98122 Messina, Italy

Paolo Daniele Maria Pigatto
Department of Dermatology and Venereology, IRCCS Istituto Ortopedico Galeazzi, 20161 Milan, Italy
Department of Biomedical, Surgical and Dental Sciences, University of Milan, 20122 Milano, Italy

Giovanni Damiani
Department of Dermatology and Venereology, IRCCS Istituto Ortopedico Galeazzi, 20161 Milan, Italy
Department of Biomedical, Surgical and Dental Sciences, University of Milan, 20122 Milano, Italy
Department of Dermatology, Case Western Reserve University, Cleveland, OH 44106, USA
Young Dermatologists Italian Network, Centro Studi GISED, 24121 Bergamo, Italy

Giuseppe Banfi
Laboratory of Experimental Biochemistry and Molecular Biology, IRCCS Istituto Ortopedico Galeazzi, 20161 Milan, Italy
Vita-Salute San Raffaele University, 20132 Milan, Italy

Giovanni Lombardi
Laboratory of Experimental Biochemistry and Molecular Biology, IRCCS Istituto Ortopedico Galeazzi, 20161 Milan, Italy
Department of Physiology and Pharmacology, Gdańsk University of Physical Education and Sport, 80336 Gdańsk, Poland

Hayato Nomura, Yuki Isokane, Ko Sunagawa, Mina Kobashi, Satoru Sugihara, Ai Kajita, Tomoko Miyake, Yoji Hirai, Osamu Yamasaki and Shin Morizane
Department of Dermatology, Okayama University Graduate School of Medicine, Dentistry, and Pharmaceutical Science, 2-5-1 Shikata-cho, Kitaku, Okayama 700-8558, Japan

Mutsumi Suganuma, Takuya Takeichi and Masashi Akiyama
Department of Dermatology, Nagoya University Graduate School of Medicine, 65 Tsurumai-cho, Showa-ku, Nagoya 466-8550, Japan

Michihiro Kono
Department of Dermatology and Plastic Surgery, Akita University Graduate School of Medicine, Hondo 1-1-1, Akita-shi, Akita 010-8543, Japan

Masahiro Kamata and Yayoi Tada
Department of Dermatology, Teikyo University School of Medicine, 2-11-1 Kaga, Itabashi-ku, Tokyo 173-8605, Japan

Sunita Keshari
Department of Life Sciences, National Central University, Taoyuan 32001, Taiwan

Arun Balasubramaniam, Binderiya Myagmardoloonjin and Indira Putri Negari
Department of Biomedical Sciences and Engineering, National Central University, Taoyuan 32001, Taiwan

Deron Raymond Herr
Department of Pharmacology, National University of Singapore, Singapore 117600, Singapore

Chun-Ming Huang
Department of Biomedical Sciences and Engineering, National Central University, Taoyuan 32001, Taiwan
Department of Dermatology, School of Medicine, University of California, San Diego, CA 92093, USA

Makoto Sugaya
Department of Dermatology, International University of Health and Welfare, Ichikawa Hospital, 6-1-14, Kounodai, Ichikawa, Chiba 272-0827, Japan

Sho Miake, Masaki Takemura and Yen Hai Vu
Department of Dermatology, Graduate School of Medical Sciences, Kyushu University, Maidashi 3-1-1, Higashiku, Fukuoka 812-8582, Japan

Takamichi Ito, Yuka Tanaka, Maho Murata and Makiko Kido-Nakahara
Department of Dermatology, Faculty of Medical Sciences, Kyushu University, Maidashi 3-1-1, Fukuoka 812-8582, Japan

Mayumi Komine
Department of Dermatology, Jichi Medical University, 3311-1 Yakushiji, Shimotsuke, Tochigi 329-0498, Japan
Department of Biochemistry, Jichi Medical University, 3311-1 Yakushiji, Shimotsuke, Tochigi 329-0498, Japan

Index

Printed in the USA
CPSIA information can be obtained
at www.ICGtesting.com
JSHW051401091023
49903JS00006B/235